Intelligent Systems Reference Library

Volume 270

Series Editors

Janusz Kacprzyk ⓘ, Polish Academy of Sciences, Warsaw, Poland

Lakhmi C. Jain, KES International, Shoreham-by-Sea, UK

The aim of this series is to publish a Reference Library, including novel advances and developments in all aspects of Intelligent Systems in an easily accessible and well-structured form. The series includes reference works, handbooks, compendia, textbooks, well-structured monographs, dictionaries, and encyclopedias. It contains well integrated knowledge and current information in the field of Intelligent Systems. The series covers the theory, applications, and design methods of Intelligent Systems. Virtually all disciplines such as engineering, computer science, avionics, business, e-commerce, environment, healthcare, physics, and life science are included. The list of topics spans all the areas of modern intelligent systems such as: Ambient intelligence, Computational intelligence, Social intelligence, Computational neuroscience, Artificial life, Virtual society, Cognitive systems, DNA and immunity-based systems, e-Learning and teaching, Human-centred computing and Machine ethics, Intelligent control, Intelligent data analysis, Knowledge-based paradigms, Knowledge management, Intelligent agents, Intelligent decision making, Intelligent network security, Interactive entertainment, Learning paradigms, Recommender systems, Robotics and Mechatronics including human-machine teaming, Self-organizing and adaptive systems, Soft computing including Neural systems, Fuzzy systems, Evolutionary computing and the Fusion of these paradigms, Perception and Vision, Web intelligence and Multimedia.

Indexed by SCOPUS, DBLP, zbMATH, SCImago.

All books published in the series are submitted for consideration in Web of Science.

Albert Ali Salah · Liane Colonna ·
Francisco Florez-Revuelta
Editors

Privacy-Aware Monitoring for Assisted Living

Ethical, Legal, and Technological Aspects of Audio- and Video-Based AAL Solutions

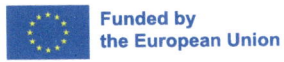

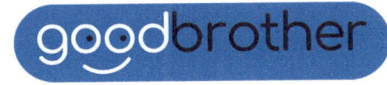

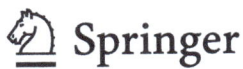

Editors
Albert Ali Salah ⓘ
Department of Information and Computing Sciences
Utrecht University
Utrecht, The Netherlands

Liane Colonna
Department of Law
Stockholm University
Stockholm, Sweden

Francisco Florez-Revuelta ⓘ
Department of Computer Technology
University of Alicante
Alicante, Spain

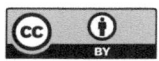

ISSN 1868-4394　　　　　　　　ISSN 1868-4408　(electronic)
Intelligent Systems Reference Library
ISBN 978-3-031-84157-6　　　　ISBN 978-3-031-84158-3　(eBook)
https://doi.org/10.1007/978-3-031-84158-3

This work was supported by European Cooperation in Science and Technology.

© The Editor(s) (if applicable) and The Author(s) 2025. This book is an open access publication.

Open Access This book is licensed under the terms of the Creative Commons Attribution 4.0 International License (http://creativecommons.org/licenses/by/4.0/), which permits use, sharing, adaptation, distribution and reproduction in any medium or format, as long as you give appropriate credit to the original author(s) and the source, provide a link to the Creative Commons license and indicate if changes were made.
The images or other third party material in this book are included in the book's Creative Commons license, unless indicated otherwise in a credit line to the material. If material is not included in the book's Creative Commons license and your intended use is not permitted by statutory regulation or exceeds the permitted use, you will need to obtain permission directly from the copyright holder.
The use of general descriptive names, registered names, trademarks, service marks, etc. in this publication does not imply, even in the absence of a specific statement, that such names are exempt from the relevant protective laws and regulations and therefore free for general use.
The publisher, the authors and the editors are safe to assume that the advice and information in this book are believed to be true and accurate at the date of publication. Neither the publisher nor the authors or the editors give a warranty, expressed or implied, with respect to the material contained herein or for any errors or omissions that may have been made. The publisher remains neutral with regard to jurisdictional claims in published maps and institutional affiliations.

This Springer imprint is published by the registered company Springer Nature Switzerland AG
The registered company address is: Gewerbestrasse 11, 6330 Cham, Switzerland

If disposing of this product, please recycle the paper.

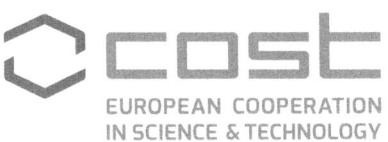

"This publication is based upon work from COST Action GoodBrother—Network on Privacy-Aware Audio- and Video-Based Applications for Active and Assisted Living (CA19121), supported by COST (European Cooperation in Science and Technology)."
"COST (European Cooperation in Science and Technology) is a funding agency for research and innovation networks. Our Actions help connect research initiatives across Europe and enable scientists to grow their ideas by sharing them with their peers. This boosts their research, career and innovation."
COST website: www.cost.eu.

Preface

Introduction

Many countries are currently grappling with significant challenges in health and social care, driven by demographic changes and mounting economic pressures that limit the resources available for public health and social care services. Active Assisted Living (AAL) technologies offer a potential solution to these pressing issues. AAL technologies are designed to enhance the health, quality of life, and overall wellbeing of older adults, as well as individuals who are impaired or frail.

These systems leverage a variety of sensors to monitor both the environment and its inhabitants. Among these sensors, cameras and microphones are becoming increasingly prevalent. They provide a direct and intuitive means of capturing and describing events, people, objects, actions, and interactions. Recent technological advancements have significantly enhanced the capabilities of these devices, enabling them to 'see' and 'hear' with remarkable precision.

While AAL technologies offer significant potential to enhance the health, quality of life, and wellbeing of older adults and individuals with impairments, their implementation comes with challenges. Addressing concerns about privacy and data protection is paramount to ensuring their acceptance and effectiveness. By prioritizing transparent communication, robust security safeguards, and user-centered design principles, AAL technologies can be successfully integrated into healthcare and social care systems, ultimately providing substantial benefits to those in need while respecting their fundamental rights.

Active Assisted Living

At the outset, it is important to clarify the concept of AAL, which is the subject of this book. AAL refers to the use of innovative and advanced Information and Communication Technologies (ICT) to create supportive and inclusive applications and environments, enabling older, impaired, or frail individuals to live independently and remain active in society.[1] There are a variety of AAL solutions that support wellbeing, quality of life, and safety, alleviate the burden of chronic diseases through continuous monitoring, contribute to more sustainable health services, and promote healthier lifestyles. AAL systems are designed to be invisible, unobtrusive, and user-friendly, learning and adapting to the needs of the assisted individuals. They overlap with fields such as Assistive Technologies, Ambient Intelligence, Pervasive Computing, and Robotics, encompassing a wide range of adaptive and intelligent ICT solutions that provide unobtrusive, effective, and ubiquitous support.

Overview and Goals

This book provides comprehensive guidance on designing privacy-aware audio- and video-based monitoring solutions for AAL. It is the culmination of a Europe-wide COST project, GoodBrother, aimed at enhancing awareness and expertise on the ethical, legal, and privacy issues associated with audio- and video-based monitoring in assisted living contexts. The project brings together a diverse group of experts from fields including computing, engineering, healthcare, design, law, ethics, and sociology, ensuring a multidisciplinary approach to these complex challenges.

This book explores how AAL technologies can be designed, developed, and deployed in a manner that prioritizes user privacy and ethical considerations. The guidance includes detailed best practices for the ethical use of audio- and video-based monitoring, strategies for maintaining transparency and accountability, and methods for ensuring that these technologies are both effective and respectful of user privacy. By addressing the multifaceted challenges of implementing AAL technologies, this book serves as an essential resource for developers, practitioners, and stakeholders committed to fostering a supportive and inclusive society through innovative technology.

The book was planned as a graduate textbook/guidebook on designing privacy-aware and ethical audio- and video-based technologies for assisting older adults. Targeting students, developers, and users of assisted living solutions, this book focuses on the crucial ethical, legal, and societal aspects of these technologies. It provides a concise conceptual grounding in the basics, it offers measures, guidelines, best practices, and a wealth of contemporary resources on assisted living.

---

[1] AGE Platform Europe. Glossary and Acronyms. (2016). Retrieved from: https://www.age-platform.eu/glossary/active-and-assisted-living-programme-aal.

Preface

Organization of the Book

This book is divided into three parts: *AAL Technologies*, *Video- and Audio-Based AAL Solutions*, and *Trustworthy AAL*, respectively. Part I, *AAL Technologies*, explores the foundational technologies that underpin AAL solutions. It covers the development and integration of various ICT designed to support the independence and wellbeing of older adults and individuals with disabilities. Readers will find detailed discussions on the latest advancements in sensor technology, smart environments, and the Internet of Things (IoT) that enable seamless and effective AAL systems.

Part II, *Video- and Audio-Based AAL Solutions*, focuses on the specific applications of video and audio technologies within AAL frameworks. It explores how these technologies can be used to monitor and assist individuals in their daily lives, ensuring their safety, health, and quality of life. Topics include fall detection and prevention, frailty and gait recognition, Activities of Daily Living (ADL) and behavior recognition, remote monitoring of vital signs, affective computing for AAL, as well as personal assistants.

Part III, *Trustworthy AAL*, addresses the critical issues of trust, privacy, and ethics in AAL systems. It provides guidance for designing and deploying monitoring solutions that respect the privacy and dignity of users. The part also covers legal frameworks, ethical and social considerations, and best practices for maintaining transparency and accountability. By focusing on building trust and ensuring the ethical use of technology, this part aims to promote the acceptance and sustainable adoption of AAL solutions.

The aim of GoodBrother was to increase the awareness on the ethical, legal, and privacy issues associated to audio- and video-based monitoring and to propose privacy-aware working solutions for assisted living, by creating an interdisciplinary community of researchers and industrial partners from different fields (computing, engineering, healthcare, law, sociology) and other stakeholders (users, policy makers, public services), stimulating new research and innovation. GoodBrother aimed to offset the "Big Brother" sense of continuous monitoring by increasing user acceptance, exploiting these new solutions, and improving market reach.

Spanning researchers and industrial stakeholders from 32 countries across the globe, the GoodBrother project focused the discussion in several areas, via dedicated working groups, such as social responsibility, privacy by design, ambient assisted living applications, and software benchmarking.

The Future of AAL

The future of AAL is poised to be transformative, driven by continuous advancements in technology and a growing emphasis on personalized, user-centered care. Emerging innovations such as artificial intelligence and advanced sensor technologies will enable AAL systems to become more adaptive and intuitive, providing real-time support tailored to individual needs. The integration of wearable devices and smart home technologies will further enhance the ability to monitor health and wellbeing seamlessly, promoting greater independence and quality of life for older adults and individuals with disabilities. Additionally, as societal awareness of the importance of ethical considerations in technology deployment grows, future AAL solutions may prioritize privacy, security, and user consent, fostering greater trust and acceptance. Collaborative efforts across disciplines will ensure that AAL technologies are not only cutting-edge, but also inclusive and accessible, paving the way for a future where everyone can benefit from enhanced support and care in their daily lives.

Utrecht, The Netherlands September 2024

Albert Ali Salah
Liane Colonna
Francisco Florez-Revuelta

Acknowledgments This work is supported by H2020 European Union program under GoodBrother COST action 19121. We thank Sara Colantonio, Gianluigi Maria Riva, and Eftim Zdravevski for their help in drafting the outline of this book.

Contents

Part I AAL Technologies

1 A Historical View of Active Assisted Living 3
Sara Colantonio, Slavisa Aleksic, Jean Calleja-Agius,
Kenneth P. Camilleri, Anto Čartolovni, Pau Climent-Pérez,
Stefania Cristina, Vladimir Despotovic, Hazım Kemal Ekenel,
Mustafa Ekrem Erakin, Francisco Florez-Revuelta,
Danila Germanese, Nicole Grech, Murat Emirzeoğlu, Ivo Iliev,
Anna Sigridur Islind, Mladan Jovanovic, Martin Kampel,
William Kearns, Andrzej Klimczuk, Lambros Lambrinos,
Jennifer Lumetzberger, Wiktor Mucha, Sophie Noiret,
Zada Pajalic, Rodrigo Pérez-Rodríguez, Galidiya Petrova,
Sintija Petrovica-Klavina, Peter Počta, Angelica Poli,
Mara Romanovska, Albert Ali Salah, Maria J. Santofimia,
Steinunn Gróa Sigurðardóttir, Susanna Spinsante,
Lacramioara Stoicu-Tivadar, Hilda Tellioğlu, and Andrej Zgank

1.1	Introduction	4
1.2	History of AAL Technology	8
1.3	A Functional View of an AAL System Architecture	10
1.4	A Taxonomy of AAL Technologies and Applications	13
1.5	Technological Underpinnings of Audio and Video Based AAL	19
	1.5.1 Video-Based Sensing Technologies	19
	1.5.2 Audio-Based Sensing Technologies	26
	1.5.3 Data Processing and Understanding for AAL	30
	1.5.4 Multimodal Data Fusion for AAL	33
1.6	Conclusions	36
	References	37

2 Machine Learning for Active Assisted Living: Core Concepts, Challenges, and Solutions 45
Eftim Zdravevski and Petre Lameski
- 2.1 Introduction to Machine Learning 45
- 2.2 Machine Learning Fundamentals 46
  - 2.2.1 Datasets 46
  - 2.2.2 Types of ML 50
  - 2.2.3 Evaluation Metrics 55
  - 2.2.4 Model Monitoring 60
- 2.3 ML and AAL Systems 60
- 2.4 ML Challenges Specific to AAL Systems 61
  - 2.4.1 Closed Set Versus Open Set Action Recognition 61
  - 2.4.2 Action Spotting Problem 63
  - 2.4.3 Class Imbalance 65
  - 2.4.4 Personalization of AAL Systems 68
  - 2.4.5 Dealing with Extra People in the Environment 69
  - 2.4.6 Multimodality of AAL Data 69
- 2.5 Conclusion 70
- References 71

3 Privacy Preservation in Audio and Video 77
Tom Bäckström, Siddharth Ravi, and Francisco Florez-Revuelta
- 3.1 Introduction 77
- 3.2 Privacy Issues in Audio and Video 78
- 3.3 Privacy Preservation in Audio 81
  - 3.3.1 Obfuscation in Speech and Audio 82
  - 3.3.2 Information Isolation 83
  - 3.3.3 Cryptography in Audio 85
  - 3.3.4 Interventions in the Acoustic Space 86
  - 3.3.5 Improving the Performance of the Trusted Task 87
- 3.4 Privacy Preservation in Video 88
  - 3.4.1 Intervention Methods 88
  - 3.4.2 Blind Vision 89
  - 3.4.3 Secure Processing 90
  - 3.4.4 Data Hiding 90
  - 3.4.5 Visual Obfuscation 91
- 3.5 Conclusion 93
- References 93

4 Data Security in AAL 99
Aleksandar Jevremovic, Slavisa Aleksic, Mladen Veinovic, and Liane Colonna
- 4.1 Introduction 100
- 4.2 Retrospective of Data Protection 102
- 4.3 Cryptological Foundations and Security Attributes of Data Protection 105

	4.3.1	Symmetric Cipher Systems	106
	4.3.2	Asymmetric Cipher Systems	107
	4.3.3	Digital Signature	108
	4.3.4	Stream and Block Cipher Algorithms	110

4.4 General System Architecture and Related Technologies 111
4.5 Technological Sovereignty and the Significance of Open Source 114
4.6 Considerations About the Life Cycle of AAL Solutions 117
    4.6.1 Fail-Secure Design 118
    4.6.2 Safe Disposal of Worn-Out and Obsolete Components 120
4.7 Legal Aspects of Data Security 120
    4.7.1 Security by Design 123
    4.7.2 Vulnerability Reporting 124
    4.7.3 Software Bill of Materials (SBOMs) 125
References 126

Part II Video- and Audio-Based AAL Solutions

5 Fall Detection 131
Jennifer Lumetzberger, Irene Ballester, and Martin Kampel
5.1 Introduction 132
5.2 Fall Statistics 132
    5.2.1 Frequency of People Falling 132
    5.2.2 Reasons for People Falling 133
    5.2.3 Importance of Early Help in Falls 134
5.3 Fall Detection 135
    5.3.1 Non-image-Based Fall Detection Methods 135
    5.3.2 Image-Based Fall Detection Methods 138
    5.3.3 Collecting Fall Detection Datasets 142
5.4 Fall Prevention 144
    5.4.1 Non-image-Based Fall Prevention 144
    5.4.2 Image-Based Fall Prevention 146
5.5 Dealing with Privacy 147
5.6 Usability 149
5.7 Conclusion 149
References 150

6 Privacy-Aware Video-Based Methods for Gait and Frailty Recognition in Active and Assisted Living Environments 155
Pau Climent-Pérez and Francisco Florez-Revuelta
6.1 Introduction 155
6.2 Potential for Automation of Frailty Assessment Scales 159
    6.2.1 Review of Frailty Scales 160
    6.2.2 Automation of Identified Frailty Scale Domains 164
6.3 Gait Analysis 166

		6.3.1	Use of Gait in Medical Studies	167
		6.3.2	Gait Analysis from Video	168
		6.3.3	Gait Analysis from Other Sensors	170
	6.4	Ecological Monitoring		171
	6.5	Privacy-Awareness		174
	6.6	Conclusion		176
	References			177
7	**Activities of Daily Living (ADL) and Behavior Recognition**			**187**
	Slavisa Aleksic, Vladimir Despotovic, and Stefania Cristina			
	7.1	Introduction		187
	7.2	Activity/Behavior Recognition		191
		7.2.1	Video-Based Approaches	191
		7.2.2	Audio-Based Approaches	195
		7.2.3	Multimodal Approaches	197
		7.2.4	Overview of Approaches	200
	7.3	Relevant Datasets		204
	7.4	Privacy Preservation		205
	References			207
8	**Remote Monitoring of Vital Signs**			**217**
	Stefania Cristina, Peter Počta, Andrej Zgank,			
	Kenneth P. Camilleri, Sara Colantonio, and Lambros Lambrinos			
	8.1	Introduction		218
	8.2	Vital Sign Monitoring		218
		8.2.1	Commonly Monitored Vital Sign Parameters	219
		8.2.2	Contact and Wearable Solutions	220
		8.2.3	Video-Based Approaches	221
		8.2.4	Audio-Based Approaches	223
		8.2.5	Multimodal Approaches	225
	8.3	Video and Audio Datasets		226
		8.3.1	Video Datasets	226
		8.3.2	Respiratory Sound Datasets	227
		8.3.3	Heart Sound Datasets	228
	8.4	Privacy Considerations in Vital Sign Monitoring		230
	8.5	Communication Technologies		231
	8.6	Trends, Challenges and Future Directions		232
	References			233

9	**Affective Computing in Active Assisted Living**	239
	Albert Ali Salah, Deniz Iren, and Heysem Kaya	
	9.1 Introduction	239
	9.2 What Is Affective Computing?	241
	9.3 Where Is AC Used in AAL?	242
	9.4 Trust and Responsible Uses of AC in AAL	246
	9.5 Legal Aspects and the AI Act	249
	9.6 Conclusions	251
	References	252
10	**A Smart Mirror to Your Health: Personalized Virtual Coaching for Active and Healthy Ageing**	259
	Maria J. Santofimia, Xavier del Toro, Cristina Bolaños, Javier Dorado, and Sara Colantonio	
	10.1 Introduction	260
	10.2 Smart Mirrors in Health and Well Being	263
	10.3 Sara: Designing a Personal Health Companion	265
	10.4 Case Studies: Impact on Active and Healthy Ageing	268
	10.4.1 Use Case 1: Personalised Risk Prediction and Prevention	268
	10.4.2 Use Case 2: Integrated Care Platform and Virtual Assistant	269
	10.4.3 Use Case 3: Health Literacy and Self-management	269
	10.5 Conclusion and Future Work	270
	References	271

Part III Trustworthy AAL

11	**Ethical Issues in AAL**	277
	Anto Čartolovni, Carina Dantas, Anamaria Malešević, and Ayşegül Ilgaz	
	11.1 Introduction	278
	11.2 Informed Consent	279
	11.3 Data Management and Access	280
	11.4 Equal Access and Distributive Justice	280
	11.5 Ethical Principles in AAL	281
	11.5.1 Autonomy	281
	11.5.2 Beneficence	282
	11.5.3 Non-maleficence	283
	11.5.4 Justice	283
	11.5.5 Fidelity	284
	11.6 Stakeholder Engagement in AAL Development and Deployment	284
	11.7 Human Dignity as a Guiding Path and Overarching Concept	285
	11.8 Conclusions	286
	References	286

12	**Smart Mirrors and Data Protection Regulation**	291
	Liane Colonna and Gianluigi M. Riva	
	12.1 Introduction	292
	12.2 Smart Mirrors	293
	12.3 Smart Mirror Characteristics	294
	12.4 Data Protection Concerns Raised by Smart Mirrors	295
	12.5 Data Protection Regulation and Smart Mirrors	300
	12.5.1 An Overview of the GDPR	300
	12.5.2 Key Factors in Applying the GDPR to Smart Mirrors	302
	12.6 The Role of "Data Protection by Design" in the Smart-Mirror Context	305
	12.7 Conclusion	307
	References	308
13	**Social and Societal Issues in AAL**	313
	Christoph Lutz, Cristina Miguel, Tamara Mujirishvili, Rodrigo Perez-Vega, and Anton Fedosov	
	13.1 Introduction	314
	13.2 Cultural Adaptation and Differences	315
	13.3 Socio-Cultural, Ethnic and Linguistic Biases	316
	13.4 Dataveillance and Normalization of Surveillance	318
	13.5 Re-shaping of Care Relationships	319
	13.6 Trust in (AAL) Technologies and Barriers to Adoption	321
	13.7 Conclusion	323
	References	325
14	**Integrating Ethics by Design and Co-design Principles in the Development of Ambient Assisted Living Technologies**	333
	Hilda Tellioğlu	
	14.1 Introduction	333
	14.2 Research Setting	335
	14.2.1 Ambient Assisted Technologies	335
	14.2.2 Co-design Practices	336
	14.2.3 Example PHOBILITYaktiv	338
	14.2.4 Ethics by Design	341
	14.3 Ethical AAL Technologies	342
	14.4 Discussion	345
	14.5 Conclusions	346
	References	347

Index 349

Contributors

Slavisa Aleksic Faculty of Digital Transformation, HTWK Leipzig, Leipzig, Germany

Irene Ballester Computer Vision Lab, TU Wien, Vienna, Austria

Cristina Bolaños Computer Architecture and Networking Group, University of Castilla-La Mancha, Ciudad Real, Spain

Tom Bäckström Department of Information and Communications Engineering, University of Aalto, Aalto, Finland

Jean Calleja-Agius Faculty of Medicine & Surgery, University of Malta, Msida, Malta

Kenneth P. Camilleri Department of Systems and Control Engineering, Faculty of Engineering, University of Malta, Msida, Malta

Anto Čartolovni Digital Healthcare Ethics Laboratory (Digit-HeaL), Catholic University of Croatia, Zagreb, Croatia

Pau Climent-Pérez University of Alicante, Alicante, Spain

Sara Colantonio Institute of Information Science and Technologies, National Research Council of Italy, Pisa, Italy

Liane Colonna Stockholm University, Stockholm, Sweden

Stefania Cristina Department of Systems and Control Engineering, Faculty of Engineering, University of Malta, Msida, Malta

Carina Dantas SHINE 2Europe, Coimbra, Portugal;
ICBAS, University of Porto, Porto, Portugal

Xavier del Toro Technology and Information Systems, University of Castilla-La Mancha, Ciudad Real, Spain

Vladimir Despotovic Department of Medical Informatics, Bioinformatics & AI, Luxembourg Institute of Health, Strassen, Luxembourg

Javier Dorado Technology and Information Systems, University of Castilla-La Mancha, Ciudad Real, Spain

Hazım Kemal Ekenel Department of Computer Engineering, Istanbul Technical University, Istanbul, Türkiye

Murat Emirzeoğlu Department of Physiotherapy and Rehabilitation, Karadeniz Technical University, Trabzon, Türkiye

Mustafa Ekrem Erakın Department of Computer Engineering, Istanbul Technical University, Istanbul, Türkiye

Anton Fedosov Institute for Interactive Technologies, University of Applied Sciences and Arts Northwestern Switzerland, Windisch, Switzerland

Francisco Florez-Revuelta Department of Computing Technology, University of Alicante, Alicante, Spain

Danila Germanese Institute of Information Science and Technologies "A.Faedo", National Research Council, Pisa, Italy

Nicole Grech Faculty of Medicine & Surgery, University of Malta, Msida, Malta

Aysegül Ilgaz Department of Public Health Nursing, Akdeniz University, Antalya, Turkey

Ivo Iliev Faculty of Electronic Engineering and Technology, Technical University of Sofia, Sofia, Bulgaria

Deniz Iren Department of Information Science, Open Universiteit, Heerlen, The Netherlands

Anna Sigridur Islind Department of Computer Science, Reykjavik University, Reykjavik, Iceland

Aleksandar Jevremovic Faculty of Informatics and Computing, Singidunum University, Belgrade, Serbia

Mladan Jovanovic Faculty of Informatics and Computing, Singidunum University, Belgrade, Serbia

Martin Kampel Computer Vision Lab, TU Wien, Vienna, Austria

Heysem Kaya Department of Information and Computing Sciences, Utrecht University, Utrecht, The Netherlands

William Kearns Department of Child and Family Studies, University of South Florida, Tampa, USA

Andrzej Klimczuk SGH Warsaw School of Economics, Warsaw, Poland

Lambros Lambrinos Department of Communication and Internet Studies, Cyprus University of Technology, Limassol, Cyprus

Petre Lameski Faculty of Computer Science and Engineering, Ss Cyril and Methodius University in Skopje, Skopje, North Macedonia

Jennifer Lumetzberger Computer Vision Lab, TU Wien, Vienna, Austria

Christoph Lutz BI Norwegian Business School, Department of Communication and Culture, Oslo, Norway

Anamaria Malešević Digital Healthcare Ethics Laboratory (Digit-HeaL), Catholic University of Croatia, Zagreb, Croatia

Cristina Miguel University of Reading, Henley Business School, Reading, UK

Wiktor Mucha Computer Vision Lab, TU Wien, Vienna, Austria

Tamara Mujirishvili Department of Computer Technology, University of Alicante, Alicante, Spain

Sophie Noiret Computer Vision Lab, TU Wien, Vienna, Austria

Zada Pajalic Institute for Nursing, Faculty of Health Sciences, VID Specialized University, Oslo, Norway

Rodrigo Perez-Vega University of Reading, Henley Business School, Reading, UK

Galidiya Petrova Biomedical Engineering, Technical University of Sofia, Sofia, Bulgaria

Sintija Petrovica-Klavina Institute of Applied Computer Systems, Riga Technical University, Riga, Latvia

Angelica Poli Department of Information Engineering, Marche Polytechnic University, Ancona, Italy

Peter Počta Department of Multimedia and Information-Communication Technology, Faculty of Electrical Engineering and Information Technology, University of Žilina, Žilina, Slovakia

Rodrigo Pérez-Rodríguez Universidad Rey Juan Carlos, Fuenlabrada, Spain

Siddharth Ravi University of Alicante, Alicante, Spain

Gianluigi M. Riva Bocconi University, Milan, Italy

Mara Romanovska Institute of Applied Computer Systems, Riga Technical University, Riga, Latvia

Albert Ali Salah Department of Information and Computing Sciences, Utrecht University, Utrecht, The Netherlands

Maria J. Santofimia Technology and Information Systems, University of Castilla-La Mancha, Ciudad Real, Spain

Steinunn Gróa Sigurðardóttir Faculty of Informatics and Computing, Singidunum University, Belgrade, Serbia

Susanna Spinsante Department of Information Engineering, Marche Polytechnic University, Ancona, Italy

Lacramioara Stoicu-Tivadar Automation and Applied Informatics, Politehnica University of Timişoara, Timişoara, Romania

Hilda Tellioğlu Faculty of Informatics, TU Wien, Vienna, Austria

Mladen Veinovic Faculty of Informatics and Computing, Singidunum University, Belgrade, Serbia

Eftim Zdravevski Faculty of Computer Science and Engineering, Ss Cyril and Methodius University in Skopje, Skopje, North Macedonia

Andrej Zgank Laboratory for Digital Signal Processing, Faculty of Electrical Engineering and Computer Science, University of Maribor, Maribor, Slovenia

Acronyms

3DES	Triple DES
AAL	Active and Assisted Living
AAL2	European Active and Assisted Living Research and Development Programme
AALIANCE2	European Next Generation Ambient Assisted Living Innovation Alliance
AAT	Ambient Assisted Technologies
AC	Affective Computing
AD	Alzheimer's Disease
ADL	Activities of Daily Living
AE	Autoencoder
AES	Advanced Encryption Algorithm
AI	Artificial Intelligence
AIoT	Artificial Intelligence of Things
ALS	Amyotrophic Lateral Sclerosis
AmI	Ambient Intelligence
ANN	Artificial Neural Network
API	Application Programming Interface
AR	Augmented Reality
ARI	Adjusted Rand Index
ASR	Automatic Speech Recognition
AT	Assistive Technologies
AUC	Area under the Curve
AUC-PR	Area Under the Precision-Recall Curve
AUC-ROC	Area Under the ROC Curve
BLE	Bluetooth Low Energy
BMI	Body Mass Index
BMVIT	Federal Ministry Republic of Austria, Climate Action, Environment, Energy, Mobility, Innovation and Technology
BoL	Beginning of Life
bpm	Beats Per Minute

CCD	Charge-coupled Device
CGA	Comprehensive Geriatric Assessment
CHF	Congestive Heart Failure
CHS	Cardiovascular Health Study
CMOS	Complementary Metal-Oxide-Semiconductor
CNN	Convolutional Neural Network
COPD	Chronic Obstructive Pulmonary Disease
CRA	Cyber Resilience Act
CRF	Conditional Random Field
CV	Computer Vision
DBN	Dynamic Bayesian Network
DES	Data Encryption Standard
DL	Deep Learning
DORA	Digital Operation Resilience Act
DoS	Denial of Service
DPbD	Data Protection by Design
DPIA	Data Protection Impact Assessment
DSP	Digital Signal Processing
DT	Decision Tree
DWT	Discrete Wavelet Transform
ECG	Electrocardiogram
EDPB	European Data Protection Board
EMA	Ecological Momentary Assessment
EMG	Electromyogram
ENISA	European Union Agency for Cybersecurity
EoL	End of Life
EU	European Union
FCR	Fault-Containment Region
FFG	Austrian Research Promotion Agency
FH	Fault Hypothesis
FHRIA	Fundamental Human Rights Impact Assessment
FI	Frailty Index
FN	False Negative
FP	False Positive
FPV	First Person Video
FSR	Force Sensing Resistor
FTC	Federal Trade Commission
GAN	Generative Adversarial Network
GCN	Graph Convolutional Network
GDPR	General Data Protection Regulation
GMM	Gaussian Mixture Model
GPS	Global Positioning System
GPU	Graphical Processing Unit
GSR	Galvanic Skin Response
HAR	Human Activity Recognition

HCI	Human-Computer Interaction
HD	Huntington's Disease
HHI	Human-Human Interaction
HMM	Hidden Markov Model
HOF	Histogram of Optical Flow
HOG	Histogram of Oriented Gradients
ICA	Independent Component Analysis
ICT	Information and Communication Technologies
IMU	Inertial Magnetic Unit
IoHT	Internet of Healthy Things
IoT	Internet of Things
IPSec	Internet Protocol Security
IR	Infrared
IS	Information Systems
KDA	Kernel Discriminant Analysis
k-NN	K-Nearest Neighbor
LBP	Local Binary Pattern
LLM	Large Language Model
LOOCV	Leave-one-out Cross Validation
LSTM	Long Short-Term Memory
MDP	Markov Decision Process
MDS-UPDRS	MDS-Unified Parkinson's Disease Rating Scale
MEI	Motion Energy Image
MFCC	Mel-Frequency Cepstral Coefficients
mHealth	Mobile Health
MHI	Motion History Image
ML	Machine Learning
mmHg	Millimetres of Mercury
MoCap	Motion Capture
MoL	Middle of Life
MS	Multiple Sclerosis
NB	Naive Bayes
NGU	Never Give Up
NIR	Near Infrared
NIST	National Institute of Standards and Technology
OSR	Open Set Recognition
PCA	Principal Component Analysis
PCBIR	Private Content-Based Image Retrieval
PD	Parkinson's Disease
PDE	Products with Digital Elements
PFF	Periprosthetic Femoral Fracture
PIR	Passive Infrared
POBA	Partial Occlusion by Background Alignment
POMA	Performance-oriented Assessment of Mobility
R&D	Research and Development

RBM	Reverse Beacon Network
REM	Rapid Eye Movement
RF	Random Forest
RFID	Radio Frequency Identification
RGB	Red Green Blue
RGB-D	Red Green Blue Depth
RI	Rand Index
RL	Reinforcement Learning
RNN	Recurrent Neural Network
ROC	Receiver Operator Characteristic
ROI	Region of Interest
RPM	Remote Patient Monitoring
RSA	Rivest Shamir Adelman
SBOMs	Software Bill of Materials
SCT	Smart Connected Toy
SFFS	Sequential Forward Floating Selection
SLAM	Simultaneous Localization and Mapping
SLM	Spatial Light Modulation
SMC	Secure Multi-party Computation
SMOTE	Synthetic Minority Over-sampling
SMPL	Skinned Multi-Person Linear Model
SOF	Study of Osteoporotic Fractures
SpO2	Periperhal Capillary Oxygen Saturation
SPPB	Short Physical Performance Battery
SSL	Secure Sockets Layer
SVM	Support Vector Machine
TCN	Temporal Convolutional Network
TN	True Negative
TP	True Positive
TUG	Timed Up and Go
USB	Universal Serial Bus
VAE	Variational Autoencoder
VGRF	Vertical Ground Reaction Forces
VPN	Virtual Private Networks
VR	Virtual Reality
WEP	Wired Equivalent Privacy
WHO	World Health Organization
WPA	Wi-Fi Protected Access

Part I
AAL Technologies

Chapter 1
A Historical View of Active Assisted Living

Sara Colantonio, Slavisa Aleksic, Jean Calleja-Agius, Kenneth P. Camilleri,
Anto Čartolovni, Pau Climent-Pérez, Stefania Cristina, Vladimir Despotovic,
Hazım Kemal Ekenel, Mustafa Ekrem Erakin, Francisco Florez-Revuelta,
Danila Germanese, Nicole Grech, Murat Emirzeoğlu, Ivo Iliev,
Anna Sigridur Islind, Mladan Jovanovic, Martin Kampel, William Kearns,
Andrzej Klimczuk, Lambros Lambrinos, Jennifer Lumetzberger,
Wiktor Mucha, Sophie Noiret, Zada Pajalic, Rodrigo Pérez-Rodríguez,
Galidiya Petrova, Sintija Petrovica-Klavina, Peter Počta, Angelica Poli,
Mara Romanovska, Albert Ali Salah, Maria J. Santofimia,
Steinunn Gróa Sigurðardóttir, Susanna Spinsante,
Lacramioara Stoicu-Tivadar, Hilda Tellioğlu, and Andrej Zgank

S. Colantonio (✉)
Institute of Information Science and Technologies, National Research Council of Italy, Pisa, Italy
e-mail: sara.colantonio@isti.cnr.it

S. Aleksic
Faculty of Digital Transformation, HTWK Leipzig, Leipzig, Germany
e-mail: slavisa.aleksic@htwk-leipzig.de

J. Calleja-Agius · N. Grech
Faculty of Medicine & Surgery, University of Malta, Msida, Malta
e-mail: jean.calleja-agius@um.edu.mt

N. Grech
e-mail: nicole.grech@gov.mt

K. P. Camilleri · S. Cristina
Department of Systems and Control Engineering, Faculty of Engineering, University of Malta, Msida, Malta
e-mail: kenneth.camilleri@um.edu.mt

S. Cristina
e-mail: stefania.cristina@um.edu.mt

A. Čartolovni
Digital Healthcare Ethics Laboratory, Catholic University of Croatia, Zagreb, Croatia
e-mail: anto.cartolovni@unicath.hr

P. Climent-Pérez
University of Alicante, Alicante, Spain
e-mail: pau.climent@ua.es

© The Author(s) 2025
A. A. Salah et al. (eds.), *Privacy-Aware Monitoring for Assisted Living*,
Intelligent Systems Reference Library 270,
https://doi.org/10.1007/978-3-031-84158-3_1

Abstract Active assisted living (AAL) aims to use innovative technologies to create supportive, inclusive, and empowering applications and environments that enable older, impaired or frail people to live independently and stay active longer in society. This chapter provides an introduction to the main concepts of AAL, provides a brief history of the evolution of such technologies, and gives a functional view of how AAL system architecture can be conceptualized. It then provides a taxonomy of AAL technologies and applications, followed by technological underpinnings of audio- and video- based AAL.

Keywords Active assisted living (AAL) · AAL taxonomy · Data sensing and processing · Computer vision · Audio-signal processing · Wearable sensing · Multimodality · Silver economy

1.1 Introduction

The concept of "Active Assisted Living" (AAL)[1] emerged in the early 2000s, by evolving the idea of assistive technologies to address the societal challenges of health, demographic change and wellbeing. Since then, numerous research and development endeavors have fueled the field, stimulated by various funding opportunities, among which the European Framework Programmes (e.g., FP7 and Horizon 2020), the

---

V. Despotovic
Department of Medical Informatics, Bioinformatics & AI, Luxembourg Institute of Health, Strassen, Luxembourg
e-mail: vladimir.Despotovic@lih.lu

H. K. Ekenel · M. E. Erakin
Department of Computer Engineering, Istanbul Technical University, Istanbul, Türkiye
e-mail: ekenel@itu.edu.tr

M. E. Erakin
e-mail: erakin20@itu.edu.tr

F. Florez-Revuelta
Department of Computer Technology, University of Alicante, Alicante, Spain
e-mail: francisco.florez@ua.es

D. Germanese
Institute of Information Science and Technologies "A.Faedo", National Research Council, Pisa, Italy
e-mail: danila.germanese@isti.cnr.it

M. Emirzeoğlu
Department of Physiotherapy and Rehabilitation, Karadeniz Technical University, Trabzon, Türkiye
e-mail: muratemirzeoglu@ktu.edu.tr

I. Iliev
Faculty of Electronic Engineering and Technology, Technical University of Sofia, Sofia, Bulgaria
e-mail: izi@tu-sofia.bg

former Active Assisted Living Joint Programme,[2] the Joint Programming Initiative More Years, Better Lives (JPI MYBL),[3] EIT Health,[4] the Innovation Partnership on

---

A. S. Islind
Department of Computer Science, Reykjavik University, Reykjavik, Iceland
e-mail: annasi@ru.is

M. Jovanovic · S. G. Sigurðardóttir
Faculty of Informatics and Computing, Singidunum University, Belgrade, Serbia
e-mail: mjovanovic@singidunum.ac.rs

S. G. Sigurðardóttir
e-mail: steinunngroa@ru.is

M. Kampel · J. Lumetzberger · W. Mucha · S. Noiret
Computer Vision Lab, TU Wien, Vienna, Austria
e-mail: martin.kampel@tuwien.ac.at

J. Lumetzberger
e-mail: jlumetzberger@cvl.tuwien.ac.at

W. Mucha
e-mail: wmucha@cvl.tuwien.ac.at

S. Noiret
e-mail: snoiret@cvl.tuwien.ac.at

W. Kearns
Department of Child and Family Studies, University of South Florida, Tampa, USA
e-mail: kearns@usf.edu

A. Klimczuk
SGH Warsaw School of Economics, Warsaw, Poland
e-mail: aklimcz@sgh.waw.pl

L. Lambrinos
Department of Communication and Internet Studies, Cyprus University of Technology, Limassol, Cyprus
e-mail: lambros.lambrinos@cut.ac.cy

Z. Pajalic
Institute for Nursing, Faculty of Health Sciences, VID Specialized University, Oslo, Norway
e-mail: Zada.pajalic@vid.no

R. Pérez-Rodríguez
Universidad Rey Juan Carlos, Fuenlabrada, Spain
e-mail: rodrigo.perez@urjc.es

G. Petrova
Biomedical Engineering, Technical University of Sofia, Sofia, Bulgaria
e-mail: gip@tu-plovdiv.bg

S. Petrovica-Klavina · M. Romanovska
Institute of Applied Computer Systems, Riga Technical University, Riga, Latvia
e-mail: Sintija.Petrovica-Klavina@rtu.lv

M. Romanovska
e-mail: Mara.Romanovska@rtu.lv

Active and Healthy Ageing,[5] and the recent European Partnership on Transforming Health and Care Systems (THCS)[6] are some of the most notable ones.

Several definitions of AAL have appeared so far in the literature [20, 44, 77, 120]. Broadly speaking, AAL can be referred to the use of innovative and advanced Information and Communication Technologies (ICT) to create supportive, inclusive and empowering applications and environments that enable older, impaired or frail people to live independently and stay active longer in society. AAL has capitalized on the growing pervasiveness and effectiveness of ICT systems to supply the persons in need with smart assistance, by responding to their necessities of autonomy, independence, comfort, security and safety. A plethora of solutions has been developed so far to respond to these core needs by

- supporting and ensuring a sustained wellbeing, quality of life and safety of people with any kind of impairment,
- alleviating the burden of chronic diseases, also by ensuring a continuous and remote monitoring and contrasting the shortage of health personnel,

---

[1] Earlier texts abbreviated "Ambient Assisted Living" as AAL, and some sources (e.g. [44]) use "Active and Assisted Living," interchangeably.
[2] http://www.aal-europe.eu/, Accessed 19 September 2024.
[3] https://jp-demographic.eu/, Accessed 19 September 2024.
[4] https://eithealth.eu/, Accessed 19 September 2024.
[5] https://ec.europa.eu/eip/ageing/home_en.html, Accessed 19 September 2024.
[6] https://www.thcspartnership.eu/, Accessed 19 September 2024.

P. Počta
Department of Multimedia and Information-Communication Technology, Faculty of Electrical Engineering and Information Technology, University of Žilina, Žilina, Slovakia
e-mail: peter.pocta@uniza.sk

A. Poli · S. Spinsante
Department of Information Engineering, Marche Polytechnic University, Ancona, Italy
e-mail: s.spinsante@staff.univpm.it

A. A. Salah
Department of Information and Computing Sciences, Utrecht University, Utrecht, The Netherlands
e-mail: a.a.salah@uu.nl

M. J. Santofimia
Technology and Information Systems, University of Castilla-La Mancha, Ciudad Real, Spain
e-mail: mariajose.santofimia@uclm.es

L. Stoicu-Tivadar
Automation and Applied Informatics, Politehnica University of Timişoara, Timişoara, Romania
e-mail: lacramioara.stoicu-tivadar@aut.upt.ro

H. Tellioğlu
Faculty of Informatics, TU Wien, Vienna, Austria
e-mail: hilda.tellioglu@tuwien.ac.at

A. Zgank
Faculty of Electrical Engineering and Computer Science, University of Maribor, Maribor, Slovenia
e-mail: andrej.zgank@um.si

- contributing towards more sustainable health, care and social services, by reducing the pressure on formal health and care infrastructures thanks to remote monitoring and tele-assistance,
- preventing aging and impaired community from social isolation,
- supporting and relieving the burden of formal and informal caregivers,
- promoting better and healthier lifestyles for the individuals at risk,
- enacting disease prevention strategies based on personalized risk assessment and continuous monitoring.

With respect to the last issue, in the middle 2010s, the so-called *Quantified Self* movement has emerged thanks to the upsurge of consumer-friendly wearable sensors (e.g., smart watches, smart bracelets or wrist bands). The idea behind this movement is to promote the self-tracking and self-monitoring of a person's health information to increase the self-awareness on her or his health status. Quantified Self and AAL technologies strongly overlap, especially when considering the lifelogging and vital signs monitoring application scenarios. Similarly, AAL can make extensive use of mobile-Health (mHealth) applications, as well as of the so-called Internet of Health Things (IoHT) to monitor and track health-related information [97]. From our viewpoint, AAL is an umbrella term that comprises the whole range of adaptive and intelligent ICT solutions that fit into the daily living and working environments, to offer unobtrusive, effective and ubiquitous support to aging, impaired or frail people. From an initial version, mainly related to indoor environments, AAL concept has broadened to include also outdoor and on-the-move facilities, to ensure the continuum of support and care, thus increasing autonomy and independence of the assisted individuals.

The application scenarios addressed by AAL are complex, due to the inherent heterogeneity of the end-user population, their living arrangements, and their physical conditions or impairment [96]. Some of the most common and effective functionalities include:

- improving safety at home by preventing accidents and incidents that might occur in an assisted environment via, for instance, fall detection systems, alarms and warnings,
- maintaining under control chronic diseases or medication compliance, with connected devices for vital data measuring as well as medication reminders,
- maintaining physical and mental abilities, with the support of intelligent mobility aids, coaching systems and brain-training activities,
- maintaining interaction with other people with dedicated apps and online community platforms,
- improving quality of life for caregivers with technology for information sharing, and better coordination,
- early detecting risks in care homes, thus reducing the number of accidents and improving communication between caregivers and their patients.

Despite aiming at diverse goals, AAL systems should share some common characteristics [19]. They are designed to provide support in daily life in a proactive, non-invasive, unobtrusive and user-friendly manner. Moreover, they are conceived to be intelligent, to be able to learn and adapt to the requirements and requests of the assisted people, and to align with their specific needs.

In this respect, the field of AAL technologies overlaps, from the technological viewpoint, with many other fields, such as those of Assistive and Supportive Technologies, Ambient Intelligence (AmI), Pervasive Computing, Personal Informatics, e-textiles, IoHT and Robotics. Indeed, depending on the embodiment, AAL can include a wide range of robots, especially physically or socially assistive robotics that help users perform certain tasks [47].

Nevertheless, to ensure the uptake of AAL in society, potential user groups must be willing to use AAL applications and to integrate them in their daily environment and lives [34]. In this respect, participatory design is a cornerstone of technology acceptance, as it consists in involving the eventual end-users in the development process. Another big contribution to acceptance comes from a clear and comprehensive consideration of ethical and legal issues related to privacy, autonomy preservation, data protection and security [45].

This chapter provides the reader firstly with an overview of the evolution in time of AAL technologies (Sect. 1.2); then, it sketches a typical functional architecture of an AAL system (Sect. 1.3), which is instrumental to introduce the main research and development (R&D) advances reviewed in this chapter and in the rest of the present volume. Then, we describe a proposal for a taxonomy of AAL applications (Sect. 1.4). Finally, the chapter will provide a detailed exposition of the technological underpinnings of audio- and video- based AAL.[7]

1.2 History of AAL Technology

The paradigm of AAL technology emerged initially with the idea to use ICT-based solutions to advance assistive technologies into a more comprehensive endeavor. Starting from tech devices able to assist people with disabilities with just one task or to ensure their safety, the goal was to evolve towards encompassing completely the living areas and the person's needs [19]. The name "Ambient and Assisted Living" emerged at that time, showing overlaps with the idea of Ambient Intelligence. Lately, as already mentioned, the concept has broadened, by addressing the needs of healthy and active aging, and disease prevention and including the support outdoor and on-the-move, thus taking the name of Active Assisted Living.

Previous works have identified three generations of AAL technologies, which correspond to assistive solutions with increasing levels of automation and technological facilities [19, 40, 106]. Considering the most recent advances in the field and the debate on ethical and legal issues, we argue that a fourth generation of AAL technologies is emerging. In this fourth wave, more advanced functionalities based on Artificial Intelligence (AI) and Robotics as well as context awareness are being fully integrated in AAL. Moreover, more attention is being paid to the co-design

---

[7] This chapter is an abridged (and edited) version of the state of the art report prepared by the GoodBrother Consortium as a whitepaper [6], led by the working group leader Sara Colantonio.

1   A Historical View of Active Assisted Living   9

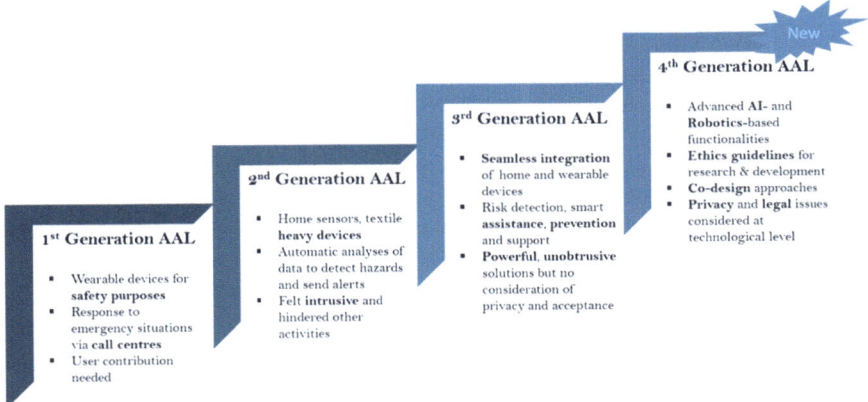

Fig. 1.1 The four generations of AAL technology. The fourth one is a brand-new wave, whose launched is testified by the "AAL Guidelines for Ethics, Data Privacy and Security", the GoodBrother initiative and the likes

process and to address the social, ethical and legal issues. Figure 1.1 illustrates these four waves of AAL technology. In the following, a very brief overview of these generations is provided.

First-Generation Technologies: The first generation of AAL technology mainly consisted of alert and alarm systems coming in the form of a pendant or alarm device. In case of an emergency, the assisted individual could press the button or pendant in order to send an alarm to a call center [106]. The first successful examples of this type of devices date back to the 1990s and include LifeAlert[8] or SafeLife Beghelli.[9] Experimental studies demonstrated that these first-generation alarms were able to ensure several benefits, such as safety and security of the assisted individuals and a reduction of stress levels of them, their families and caregivers [105]. On the other hand, they exhibited a number of limitations, as the assisted individual needed to remember to carry or wear the device and to be able to press the button.

Second-Generation Technologies: The second generation of AAL technology was more technologically advanced as it integrated sensors able to perceive risky conditions and react accordingly, as in case of environmental hazards [105]. An example of these solutions, particularly useful for older adults with mild cognitive impairment, was the device able to detect a gas leak and send an automatic alarm by contacting the appropriate authorities [105]. These technologies emerged by the end of 90s, early 2000s, and some of them are available on the market.

Third-Generation Technologies: The third generation of AAL technology has been boosted by the advancements of ICT moving towards a more comprehensive concept of AAL. The solutions in this case are complex systems that integrate diverse

---

[8] https://www.lifealert.com/.

[9] https://www.beghelli.it/salvalavita.

sensors and computing facilities, in some cases seamlessly incorporated into home appliances, to monitor the home environment for any types of risk or accident as well as to track the activity and health status of the assisted person. In this wave, the technologies are conceived to not only detect and report problems, but also to prevent worst scenarios by using preventative and prediction strategies. Moreover, they include actuators to provide the assisted individuals with assistance, and smart interfaces to provide them with information, support, and encouragement [25, 57, 80]. In the last years, there has been an explosion of these third-wave AAL solutions. Some of the products currently available are included in the AAL Products Catalogue[10] online, categorized according to the AAL applications they support, as well as the aspects of the quality of life they address.

Fourth-Generation Technologies: We argue that a new generation of AAL technology has started. The technological advances and the successes of the most recent Computer Vision (CV) and Signal Processing techniques (based mainly on Deep Learning) has strongly boosted the field of AAL. More powerful and effective solutions are being developed and experimented, as, for instance, those based on conversational agents and robotic assistants. Furthermore, in consideration of this increasing power and pervasiveness of technological solutions, the scientific communities, policy makers and funding bodies have started discussing strategies and approaches to ensure that such solutions respond to the highest ethical, legal and privacy standards and requirements. The AAL Programme has issued the "AAL Guidelines for Ethics, Data Privacy and Security" [1], with which "AAL goes one step further and demands more than just legal and ethical compliance, – it proposes Ethical Excellence, by fostering the implementation of the ethical dialogue and integrating relevant values in an iterative process of discussion. And applies this method not only during projects' lifetime but also for solutions already in the market". In this respect, the co-design of an AAL solution with the end-users is currently considered as an indispensable step that accompanies the whole development process [109]. Moreover, the issues pertaining to privacy preservation, especially in the case of audio and video data, have started to be handled also at the technological level, with different approaches now appearing in the literature [32, 42], as extensively surveyed in a white paper published by the GoodBrother COST Action[11] [5].

1.3 A Functional View of an AAL System Architecture

An AAL system can serve several functions or application scenarios, by integrating different ICT and sensor technologies to address the needs of diverse end-users [29, 96]. Consequently, an AAL system can come in different forms and with different architectures. Previous works [41] have attempted to find uniformities in existing

---

[10] https://www.aal-products.com/, Accessed 25 September 2024.
[11] https://www.cost.eu/actions/CA19121/, Accessed 25 September 2024.

solutions towards a standard design strategy. Nevertheless, diving in depth into the technical details of AAL software is over-encompassing and out of the scope of this chapter. A more high-level, functional view of the typical architecture of an AAL system is much more pertinent as it allows the reader to have an overview of how an AAL system functions and interacts with the end-users.

Essentially, a functional view of an AAL system derives from the compulsory components and functionalities it encompasses. Foremost, the system should incorporate sensor technologies that enable the acquisition of useful data about the ambient settings and the environment as well as the psychophysical conditions and the activities of the assisted individuals. The sensor technologies constitute the *sensing* or *perception* layer of the system. Dedicated algorithms process the data acquired by the sensors with the goal to understand, detect or measure the conditions of interest, for instance to recognize the activities of the assisted person to identify a risky situation (e.g., a fall) or to assist her in performing a task (e.g., dressing up). These algorithms compose the *data-processing* or *understanding layer* of an AAL system. The data can be stored locally and the algorithms can be embedded in the living environment or in mobile devices (this situation is currently referred to as "computing at the edge" or "edge processing/computing") or the processing layer can be located on distant servers on the cloud. Currently, the data processing layer is often a mixture of algorithms at the edge and on the cloud. In accordance with the information inferred by interpreting the sensed data, the AAL system can provided the end-users with feedback, for instance on suggestions on what to do next when performing a task, alarms or alerts when a risky situation is detected, or engaging them in a game. This happens through the *actuator/application* or *interaction* layer. This layer comprises the user interfaces and may require additional computing facilities to support the interactions, such as planning and controlling [14]. Figure 1.2 shows the three layers and their components. As shown, the sensor layer can be composed of simple smart and connected devices (i.e., the so-called Internet-of-Things, IoT) or it can correspond to a more complex sensor network composed by environmental sensors, intelligent devices, video cameras, or audio-based home assistants [29].

Environmental and appliance sensors can acquire information about temperature, humidity, air quality as well as the status of the appliance. Moreover, non-invasive sensors, such as cameras or infrared sensors, have been integrated in various devices (i.e., the so-called "smart objects", or "smart devices") and appliances (e.g., mirrors, TVs, rings, bracelets, watches), to monitor individuals in a non-obtrusive and easily acceptable manner, without affecting their normal activities. Accelerometers, gyroscopes, infrared or radar sensors can be embedded into smartphones or wearable devices, such as smart watches, fitness bands, clothing and fabrics to continuously monitoring people in both indoor and outdoor applications. Other medical devices (e.g., pulse oximeters, blood pressure monitors) can be connected to the network, thus allowing for the automatic transfer of vital parameters. This whole set of smart and connected devices used to monitor the vital parameters of an individual currently goes under the name of Internet of Health Things (IoHT).

The variety of technologies automatically implies a greater complexity of data, as they can change considerably in terms of size, heterogeneity, and sampling frequency.

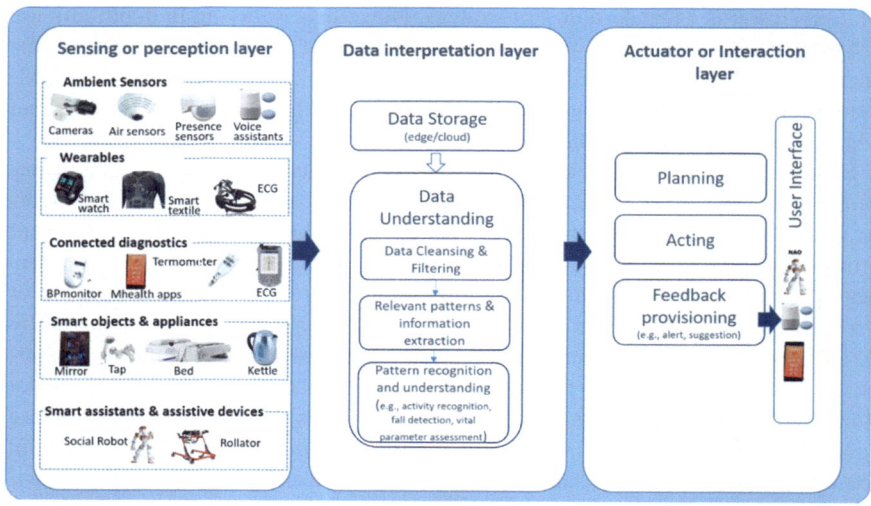

Fig. 1.2 A functional view of the main components of an AAL system. The various sensors networked in the sensing layer need a suitable orchestration to regulate data recording and storage. The algorithms in the data-understanding layer can work on data coming from a single sensor or on multiple sensors. The user interface could be embedded in any type of smart appliance (i.e., could be tangible or intangible)

Consequently, several issues related to data management are also relevant in AAL technology (e.g., communication protocols, security controls, energy consumption, failure detection, interoperability among diverse vendor devices, and so on).

Among the various typologies introduced above, the video and audio sensors are among the most powerful ones in terms of the information they convey. For instance, a single camera placed in a room can record most of the activities performed in the room, thus replacing many other non-visual sensors. As the costs of cameras have significantly dropped, a plethora of works have used cameras and computer vision techniques to address most of the AAL applications scenarios, boosting notably the field. Currently, video-based applications are able to recognize and monitor the activities, the movements, and the overall conditions of the assisted individuals as well as to assess their vital parameters (e.g., heart rate, respiratory rate). Similarly, audio sensors have a potential to become one of the most important modalities for interaction with AAL systems, as they can have a large range of sensing, do not require physical presence at a particular location and are physically intangible. Moreover, using voice is a more natural way of interaction than tactile interfaces.

Overall, audio and video-based sensors appear as less obtrusive with respect to the hindrance other wearable sensors can cause to one's activities. Nevertheless, they are often perceived as the most intrusive technologies from the viewpoint of the privacy of the monitored individuals. This is due to the richness of the information these technologies convey and the intimate setting where they are inserted.

In the following section, we propose a first attempt to categorize the various axes that characterize an AAL system.

1.4 A Taxonomy of AAL Technologies and Applications

Considering the plethora of diverse systems developed in the last decades, systematizing the various AAL technologies and applications is a challenging endeavor, which has been undertaken so far only partially, by providing only very limited classification schemes. Indeed, while several scoping reviews or scientific surveys have analyzed the existing literature in the field of AAL, only a couple of attempts produced an AAL taxonomy and both of them considered mainly the AAL application scenarios.

In 2014, the project TAALXONOMY,[12] funded by the Austrian Research Promotion Agency (FFG), proposed a taxonomy for the practical and effective classification of AAL products and services, by taking into account international definitions, initiatives and standards as well as feedback from relevant stakeholders, users and experts. Nevertheless, the TAALXONOMY classification scheme[13] mainly distinguishes the various living environments and life aspects that are addressed by the AAL system or service. The primary categorization axis is according to the application scope and groups AAL systems into "Health & Care", "Living & Buildings", "Safety & Security", "Mobility & Transport", "Work & Training", "Vitality & Abilities", "Leisure & Culture", and "Information & Communication" classes. Within each of these classes, a secondary classification is applied based on the field of application. For instance, the "Health & Care" class is further split in "Health Care and Prevention", "Body and Vital Data", "Telecare and Telehealth", "Electronic Health Record", "Nutrition & Diet", "Personal Hygiene", "Therapy", "Drugs and Pharmaceuticals", and "Care".

The TAALXONOMY classification scheme has served the creation of the AAL Products Catalogue[14] online catalogue, put together by the Department of Strategic Management, Marketing and Tourism from the University of Innsbruck and EURAC Bolzano. "AAL Products" is conceived to give solution providers the opportunity to advertise their AAL solutions cost-free, thus enhancing their visibility. Moreover, it provides the visitors with an overview of assistive- and smart-technology products and services available on the market.

Another AAL taxonomy appears in the work by Byrne et al. [21], which provides a classification framework based on four core categories: "smart homes", "intelligent life assistants", "wearables", and "robotics". Each of these has distinctive subclasses that categorize AAL systems in accordance with their primary function. For

---

[12] https://www.taalxonomy.eu/en/, Accessed 25 September 2024.
[13] https://www.taalxonomy.eu/wp-content/uploads/Downloads/D4.1-ANNEX-TAALXONOMY-final-oeffentlich.xlsx, Accessed 25 September 2024.
[14] https://www.aal-products.com/index.php/frontend/start?categorie=-1, Accessed 25 September 2024.

instance, "Smart Homes" are further distinguished in "General Health Monitoring" and "Platforms"; whilst "Intelligent Life Assistants" are further split into "Wandering Prevention Tools", "Electronic Home Control Systems" and "Fall Detection Systems".

The GoodBrother Consortium has worked on an AAL taxonomy with the idea to distinguish the various technological facilities, ICT components, main functionalities and application scopes of an AAL system. The idea of such a taxonomy is to illustrate the wide spectrum of options that characterize assistive and supportive technologies and systems. The resulting scheme is a tree-like structure that is described in the following paragraphs, starting from the root and the primary branches moving towards the leaves.

An AAL application or system is characterized by its "Technological underpinnings" and "Assistive & supportive undertakings", as shown in Fig. 1.3. The "Technological underpinnings" include the ICT facilities for "Data acquisition" and "Data processing & understanding" as well as the "Enabling infrastructure" and the facilities for the "Human-computer interaction". An AAL application can implement one or more "Assistive & supportive scopes", which can be characterised by defining their "End-user & beneficiaries", the "Ambient settings" where the application is deployed, the "Care needs" that the application addresses, the "Assistive and/or supportive functionalities" it provides, the "Other involved actors" if any, and the type of the "Output & feedback provided" during the interaction with the end-users.

Considered in more detail, "Data acquisition" can be further specialized as shown in Fig. 1.4. More specifically, it encompasses diverse modalities for acquiring data about the end-users and the environment where they live, work or move. Reflecting the major interest of GoodBrother Consortium in video- and audio-based AAL, among the "Data sensing devices", we highlight video and audio sensors. "Video and image sensors" include "RGB cameras", "Depth sensors", "Thermal cameras" and "Multispectral cameras" (in this we also include hyperspectral ones). Among the "Other types of sensors", we include the various sensors that use different modalities to acquire data, such as gyroscopes and accelerometers that fall within "Motion-based" sensors or Galvanic Skin Response sensors that fall within the "Electrodermal" sensors, and others.

Sensor devices can be deployed in various modalities: they can be installed in the environment (e.g., on the ceiling); they can be worn by the user when they are integrated into wearables; they can be integrated into social robots or home assistants (e.g., Google Home or Amazon Alexa), or they can be embedded in smart appliances (e.g., in the fridge or behind a smart mirror) or integrated into the smart phone. Data can come also in the form of manual input from the users, via a mobile or tablet applications, by replying to questionnaires, or filling forms or from diagnostic examinations.

"Data processing & understanding" encompasses methods and technologies belonging to disciplines such as CV, Signal Processing, Multimodal and Big data analytics, Artificial Intelligence and Machine Learning. These include a wide range of methods, whose listing is out of the scope of this chapter. The "Computing infrastructure" comprises all the ICT facilities for the storage, the transmission and the

1 A Historical View of Active Assisted Living

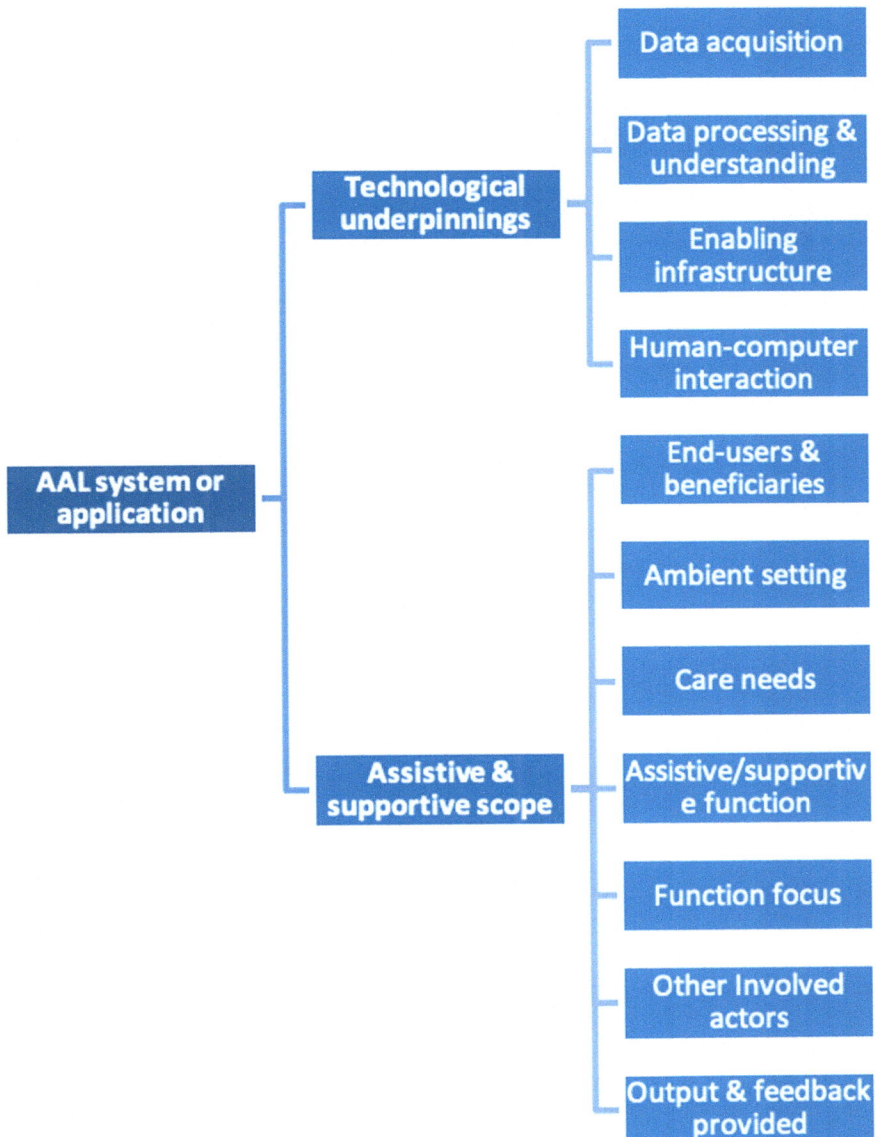

Fig. 1.3 The primary layers of the proposed AAL taxonomy

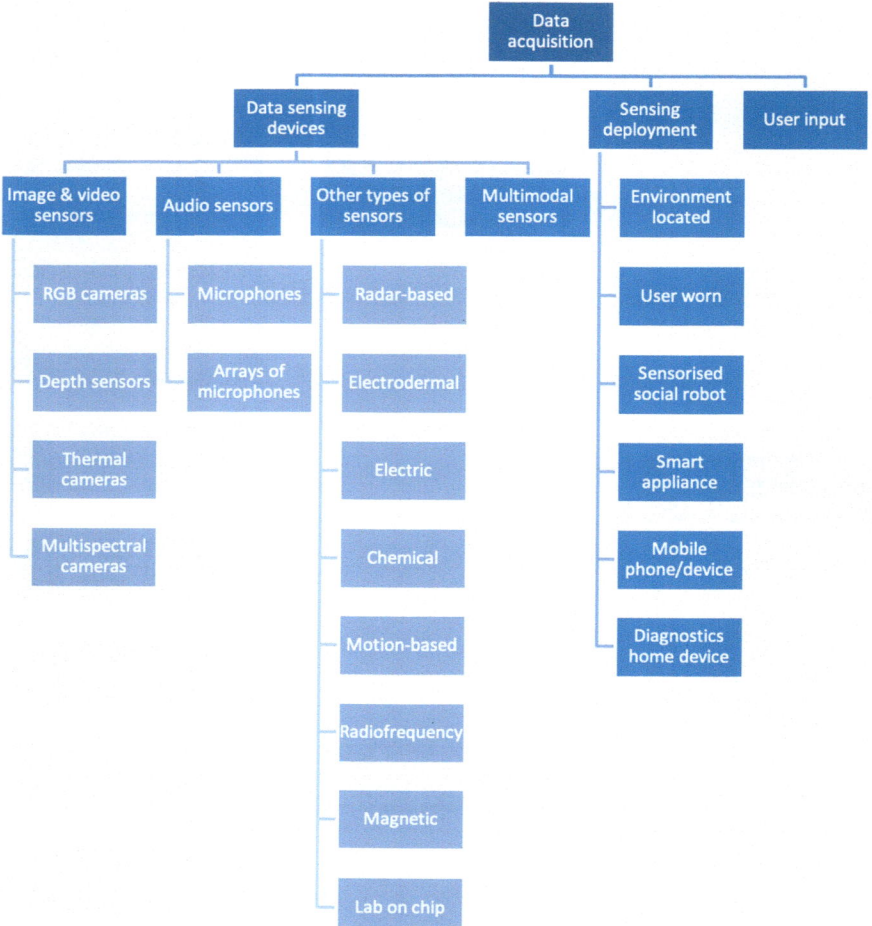

Fig. 1.4 The specialization of data acquisition

communication of data, as well as for orchestrating the sensor devices and the computing resources. Computing localization may be "on-site," or on the cloud. Finally, "Human-computer interaction" comprises the interfaces through which the support and feedback are provided to and the commands or inputs are received from the end-users. Figure 1.5 further summarizes this specialization.

When considering the "Assistive & supportive scope", an AAL system can address various types of "End-users & beneficiaries". These include frail or impaired individuals, chronic and multi-morbidity patients, and aging healthy subjects. Among the beneficiaries, we can also include formal and informal caregivers, as the assistive and supportive environments can help them by alleviating their work and burden.

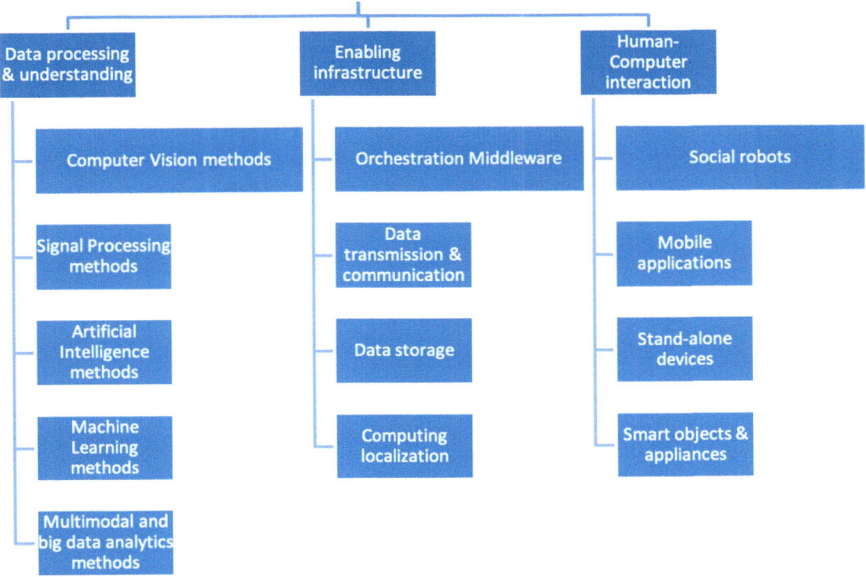

Fig. 1.5 The underpinnings of "Data processing & understanding", "Computing infrastructure" and the "Human-computer interaction" categories

Moreover, Clinicians and General Practitioners can be addressed as end-users with the provision of information and analyses of physical, cognitive and behavior information of chronic patients recorded remotely.

The "Care needs" addressed by an AAL application include the primary prevention, for preventing diseases for at-risk subjects, the diagnosis or risk detection for the detection of disease exacerbation events, therapy or treatment for enacting and monitoring compliance, or tertiary prevention, to improve quality of life and reduce disease symptoms. Accordingly, the assistive or supportive function can be monitoring (e.g., behavior or vital signs), detecting or recognizing (e.g., disease exacerbation, risks or falls), preventing (e.g., disease worsening or accidents), assisting (e.g., in the daily-life activities), training or supporting rehabilitation (e.g., through exergames). The focus of such function ("Function focus") can be any of the various assets of health and wellbeing, including psychophysical conditions, with vital signs (e.g., cardiovascular parameters, breathing patterns) and emotional state (e.g., stress, anxiety, fatigue, or depression), lifestyle (e.g., physical activity, and food intake) sleep hygiene, sensorimotor and cognitive conditions, social interactions or the Activities of Daily Living (ADLs). The "Output and feedback" that can be provided to the end-users include alarms and alerts (e.g., when a fall or an exacerbation event is detected), suggestions or advice (e.g., on lifestyle), engagement in social interactions or exergames, reminders for drug intake, support in performing any task of daily living, support in out-door activities. The "Ambient settings" can, indeed, be indoor or

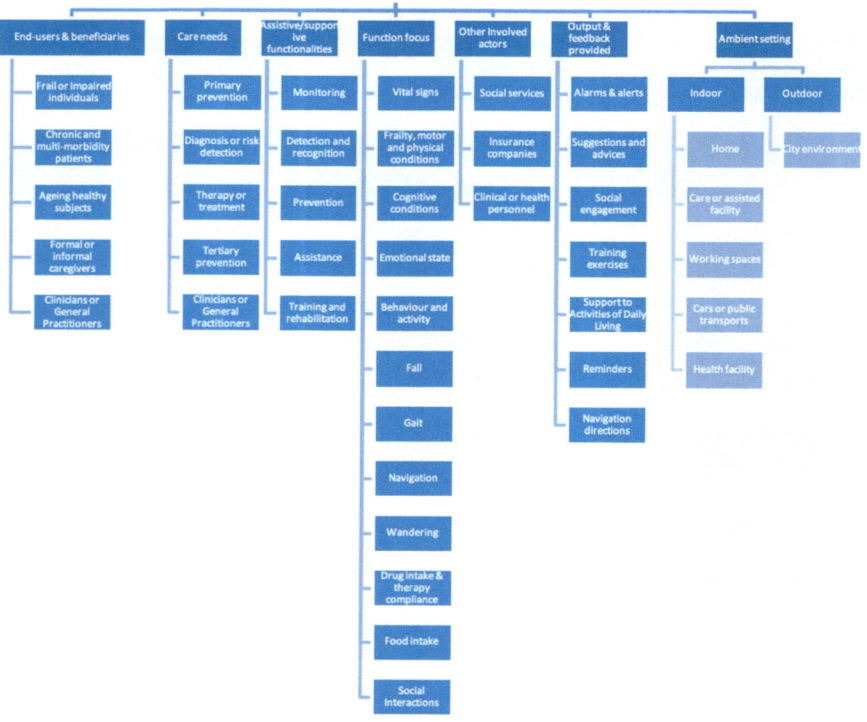

Fig. 1.6 Detail structure of the subcategories under "Assistive & supportive scope"

outdoor. We also include in the scheme "Other actors", including in this category the other professionals that intervene in the caring or assistive process. Figure 1.6 details the various sub-categories listed above.

An AAL system or application can encompass various options of those included in the taxonomy: for instance, it may address older adults suffering from Moderate Cognitive Impairment, by monitoring their vital signs and emotional state, engaging them in cognitive-training games, supporting them in ADLs and providing them with suggestions on physical activities and food intake. This might be done by integrating various sensing modalities and exploiting several data interpretation methods.

In this chapter, we concentrate on AAL applications based on video and audio data. In this respect, we document the recent advances in the technological underpinnings related to video and audio data sensing and processing (Sect. 1.5).

1   A Historical View of Active Assisted Living   19

1.5   Technological Underpinnings of Audio and Video Based AAL

This section summarizes the state of the art of the technological underpinnings of video- and audio-based AAL. Firstly, an overview of the various video-based sensing technologies is provided in Sect. 1.5.1, by describing the main types of sensors used in AAL. A similar overview of the sensing technologies for audio data is presented afterwards in Sect. 1.5.2.

1.5.1   Video-Based Sensing Technologies

Nowadays, monitoring and behavior analysis tasks can be carried out by a variety of image-based technologies. These technologies can be classified by the place where they are installed, such as indoors or outdoors, wearables or embedded systems, but can also be divided by their mechanical capacities, such as bullet type, omni-directional or pan-tilt-zoom cameras, or by their in-built features, such as motion detection or night vision.

Apart from the shape, angle and environment also the underlying camera technology varies. Not only RGB (Red, Green, Blue) cameras, which are highly controversial for their usage in AAL due to their lack of privacy protection, but also more privacy-aware solutions such as depth and infrared cameras have evolved in this area. While depth sensors measure distances from objects to the sensor, infrared (IR) sensors compute the temperature generated from objects. In the upcoming subsections, different image-based technologies are explained in more depth. Some of them are depicted in Fig. 1.7.

1.5.1.1   RGB Cameras

For humans, images and video are straightforward to interpret, as they reproduce the way we see the world. Digital cameras replace the light-sensitive film of analogue cameras of the past, by a digital matrix of sensors, either as a charge-coupled device (CCD) or an active-pixel sensor (CMOS). These matrices contain sensors encoding the RGB signals received when the shutter is open for a fraction of a second. This process works similar to how the human eye forms images in the retina, in the back of the eye, using physiological structures called cones and rods, which are specialized in capturing different wavelengths of light.

The product of such a process in a digital camera thus produces images with a value representing the intensity of the light received in the picture element (pixel) at each coordinate of the sensor matrix. This is what the computer 'perceives' from a camera connected to it, just a bunch of numbers, representing pixel intensities. This type of representation is very high dimensional and has no semantics associated with

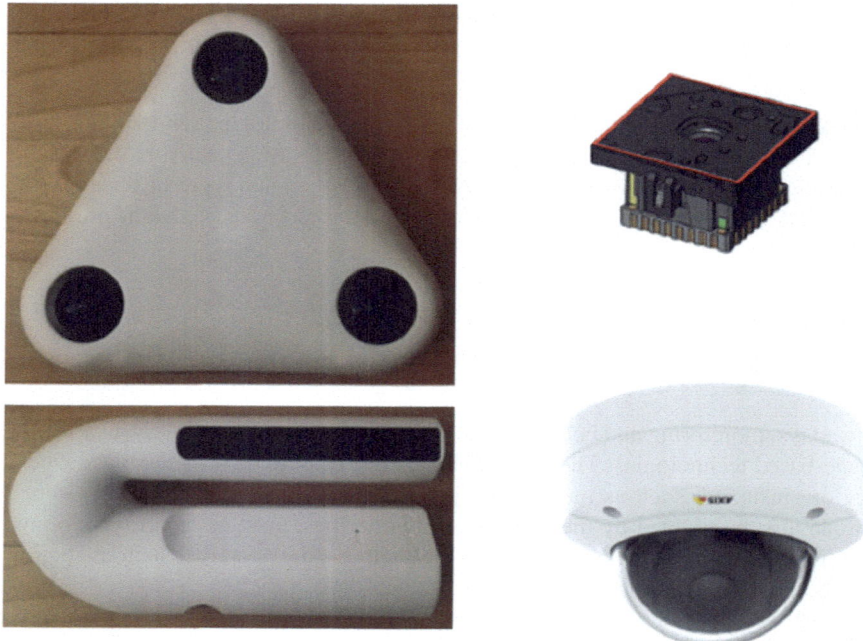

Fig. 1.7 Different camera types used in AAL applications: top left—Omni-directional camera, top right—Thermal camera, bottom left—depth sensor, (d) bottom right—RGB dome camera

it, therefore the analysis is very complex. Computer vision (CV) aims at making it possible for computers to interpret such rich information and infer useful knowledge from it. In the past, this was done via filtering, hand-crafted feature extraction and robust algorithms, such as Support Vector Machine (SVMs) or Random Forest (RF) among others. At the present, Artificial Neural Networks (ANN) are used for this process, which have proven to be very good at this task, often improving previous attempts, and even outperforming humans in some specific scenarios. Furthermore, humans have the ability to estimate depth thanks to the use of binocular vision, namely having two eyes separated by some distance. The different appearance of objects on the images, mainly in the relative horizontal position, received by the brain from each eye, helps it determine the distance of relevant objects.

Likewise, in stereoscopic CV it is possible to use several calibrated cameras to obtain pairs (or sets) of images and estimate the so-called "disparity maps" of objects appearing in the scene via "triangulation" of matching points. Another possibility is to use structured light patterns and check the deviation of the light as it rebounds in observed objects [124]. These light patterns can be visible, or be emitted by an infrared (IR) light source, in which case, an additional IR sensor is required in the setting. Using this setup (common in Microsoft Kinect, ASUS xtion, Orbbec Astra and similar devices), an additional "channel" is received, thus forming RGB-D (D for depth) images.

Within the AAL field, the most relevant applications as collected in Planinc et al. [86] are:

- behavior analysis or understanding: specific applications include detecting initiated activities to follow along and give cues for correct finalization when the person is disoriented or leaves the activity due to forgetfulness, or detecting patterns of long-term behaviors in the performance of activities of daily living (ADLs).
- fall detection and prevention (gait analysis): detecting falling people, but also analyze gait as an important marker for cognitive impairment, and physical decline, leading to falls in the future.
- motor rehabilitation: programs for older people and physical injury recovery therapies, aided by pose estimation, to check the correctness of exercise performance, as well as evaluate the range of mobility.
- vital sign and remote monitoring: including but not limited to heart rate monitoring via amplification of color changes in the skin as part of normal blood circulation.

Some of these applications are reviewed in detail in other chapters in this book, such as activities of daily living [7] (Chap. 7), fall detection and prevention [73] (Chap. 5), and remote monitoring of vital signs [36] (Chap. 8).

Until recently, RGB-D and stereoscopic vision were considered essential for assisting with tasks like 3D shape reconstruction. For example, RGB-D technology enabled the retrieval of skeletal data, representing a person's body pose as a set of 15–20 joints, depending on the sensor model and brand. Pose estimation from skeletal data is highly relevant in AAL, as it serves as a foundation for human motion analysis, which is important for activity recognition, gait analysis, and fall detection. Nonetheless, with the use of deep neural networks it has been possible to use monocular images for these tasks. Examples of this are the OpenPose [22] and LCRNet [98] networks, providing skeletal data as body joint coordinates (in 2D and 2D/3D respectively); or the DensePose [51] and FrankMocap [99] networks, developed at Facebook, Inc. The former provides an IUV image, consisting of three channels, each providing information at the pixel level about the body part index (I), and the (u, v) coordinates within the body part surface of each pixel (U, V channels). By contrast, the latter uses the SMPL (Skinned Multi-Person Linear Model) human body model [67, 72], developed at the Max Planck Institute and fits it on the detected body pose and shape (i.e., body variations, such as waist circumference, and so on). Example outputs of these networks are shown in Fig. 1.8.

1.5.1.2 Depth Sensors

As pointed out by Planinc et al. [86], advances in the development of 3D sensors motivate their use instead of cameras for wearable sensors, since they provide advantages like privacy protection and improved robustness when it comes to behavior mod-

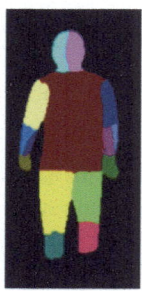 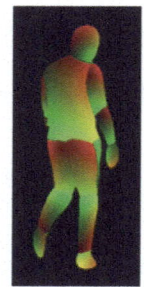 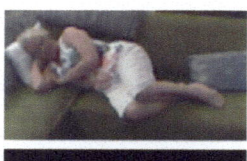 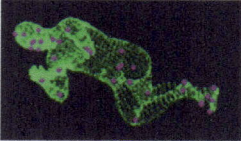

Fig. 1.8 (left) Body part indices (colorized for improved visualisation) of a DensePose network output image; (right) the original output of DensePose also contains U and V coordinates of the inferred body part surface (shown as red-to-green gradients)

eling, gesture recognition or activity recognition. In contrast to RGB based analysis, depth-based approaches do not process RGB color images, but depth of range images measuring distance from objects to the sensor. Depth images do not visualize the scene with colors, but the gray level indicates the distance of the objects and its surroundings to the sensor. The darker the color, the closer the object is to the sensor. On the other hand, brighter colors are used for objects at a higher distance. Black holes within the depth image indicate reflecting or absorbing areas where no valid depth measurement is available and are caused due to the functionality of the sensor. In contrast to RGB based approaches, only the silhouette is detected and thus no conclusions whether the person is wearing clothes or the emotional state can be obtained since neither the clothes, nor the face are visible. Hence, the appearance of the person is fully protected. However, this is only the case if processing is solely based on depth images.

RGB-D based approaches combine depth information together with appearance information in order to obtain and combine more details. Although these approaches limit the privacy of older adults, color information can be taken into consideration, thus permitting to perform a more in-depth analysis. With the introduction of the Microsoft Kinect in 2010, depth sensors have become more popular, and other sensors, such as Intel RealSense were marketed[15].

The functionality of the Kinect is based on structured light imaging, where the projector emits a pre-defined IR light pattern to the scene [46, 53]. Due to the spatial arrangement of the pattern and its varying sizes as well as distortions depending on the distance to the camera, the depth camera captures the light pattern and an on-board chip calculates a depth map.

The main advantages of depth-based sensors, especially within the context of AAL, can be summarized as follows:

- No additional light source needed: due to the use of infrared light, sensors also work during the night (e.g., when falls of older adults occur),

---

[15] Kinect was discontinued since July 2023, as of September 2024.

- Sensor is robust to changing lighting conditions: switching the lights on and off does not affect the results of the depth images. However, direct sunlight interferes with the projected infrared pattern and thus, no depth value can be calculated. This restricts the use of the sensors to indoor environments only,
- No calibrated camera setup is needed: in contrast to the use of a calibrated multiple camera setup in order to calculate a 3D reconstruction, no calibration is needed,
- Standard algorithms can be applied to depth information: standard algorithms for CV (e.g., foreground/background segmentation, tracking) can be applied to depth data directly,
- Protection of privacy: if only depth information is processed, privacy is protected since the appearance of the person is not recognized in depth images. However, if a combined analysis of RGB and depth images is performed, privacy is not protected.

Different types of information are extracted from depth data in order to carry out specific tasks. Skeletal data, for instance, is used to extract body parts and skeleton joints in order to estimate a person's pose [103]. Methods operating on depth maps frequently use histogram-based features and supervised learning for person detection [58, 108, 119]. Another approach is to first re-project depth map pixels to world coordinates and to operate on the resulting point cloud. One application for this method is the estimation of a person's proportion based on their height [61]. A reason why methods operating on point clouds are slow is the large number of points (up to 300 K) and the fact that clustering is a complex task. Sub-sampling the point cloud can alleviate this problem [56]. An alternative are so-called plan-view maps, two-dimensional representations of the scene as viewed from the top and under orthographic projection [16].

1.5.1.3 Low-Resolution Thermal Sensors

In the last decade, thermal vision systems based on low-cost IR array sensors provoked the interest of the researchers and became attractive in many AAL scenarios. These scenarios focus on

1. looking at people in their home for detecting possible emergency situations (see Fig. 1.9)
2. monitoring indoor people's presence (occupation) in buildings
3. detecting stationary position or tracking moving people in a room or building
4. fall detection and detection of unusual activity for older adults in toilets, bathrooms, changing rooms, etc.

The use of low-resolution IR arrays comes with the following benefits: privacy preservation, low power consumption (passive device), low price, insensitivity to ambient lighting level and changes, operation in total darkness, fast response time, easy deployment and easy image processing. These sensors are less invasive and more convenient to use in indoor environments. The IR array sensors measure the

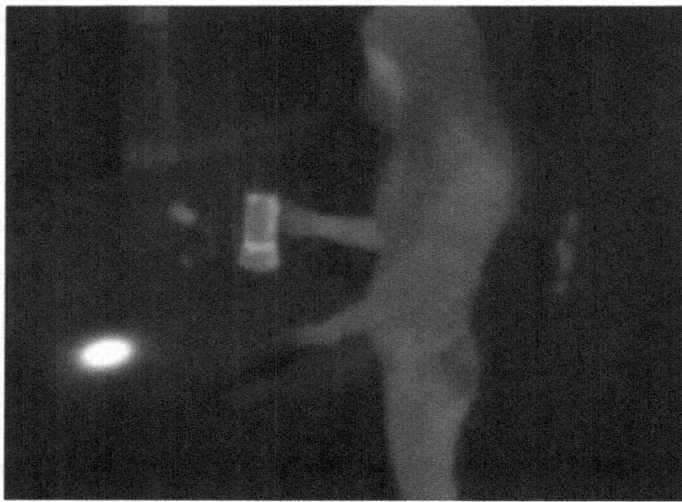

Fig. 1.9 Raw thermal image showing a switched-on stove and a person in the kitchen

heat generated from the human body or other objects and visualize it on a low-resolution IR matrix. Low-resolution IR thermal arrays typically have a resolution of 8 × 8, 4 × 16, 16 × 16 or 24 × 32 pixels.

Several studies have explored various combinations of sensing modalities, methods, processing techniques, and machine learning approaches for detecting, localising, and counting individuals inside rooms or buildings using low-cost, low-resolution IR sensor arrays (e.g., 8 × 8 pixels). Jeong et al. [59] introduced a probabilistic method with pre- and post-processing techniques to detect humans based on heat signatures from a thermal IR sensor array system. Similar approaches have been developed by Basu and Rowe [13] and Trofimova et al. [115], showing promising results in human detection.

In addition to single-person detection, low-resolution IR sensor arrays have been applied to estimate the flow of people [79], using threshold-based and temperature filtering techniques. Maaspuro [75] explored the use of IR sensor arrays for doorway occupancy counting, employing a Kalman filter tracking algorithm. Singh and Aksanli [104] demonstrated how careful algorithm selection can yield highly accurate results for detecting the presence of individuals, with the best outcomes achieved when sensors are mounted on the ceiling. They also addressed static activity detection, such as sitting or standing, by combining data pre-processing techniques and machine learning methods to successfully identify four static activities.

In the AAL context, several fall detection methods using thermal IR sensor arrays have been developed with a focus on privacy preservation. Hayashida et al. [54] used a thermal camera to capture falls and developed a heuristic recognition algorithm. Spasova et al. [107] proposed a real-time, privacy-preserving fall detection algorithm that uses geometric properties of the human silhouette and a support vector machine,

1 A Historical View of Active Assisted Living

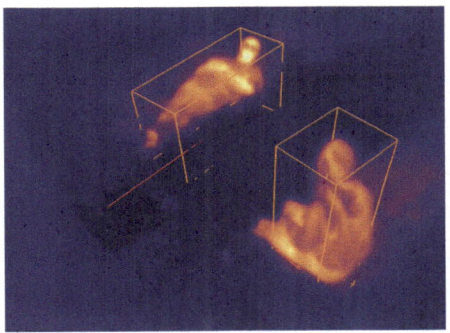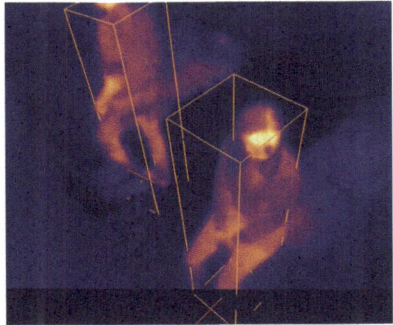

Fig. 1.10 Example visualizations of raw IR data of a person lying on the floor (left) and standing (right)

leveraging both infrared and visible light imagery. Additionally, in [121] further improved fall detection using a 24 × 32 pixel thermal sensor, building on earlier work [113].

Figure 1.10 shows from different camera angles what images with this resolution look like. The algorithm is based on a pipeline composed of the following steps: preprocessing, feature extraction and classification. The collected dataset includes two sensor-mounting scenarios: overhead and sideways placement. Recent experiments with very low resolution photoreceptors show that it may be possible to solve a range of tasks with these sensors, but the camera placement is a very important parameter, and intuitive designs by humans actually do not work [9]. The solution is to optimize the sensor placement with algorithms.

1.5.1.4 Wearable Cameras: First Person or Egocentric Vision

As explored above, cameras can be placed in the environment, or, conversely, they can be placed on the user, i.e., as wearable cameras, mounted on a belt around the chest, or a lanyard; or as part of "smart glasses" or similar head-mounted devices. Methodologies dealing with footage from such cameras receive multiple names, such as "egovision", "egocentric vision" and also "first-person video" (FPV). One drawback of wall-mounted cameras is that the user's own body, such as the torso, can obstruct the view of the activity being performed, making it difficult for the camera to capture the action [83]. For instance, if the user opens a refrigerator door or interacts with a moving part of an appliance, certain body parts may block the camera's view during the activity. However, these types of occlusions can be avoided when cameras are worn by the user. Additionally, objects being manipulated, as well as the hands, remain visible, which is particularly beneficial given that most ADLs involve the upper extremities.

Historically, methods for activity recognition from wearable cameras have been divided into "object-based" (context of visible objects being used to recognize the activity), and "motion-based" where physical features (magnitude, angle, frequency) of motions are used to determine the types of actions being performed. Both methods have disadvantages, as noted in the review by Nguyen et al. [83], namely, missing detections of relevant objects and types of actions involving small movements of the limbs implied in the action, respectively. It is worth noting, however, that both types are not mutually exclusive and can be combined. The way these two proposed modalities of action recognition are combined can be via a hierarchical framework, as done by Betancourt et al. [15], in which "hand detection" or "motion pattern detection" are at a lower level of "basic scene understanding", and higher levels correspond to subject-object interactions involving detections of relevant objects, and other contextual information. Nonetheless, this split between modalities was more relevant or clear before the advent of end-to-end differentiable (trainable) deep neural network methodologies, in which all elements (subnets) of the model may contribute to the inference of the type of action being performed. Some branches of the model might be specialized in certain tasks, but the contribution to the final decision is not clear-cut, or at least, not as much as with previous methodologies. The reader is referred to the review by Bandini et al. [12], which shows examples of this.

Finally, for further reading of the latest advancements in action recognition for the purposes of lifelogging, from wall-mounted as well as wearable cameras, Climent-Pérez et al. offer a literature review exploring existing video-based technologies in the AAL context [31], with a focus on methods whose outputs can be assembled into a lifelog for the user, that is then able to share it, according to their needs, with healthcare providers, caregivers or social workers of their choice. Plizzari et al. [87] explore how egocentric vision can enhance daily life by enabling tasks such as localization, scene understanding, action recognition, and social interaction. The paper provides a detailed review of the current technologies and research tasks related to egocentric vision, identifies limitations in existing systems, and highlights the gap between current methods and future applications. The survey also examines key areas for future exploration, including gaze prediction, body pose estimation, and privacy concerns, as well as the need for more robust hardware to realize the potential of egocentric vision in everyday use.

1.5.2 Audio-Based Sensing Technologies

Though CV has brought the largest advances in AAL, it often requires installation of video cameras at user's homes, which may be considered intrusive and thus refused by the targeted population. Furthermore, video processing is extremely sensitive to light conditions that may vary substantially at different positions in a home [26]. In this context, audio-based technology can be seamlessly integrated into the user's environment and has a potential to become one of the most important modalities for interaction with AAL systems. It has a large range of sensing, does not require physical presence at a particular location and it is physically intangible [88]. Using voice is a more natural way of interaction than tactile interfaces. Despite these advantages, audio technologies still remain rarely deployed in real settings, partly because the audio analysis in the presence of ambient noise is a challenging task [118]. Nevertheless, with the recent advancement of audio technologies and their integration in mobile and Internet of Things (IoT) devices, the use of audio signals in AAL becomes feasible [11], with applications in human activity recognition (HAR) [26, 88], fall detection and fall prevention [27, 117], food intake monitoring [76, 91], emotional state recognition [23, 62], and so on.

Monitoring and behavior analysis in the context of an acoustical environment can be realized these days by two different technologies, i.e., conventional microphones and their arrays or specific acoustical sensors. These technologies can be divided into two categories according to a frequency range, which they operate in, namely a human audible frequency range (20 Hz–20 kHz) and a human inaudible frequency range (all frequencies outside of the human audible frequency range). When it comes to the specific acoustical sensors, they are represented by surface acoustic sensors, floor acoustic sensors, ultrasonic sensors and throat microphones or laryngophones. In the upcoming sections, the technologies deployed for monitoring and behavior analysis in the context of an acoustical environment are described in more detail.

1.5.2.1 Microphone and Microphone Arrays

A standard microphone is an electroacoustic device, which converts sound waves into an electrical signal. The sound waves produced by an audio source propagate through the air and cause slight changes in air pressure around the microphone, whose task is to detect them. The general principle has many similarities with a human ear, as they share the same objective. The sound waves produce motion of the outer part of a microphone (i.e., diaphragm). In the next part of a microphone, this motion is converted to an electrical signal proportional to the sound waves.

The way a microphone converts motion into an electrical signal depends on its type. Two main types are dynamic and condenser microphones. Electromagnetic induction is used in dynamic microphones. The diaphragm is attached to an induction coil, which is placed in a magnetic field. The coil movement induces an electrical current representing the audio signal. The dynamic microphone design results in an inexpensive and robust device. The condenser microphone is based on the change of electric charge. The diaphragm is in the form of a plate of a capacitor. The diaphragm's movement alters the distance between plates and consequently changes the electric charge, which presents the audio signal. The condenser microphones have better sensitivity due to their design. They require a power source needed for the capacitor plates to operate.

The level of small air pressure changes also corresponds to the low electrical signal level produced on a direct output of a microphone. Thus, additional signal processing is necessary, where a separate amplification unit (i.e., preamplifier) is

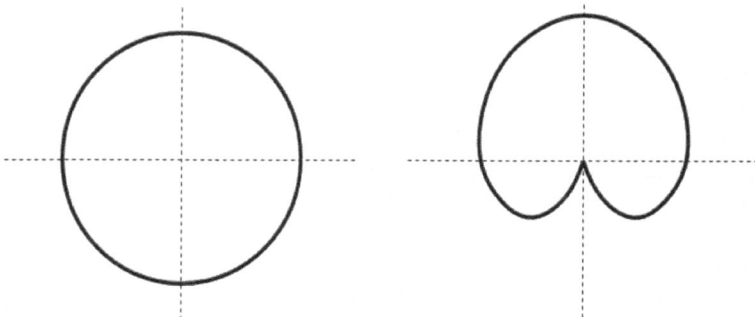

Fig. 1.11 Omni-directional (left) and cardioid (right) microphone polar patterns

applied. The goal is to increase the level of the captured electrical signal without achieving the same effect on the coexistent audio noise signal.

Microphone polar pattern is an important parameter (Fig. 1.11), which shows its directional sensitivity projected on a polar plane. It depends on the device design. Frequent polar patterns are omni-directional, bi-directional, cardioid, subcardioid, hypercardioid, supercardioid, and shotgun. Which polar pattern is the most suitable one highly depends on the usage scenarios. Different AAL applications and systems prefer various microphone polar patterns.

Another important characteristic of a microphone is its quality. If advanced audio technologies are used in an AAL system, such as spoken language technology interfaces, audio quality plays a significant role. Some parameters defining the microphone quality are the frequency range, sensitivity, level of total harmonic distortions, etc.

Microphones can be found in many devices, as speech presents a natural way of human interaction. One of the most omnipresent devices nowadays are mobile phones. They usually have one primary microphone and additional secondary microphones to improve the captured audio signal. In other scenarios, two microphones are also used for stereo recordings.

An audio device hosting more than one primary microphone is called a microphone array. Several microphones are operating in parallel, all capturing audio signals simultaneously, producing a multichannel signal on direct output. Microphones in an array are placed in different patterns, which also influences the task they are best used for. The raw audio signal needs to be processed to benefit from the array setup. Digital signal processing is carried out on a digital signal processing (DSP) board or a computer. Modules responsible for this provide the system with advanced functionalities such as virtual polar patterns, beamforming, source localization, local echo cancellation, and noise reduction. Microphone arrays are essential for various AAL applications as they can better capture audio in a real-life environment.

1.5.2.2 Specific Acoustic Sensors

Surface acoustic sensors detect the mechanical waves that propagate through or on the surface of the solid materials. They typically use piezoelectric effect to convert the wave into an electric signal, such that changes made to the mechanical wave are reflected in the output electric signal. Surface acoustic sensors mostly work as passive sensors, which makes them power-efficient and reduces the production and operation costs. However, they are sensitive to coupling between surface material and the sensor and may require periodical sensor calibration. Surface acoustic sensors can be used for fall detection or for detecting the activities of daily living in a household that cause vibrations on the ground surface, such as object dropping, falling [8] or walking [85].

Floor acoustic sensors are special types of surface acoustic sensors used for detection of human falls. They are positioned on the floor surface, in the vicinity of the sound source and capture direct sound waves without reflection from the surface. They usually consist of an inner resonant container with a microphone located inside, that captures the vibration of the surface. A membrane at the bottom of the container touches the floor and enables acoustic coupling with the surface. Inner container is surrounded by an outer container (capsule) and acoustically isolated, to decrease the intensity of acoustic waves that propagate through air [90].

Ultrasonic sensors are piezoelectric transducers that actively send and receive ultrasonic pulses and measure the signal propagation time to and from the measured object. They operate by converting an electrical signal into mechanical vibrations and vice versa. Since the operation frequency is outside the human audible range (i.e., from 20 kHz to 200 MHz, typically at 40 kHz), they can be considered unobtrusive. Depending on the sensor and object properties, the effective sensor range is between several centimeters and several meters. The sensor that works at the frequency of 40 kHz can typically sense objects at a distance of up to 2 m [48]. Ultrasonic sensors can be used for fall detection [81], detecting activities of daily living such as standing or sitting [50], or even in-air gestures [92] and respiratory rate [95] when operating in a close range mode.

Throat microphones, or laryngophones, are contact microphones that absorb audio vibrations generated by the larynx directly from the user's throat using the neck-mounted sensors. While standard microphones pick up sound vibrations that propagate through the air, capturing at the same time background noise, throat microphones capture only vibrations from the throat, ignoring background noise and wind turbulence. Therefore, they can be used in extremely noisy or windy environments (e.g., while riding a motorcycle). Moreover, they are able to capture whispers, making them suitable for use in situations where silent communication is required (e.g., military or law enforcement operations). Since they are positioned on the human's neck, they can be used without obstructing helmets or respiratory protection. However, the nasal sounds and sounds generated by the tongue and lips are muffled. In the context of the AAL applications throat microphones are used for monitoring of chewing and swallowing [102] and in food intake monitoring [17].

1.5.3 Data Processing and Understanding for AAL

The data acquired by the video and audio-sensing layer are processed to perform specific tasks, such as detecting and recognizing relevant objects, detecting movements and incidents, measuring vital parameters, or analyzing gait. In this respect, AAL solutions relies on methods and technologies coming from several connected disciplines working on data processing and understanding as well as inference and problem solving, such as CV, Signal Processing, Internet of Everything and IoHT, Computational Physiology, Machine Learning and Artificial Intelligence.

As already sketched within the functional architecture of an AAL system shown in Fig. 1.2, the typical pipeline for data processing can be summarized as shown in Fig. 1.12 [111, 112, 123].

The data-cleaning step aims to improve the quality of the collected data by removing noise, harmonizing the data or selecting specific parts of the data. This step is also usually referred to as a pre-processing step. To extract the relevant information or patterns from the data, a segmentation step is often performed. This consists in identifying and selecting only the regions of interest in an image (e.g., a person's face or silhouette) or a signal (i.e., a word or a sentence in an audio signal). Once the relevant patterns are selected, these are usually described by computing a number of parameters, called features, which express and measure significant characteristics of the pattern. Such features are also usually referred to as hand-crafted features, as they are selected according to the knowledge of task to be performed.

In some cases, the features are extracted before segmentation to perform the segmentation itself. In other cases, the features are extracted without segmenting the data. The features are processed by "intelligent" algorithms that are able to recognize the detected patterns to perform a specific task, such as recognizing a fall or a vocal command. In some easy tasks, this latter step can rely on simple rules,

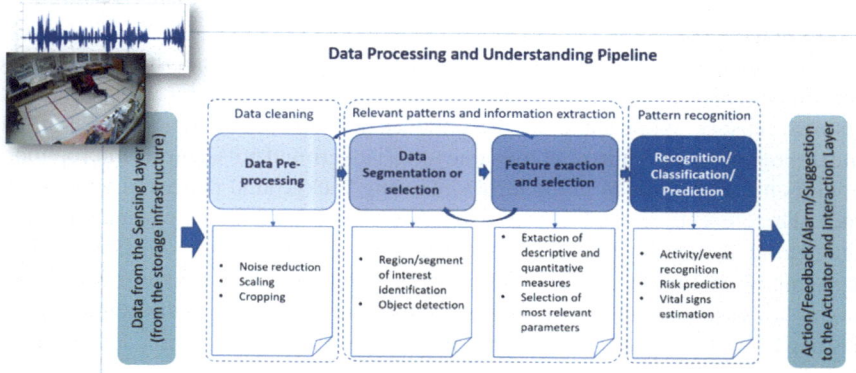

Fig. 1.12 A simplified version of the video and audio-data processing pipeline

based on threshold applied to the features' values. In most of the cases, it requires more complex solutions based on advanced statistical or data-inductive models [29].

As said, this pipeline is a high-level and simplified vision of the data-processing chain. In practice, more iterations of the steps might be required (e.g., activity recognition may require person recognition and tracking) or each step should be further adapted to respect the data typology (e.g., when processing time-series or multimodal data). For instance, the last recognition step, based on data-inductive methods, might be required to recognize the relevant objects in an image or sentences in an audio signal.

Data-inductive methods are those methods able to learn directly from the data the significant pattern relationships that are relevant to perform a specific task. These methods gather under the discipline known as Machine Learning (ML). Among the several definitions proposed for ML so far, the most renowned one is by Mitchell: "ML is the science that is concerned with the question of how to construct computer programs that automatically improve with experience" [78]. The peculiarity of ML methods is their ability to discover patterns and information from a set of data or examples. This ability enables them to learn autonomously how to recognize categories, perceive stimuli, predict trends, make decisions and apprehend behaviors. Simply speaking, ML methods are not specifically programmed to solve a task, but learn how to solve it based on the data available. ML is at the core of Knowledge Discovery and Data Mining as well as the most recent Big Data analytics.

In AAL, some of the most commonly used ML methods comprise Support Vector Machines (SVMs), k-Nearest Neighbor (k-NN), Artificial Neural Networks (ANN), Naïve-Bayes (NB), Decision Trees (DTs) and, among the latter, the Random Forest (RF) [18, 123]. The listed methods are all supervised methods, which are trained by providing them with the expected outcomes (e.g., the expected class for a given example). SVMs and k-NN are instance-based methods, as they group data into sets of similar cases and any new instance of data is compared (using a similarity measure) against the representative case of each set to find the best match and make a classification or prediction. NB is a Bayesian method that requires the knowledge of a-priori and conditional probabilities of the data to apply the Bayes' Theorem. DT and RF are tree-based methods, which build a sort of decision-making diagram, in the form of a tree, based on conditions on the data values. The prediction for a new instance of the data is obtained following the tree structure until a leaf is reached. The RT is an ensemble version of DT, which combines a large number of DTs to solve a task.

ANNs are connected networks of nodes, whose inspiration comes from the biological networks of neurons. ANNs are structured in layers of nodes (neurons) and the output of each layer goes in input to the following layer. Each node applies an activation function to the weighted sum of its input. Moving from the first layer to the last one, an ANN maps the input data to the output label of a class [39].

In the last decade, boosted by the data deluge, ML has made significant steps forward. A particular type of ANNs, the so-called Convolution Neural Networks (CNNs), has demonstrated to perform unprecedentedly well, especially when solving perception tasks, such as vision, object recognition and natural language processing [69]. Considering the depth in terms of number of layers of this type of networks, the term Deep Learning (DL) has emerged when referring to them. DL has emerged in opposition to the shallow learning, which is the traditional learning approach of ML methods. DL methods are able to learn the main features that allow for the distinction of the relevant patterns, in this respect they are also referred to as Representation Learning. More precisely, DL methods and CNNs permit to simplify the data-processing pipeline seen before in Fig. 1.12, as they do not necessarily require to segment the data and extract significant features, but they directly process the input (pre-processed) data to provide a result. In practice, they do not require the extraction of handcrafted features, as they identify on their own the relevant structures in the data and the characteristics of these structures. Being deep, CNNs and DL methods require seeing many data points (i.e., a lot of examples) in order to be accurate and effective, as they need to set the values of a huge number of internal parameters (namely, the network architecture and the parameters of training process). Most of the more recent works on video- and audio-data processing for AAL rely on the use of DL methods as they ensure very high performances (see [94] for an extensive review).

The various methods strongly depend on the task that should be performed (e.g., fall detection, vital signs monitoring, activity recognition, ...). For this reason, revising the various solutions proposed in the literature is out of scope for this chapter. The most recent advances are extensively presented in [6].

In the following, we discuss briefly some of the most common challenges that affect the data processing methods for video and audio understanding.

1.5.3.1 Main Challenges for Data Processing

The previous sections on audio and video data sensing have already highlighted some of the technical challenges related to each specific data modality. In this section, the most cogent challenges related to the task of interpreting the sensed data are discussed [29, 116]:

- **Lack of available datasets**: This has been affecting the AAL field for years, until the recent few years when some datasets are being publicly appearing and shared within the research community. Nevertheless, this is true for video-based AAL, while for applications based on audio the challenge is still there. Moreover, the datasets available either are of limited size or are obtained by simulating real-life events (e.g., falls are simulated in the lab or using dolls in case of audio-based datasets). Therefore, it is necessary to develop systems that are able to work with insufficient training data, using techniques based on oversampling, semi-supervised learning, anomaly detection or one-class classification.
- **Need for data annotation and labeling**: Another problem that affects data is the availability of quality annotation that can be used as ground-truth to train the ML methods. In this respect, unsupervised or semi-supervised techniques might be useful to overcome the issue, as they are based on ML methods that autonomously

discover how data gather into homogeneous classes [39]. Unsupervised methods are particularly beneficial when the problem is framed as an anomaly detection problem, such as, for instance, when detecting an abnormal usage of home appliances, detecting a fall, or detecting the worsening of a vital parameter tracked over time. Nevertheless, in this respect, such methods may require a huge amount of "normal" data representing all the possible normal situations, which might be difficult to obtain in experimental settings. This can cause the method to produce a high number of false alarms, when deployed in practice.

- **Class imbalance**: Risky or adverse events are usually and fortunately less common that normal conditions. This means that the most relevant events that are to be detected are usually less frequent and represented in the datasets. This may challenge the recognition methods, unless specific approaches are adopted. These may rely on data augmentation, class weighting techniques or anomaly detection methods (see Chap. 2 in this volume [122]).
- **Privacy concerns**: Audio and video data acquired for AAL purposes are negatively perceived by the assisted person with respect to privacy preservation. The feeling of intrusion also depends on the location of the audio and video sensor. Privacy-preserving methods based on specific processing techniques are highly desirable (see Chap. 3 in this volume [10]).
- **Ethical concerns**: Most of the newest methods to understand the content of audio and video data in AAL are based on DL. These methods ensure very high performances in terms of accuracy in the recognition, prediction and classification tasks. However, they can be very complex models, with a huge number of layers and complex computing modules, whose inner functioning is not easily understandable. For this reason, they are often referred to as "black boxes" or "opaque models". The European Commission and the High Level Expert Group appointed by the Commission have produced important guidelines to steer an ethical development of DL and AI models, especially when the impact of such models may affect directly citizens, as in the eHealth and AAL domains [4]. One of main principles promoted by these guidelines pertain to the transparency of decision based on AI and DL methods, which directly entails the possibility to explain why the methods have provided a certain output. This has led to a renewed interest the so-called "explainable AI". Several methods have been proposed in the literature and will be discussed later in this chapter. Explaining the results from an AI method is the first step to make this method trustworthy and, hence, promote its acceptability by end-users.

1.5.4 Multimodal Data Fusion for AAL

In this section, we introduce two technological approaches for fusing multimodal sensing data. Firstly, we survey how thermal and depth data can be combined. Secondly, we show how radar is used for data fusion.

1.5.4.1 Combining Thermal and Depth Data

Depth and thermal sensors have advantages over traditional cameras in application fields such as AAL, which involves continuous monitoring of people that should be unobtrusive and privacy-preserving [2, 103]. This is because depth and thermal sensors require no external illumination, working even in darkness, and do not expose colors or textures, making it harder to identify people. Images of depth sensors encode the scene geometry whereas thermal images encode surface temperatures. Both technologies have been described separately in Sect. 1.5.1, but they are also complementary for solving person-centric vision tasks, as people are clearly visible in thermal images, facilitating detection and segmentation. Yet there is little research on this matter, presumably because thermal sensors that are inexpensive and produce images of sufficient quality have become available only recently.

Pramerdorfer et al. [89] address a research gap by first evaluating the data quality of two commonly available depth and thermal sensors, and then deriving empirical noise models. Their primary contribution is a method for synthesizing realistic depth and thermal images, leveraging 3D data modeling and the derived noise models. This approach was used to generate a dataset of 40,000 image pairs.

The value of synthetic data is demonstrated by training CNNs [55] for scene state classification and evaluating their generalization performance on real-world data. Pramerdorfer et al. also present their own dataset of 8,000 image pairs [89]. Both datasets are publicly available to foster further research on (synthetic) depth- and thermal-based vision tasks.[16]

The potential of combining synthetic depth data and machine learning was first highlighted by Shotton et al. [103] for human pose estimation. Similar approaches were adopted by Abobakr et al. [2] for fall detection and by Oberweger et al. [84] for hand pose estimation. Improving the realism of synthetic data and its generalization to real data requires accurate sensor noise modeling.

Khoshelham developed a basic noise model for the Microsoft Kinect depth sensor [65], which was later extended in [82]. Thermal data, on the other hand, has been less explored. For instance, Quero et al. [93] employed a thermal sensor for CNN-based fall detection. Kniaz et al. used a generative adversarial network (GAN) to generate thermal images from color images [66]. In contrast, Pramerdorfer et al.'s approach requires no color images and appears to produce more realistic thermal images based on visual inspection [89]. According to them, the only works utilizing both depth and thermal data are [52] and [110], which focus on person tracking using particle filters on real data, whereas Pramerdorfer et al. emphasize synthetic data and image classification using CNNs.

Currently, no commercially available hardware combines depth and thermal sensors. As a result, Pramerdorfer et al. designed and built such a device using off-the-shelf sensors and 3D printing [89].

---

[16] https://cvl.tuwien.ac.at/research/cvl-databases/sdt-icip/, last accessed 29/07/2024.

1.5.4.2 Radar Data Visualization and Fusion

In addition to the typical image-based technologies such as RGB, depth or thermal (see Sect. 1.5.1), radar data can also be visualized like an image, using point clouds to illustrate the rough shape of a person. Cippitelli et al. present a review on radar and RGB-D sensors for fall detection in which challenges of both individual technologies are investigated [30].

Challenges related to radar technology include:

- strong scatterers and clutter indoors, generating multi-path and ghost targets or obscuring the person to be monitored; can also be a problem in RGB-D,
- pets can cause false alarms, can also be a problem in RGB-D,
- compliance of selected radar wave forms with telecommunication directives, leading to constraints in band width and transmitted power,
- location of radar sensor can change attenuation of radar Doppler signature; less problems on the ceiling than on the wall.

Application areas of radar vary from multi-human detection [28, 68], gesture recognition [3, 49, 64, 70], localization [71], to sleep and vital signs monitoring and much more. Unlike (standard RGB) cameras, radar is able to detect falls in a privacy-preserving way. This facilitates the use of radar technology in the end-user's homes as well as in care facilities and hospitals. Moreover, radar allows to measure vital signs of newborns and to detect burned people due to its non-invasive nature [63].

Diraco et al. [38] achieve sensitivity and specificity greater than 97% and 90% in fall detection by using a micro-motion signature and unsupervised learning. The highest accuracy is achieved in correspondence of ADLs/postures without too much movement (not further specified), such as, sleeping/resting, post fall, and watching TV. Thus, activities like cooking (standing posture) are more difficult to detect in comparison to the other ADLs. The same applies, although at a lesser extent, in the case of the eating activity, due to some occurrence of chest oscillations. Some differences are found also in dependence of the monitored subject's orientation. When more people are present in the sensor's field of view (in addition to the monitored subject), the movement compensation strategy is robust enough as long as the distance between the monitored subject (i.e., the person closer to the radar) and the other people is greater than 0.5 m.

Erol et al. use range information integrated with a fall detection algorithm to distinguish an actual fall from a sitting motion [43]. Both movements cause a high Doppler frequency, so distinguishing between them leads to a reduced false alarm rate. Although the Doppler time-frequency signatures of the two motions can be similar, the range extent of a fall is considerably higher than that of a sit. This varies according to the type and the depth of the base of the furniture the person is sitting on.

1.6 Conclusions

The global population is ageing. Given that age is the primary risk factor for many diseases and coupled with the concomitant advances in healthcare technologies and modern medicine permitting individuals to live longer with chronic conditions, the introduction of AAL is inescapable. While AAL technologies offer hope in addressing economic challenges to healthcare and the prospect of prolonging independent living thereby improving life quality, the underlying social [74] (see Chap. 13 in this volume), ethical concerns [24] (Chap. 11) and legal issues [35] (Chap. 12), cannot be overlooked.

It could be argued that as all technologies need to pass certain regulatory processes, the legal aspects pertinent to AAL have been addressed. The relevant regulations such as the GDPR cover the collection, use, processing and sharing of personal data. Consumer protection laws deal with the safety of components used in these technologies. Yet as technologies advance, the laws must stay abreast of such progress. A framework for which further research can be performed is presented in this chapter. We conclude that AAL technologies require a legal system that both promotes their development while at the same time safeguards against risks posed by the technology. Here, it is clear that the law is failing to provide a speed of adoption commensurate with the development of the technology. Not only are there serious uncertainties in the application of existing legal frameworks to AAL technologies, but there is also a lack of appropriate legal restrictions and precautions to control some of the risks posed by lifelogging technologies. It is recommended that a more holistic approach to the regulation of AAL technologies is taken, one that integrates deeper technological and international perspectives than the current legal framework represents. The more nebulous aspects of AAL application lie with the ethics of their implementation. AAL technologies are by their nature intrusive. They can also be deemed to be overprotective which can subtly erode respect for autonomy. The benefits brought by AAL need to be carefully weighed against the risks and the risk/benefit ratio assessed on a regular basis as individuals age and applications of technology change. An ethical approach and a thorough understanding of all ethical principles relevant to surveillance/monitoring architectures are essential.

AAL poses many challenges, raising questions which will affect immediate acceptance and long-term usage. Furthermore, issues emerge from social inequalities and their potential exacerbation by AAL, accentuating the existing access gap between high and low-income countries. Ethics should be incorporated at the AAL design (or co-design, see Chap. 14 in this volume [114]) stage, taking all of these aspects into account and evaluating (i) beneficence, (ii) non-maleficence i.e., a risk/benefit analysis (iii) respect for autonomy, and (iv) protection of confidential information and data that may reveal personal and sensitive attributes.

The social issues are related with the impact of AAL technologies before and after their adoption [74] (Chap. 13 in this volume). Some are rooted in the collective understandings of the technology at hand, whereby users can relate audio-video based AAL to activities such as surveillance practices. One of the prominent social and design challenges will be facilitation of the workflow and avoiding the sense of additional technological burden. Taking care of that will directly impact institutional and individual adoption of AAL.

Future AAL technologies need to consider all aspects of equality such as gender, race, age and social disadvantages and avoid increasing loneliness and isolation among, e.g. older and frail people. Finally, the current power asymmetries between the target and general populations should not be underestimated nor should the discrepant needs and motivations of the target group and those developing and deploying AAL systems. These differences could lead to governance challenges, serious ethical questions, and potential misuse of the technology.

At the core of many AAL technologies lie machine learning approaches [122] (Chap. 2 in this volume), and progress in this domain will improve accuracy and reliability of the AAL core components, leading to trustworthy applications in areas like fall detection and prevention [73] (Chap. 5), gait and frailty recognition [33] (Chap. 6), recognition of activities of daily living [7] (Chap. 7), remote monitoring of vital signs [36] (Chap. 8), smart mirrors [101] (Chap. 10), and long-term sensing of user affective states [100] (Chap. 9). Furthermore, improvements in data security [60] (Chap. 4) and privacy preserving algorithms [10] (Chap. 3) will contribute to wider adoption of AAL technologies. We firmly believe that the technical and non-technical challenges in AAL are surmountable, and this area holds great promise for the future.

Acknowledgements This publication is based upon work from COST Action GoodBrother—Network on Privacy-Aware Audio- and Video-Based Applications for Active and Assisted Living (CA19121), supported by COST (European Cooperation in Science and Technology). We thank M. Atanasov for his contributions.

References

1. AAL Program: AAL guidelines for ethics, data privacy and security (2020). http://www.aal-europe.eu/wp-content/uploads/2020/08/AAL-guidelines-for-ethics-final-V2.pdf. Last accessed: 28/07/2024
2. Abobakr, A., Hossny, M., Nahavandi, S.: A skeleton-free fall detection system from depth images using random decision forest. IEEE Syst. J. **12**(3), 2994–3005 (2017)
3. Ahmed, S., Khan, F., Ghaffar, A., Hussain, F., Cho, S.: Finger-counting-based gesture recognition within cars using impulse radar with convolutional neural network. Sensors **19** (2019)
4. AI Act: Proposal for a regulation of the European parliament and of the council laying down harmonised rules on artificial intelligence (artificial intelligence act) and amending certain union legislative acts. Official Journal (2021). https://eur-lex.europa.eu/legal-content/EN/TXT/?uri=CELEX:52021PC0206. Last accessed: 28/07/2024
5. Ake-Kob, A., Blazeviciene, A., Colonna, L., Cartolovni, A., Dantas, C., Fedosov, A., Florez-Revuelta, F., Fosch-Villaronga, E., He, Z., Klimczuk, A., et al.: State of the art on ethical, legal, and social issues linked to audio-and video-based AAL solutions. Whitepaper of COST Action GoodBrother—Network on Privacy-Aware Audio- and Video-Based Applications for Active and Assisted Living (2021)

6. Aleksic, S., Atanasov, M., Agius, J.C., Camilleri, K., Cartolovni, A., Climent-Peerez, P., Colantonio, S., Cristina, S., Despotovic, V., Ekenel, H.K., et al.: State of the art of audio-and video-based solutions for AAL. arXiv:2207.01487 (2022)
7. Aleksic, S., Despotovic, V., Cristina, S.: Activities of daily living (ADL) and behavior recognition. In: Salah, A.A., Colonna, L., Florez-Revuelta, F. (eds.) Privacy-Aware Monitoring for Assisted Living. Springer, Cham (2025)
8. Alwan, M., Rajendran, P., Kell, S., Mack, D., et al.: A smart and passive floor-vibration based fall detector for elderly. In: Proceedings of the 2nd International Conference on Information Communication Technologies, vol. 1, pp. 1003–1007 (2006)
9. Atanov, A., Fu, J., Singh, R., Yu, I., Spielberg, A., Zamir, A.: Solving vision tasks with simple photoreceptors instead of cameras. In: Proc. ECCV (2024)
10. Bäckström, T., Ravi, S., Florez-Revuelta, F.: Privacy preservation in audio and video. In: Salah, A.A., Colonna, L., Florez-Revuelta, F. (eds.) Privacy-Aware Monitoring for Assisted Living. Springer, Cham (2025)
11. Bai, Y., Lu, L., Cheng, J., Liu, J., Chen, Y., Yu, J.: Acoustic-based sensing and applications: A survey. Comput. Netw. **181**, 107,447 (2020)
12. Bandini, A., Zariffa, J.: Analysis of the hands in egocentric vision: a survey. IEEE Trans. Pattern Anal. Mach. Intell. **45**(6), 6846–6866 (2020)
13. Basu, C., Rowe, A.: Tracking motion and proxemics using thermal-sensor array. arXiv:1511.08166 (2015)
14. Becker, M.: Software architecture trends and promising technology for ambient assisted living systems. In: Schloss-Dagstuhl-Leibniz Zentrum für Informatik, pp. 1–18 (2008)
15. Betancourt, A., Morerio, P., Marcenaro, L., Barakova, E., Rauterberg, M., Regazzoni, C.: Towards a unified framework for hand-based methods in first person vision. In: 2015 IEEE International Conference on Multimedia & Expo Workshops (ICMEW), pp. 1–6 (2015)
16. Beymer, D.: Person counting using stereo. In: Proceedings of the Workshop on Human Motion, pp. 127–133 (2000)
17. Bi, Y., Lv, M., Song, C., Xu, W., Guan, N., Yi, W.: AutoDietary: a wearable acoustic sensor system for food intake recognition in daily life. IEEE Sens. J. **16**(3), 806–816 (2016)
18. Bishop, C.: Pattern Recognition and Machine Learning. Springer, Berlin/Heidelberg, Germany (2006)
19. Blackman, S., Matlo, C., Bobrovitskiy, C., Waldoch, A., Fang, M.L., Jackson, P., Mihailidis, A., Nygård, L., Astell, A., Sixsmith, A.: Ambient assisted living technologies for aging well: a scoping review. J. Intell. Syst. **25**(1), 55–69 (2016)
20. van den Broek, G., Cavallo, F., Wehrmann, C.: AALIANCE Ambient Assisted Living Roadmap, vol. 6. IOS Press (2010)
21. Byrne, C.A., Collier, R., O'Hare, G.M.: A review and classification of assisted living systems. Information **9**(7), 182 (2018)
22. Cao, Z., Hidalgo, G., Simon, T., Wei, S., Sheikh, Y.: OpenPose: realtime multi-person 2D pose estimation using part affinity fields. IEEE Trans. Pattern Anal. Mach. Intell. **43**(1), 172–186 (2019)
23. Carolis, B.D., Ferilli, S., Palestra, G., Redavid, D.: Emotion-recognition from speech-based interaction in AAL environment. In: Proceedings of the Second Italian Workshop on Artificial Intelligence for Ambient Assisted Living co-located with 15th International Conference of the Italian Association for Artificial Intelligence (2016)
24. Čartolovni, A., Dantas, C., Malešević, A., Ilgaz, A.: Ethical issues in AAL. In: Salah, A.A., Colonna, L., Florez-Revuelta, F. (eds.) Privacy-Aware Monitoring for Assisted Living. Springer, Cham (2025)
25. Chaaraoui, A., Padilla-López, J., Ferrández-Pastor, F., Nieto-Hidalgo, M., Flórez-Revuelta, F.: A vision-based system for intelligent monitoring: human behaviour analysis and privacy by design. Sensors **14**(5), 8895–8925 (2014)
26. Chahuara, P., Fleury, A., Portet, F., Vacher, M.: On-line human activity recognition from audio and home automation sensors: comparison of sequential and non-sequential models in realistic smart homes. J. Ambient Intell. Smart Environ. **8**, 399–422 (2016)

27. Cheffena, M.: Fall detection using smartphone audio features. IEEE J. Biomed. Health Inform. **20**(4), 1073–1080 (2016)
28. Choi, J., Nam, S., Cho, S.: Multi-human detection algorithm based on an impulse radio ultra-wideband radar system. IEEE Access **4**, 10300–10309 (2016)
29. Cicirelli, G., Marani, R., Petitti, A., Milella, A., D'Orazio, T.: Ambient assisted living: a review of technologies, methodologies and future perspectives for healthy aging of population. Sensors **21**(10), 3549 (2021)
30. Cippitelli, E., Fioranelli, F., Gambi, E., Spinsante, S.: Radar and RGB-depth sensors for fall detection: a review. IEEE Sens. J. **17**, 3585–3604 (2017)
31. Climent-Perez, P., Spinsante, S., Mihailidis, A., Florez-Revuelta, F.: A review on video-based active and assisted living technologies for automated lifelogging. Expert Syst. Appl. **139**, 112,847 (2020)
32. Climent-Pérez, P., Florez-Revuelta, F.: Protection of visual privacy in videos acquired with RGB cameras for active and assisted living applications. Multimed. Tools Appl. 1–16 (2021)
33. Climent-Pérez, P., Florez-Revuelta, F.: Privacy-aware video-based methods for gait and frailty recognition in active and assisted living environments. In: Salah, A.A., Colonna, L., Florez-Revuelta, F. (eds.) Privacy-Aware Monitoring for Assisted Living. Springer, Cham (2025)
34. Colantonio, S., Coppini, G., Giorgi, D., Morales, M.A., Pascali, M.A.: Computer vision for ambient assisted living: monitoring systems for personalized healthcare and wellness that are robust in the real world and accepted by users, careers, and society. In: Computer Vision for Assistive Healthcare, pp. 147–182. Elsevier (2018)
35. Colonna, L., Riva, G.M.: The legal and regulatory issues in AAL: the case of smart mirrors. In: Salah, A.A., Colonna, L., Florez-Revuelta, F. (eds.) Privacy-Aware Monitoring for Assisted Living. Springer, Cham (2025)
36. Cristina, S., Počta, P., Zgank, A., Camilleri, K.P., Colantonio, S., Lambrinos, L.: Remote monitoring of vital signs. In: Salah, A.A., Colonna, L., Florez-Revuelta, F. (eds.) Privacy-Aware Monitoring for Assisted Living. Springer, Cham (2025)
37. Das, S., Dai, R., Koperski, M., Minciullo, L., Garattoni, L., Bremond, F., Francesca, G.: Toyota smarthome: real-world activities of daily living. In: Proceedings of the IEEE/CVF International Conference on Computer Vision, pp. 833–842 (2019)
38. Diraco, G., Leone, A., Siciliano, P.: A radar-based smart sensor for unobtrusive elderly monitoring in ambient assisted living applications. Biosensors **7**(55) (2017)
39. Domingos, P.: A few useful things to know about machine learning. Commun. ACM **55**(10), 78–87 (2012)
40. Doughty, K., Cameron, K., Garner, P.: Three generations of telecare of the elderly. J. Telemed. Telecare **2**, 71–80 (1996)
41. El Murabet, A., Abtoy, A., Touhafi, A., Tahiri, A.: Ambient assisted living system's models and architectures: a survey of the state of the art. J. King Saud Univ. Comput. Inform. Sci. **32**(1), 1–10 (2020)
42. Elahi, H., Castiglione, A., Wang, G., Geman, O.: A human-centered artificial intelligence approach for privacy protection of elderly app users in smart cities. Neurocomputing **444**, 189–202 (2021)
43. Erol, B., Amin, M., Zhou, Z., Zhang, J.: Range information for reducing fall false alarms in assisted living. In: 2016 IEEE Radar Conference (RadarConf), pp. 1–6 (2016)
44. Florez-Revuelta, F., Chaaraoui, A.A.: Active and Assisted Living: Technologies and Applications. The Institution of Engineering and Technology (2016)
45. Florez-Revuelta, F., Mihailidis, A., Ziefle, M., Colonna, L., Spinsante, S.: Privacy-aware and acceptable lifelogging services for older and frail people: The PAAL project. In: IEEE 8th International Conference on Consumer Electronics-Berlin (ICCE-Berlin), pp. 1–4 (2018)
46. Fofi, D., Sliwa, T., Voisin, Y.: A comparative survey on invisible structured light. In: Price, J., Meriaudeau, F. (eds.) Electronic Imaging 2004, pp. 90–98. SPIE (2004)
47. Fosch-Villaronga, E., Drukarch, H.: On healthcare robots: concepts, definitions, and considerations for healthcare robot governance. arXiv:2106.03468 (2021)

48. Fu, Y.: Sensor applications for human activity recognition in smart environments. Ph.D. thesis, Darmstadt University of Technology (2020). https://d-nb.info/1230554467/34. Last accessed: 23/02/2022
49. Ghaffar, A., Khan, F., Cho, S.: Hand pointing gestures based digital menu board implementation using IR-UWB transceivers. IEEE Access **7**, 1–1 (2019)
50. Ghosh, A., Chakraborty, D., Prasad, D., Saha, M., Saha, S.: Can we recognize multiple human group activities using ultrasonic sensors? In: Proceedings of the 10th International Conference on Communication Systems Networks (COMSNETS), pp. 557–560 (2018)
51. Güler, R., Neverova, N., Kokkinos, I.: DensePose: dense human pose estimation in the wild. In: Proceedings of the IEEE Conference on Computer Vision and Pattern Recognition, pp. 7297–7306 (2018)
52. Halima, I., Laferté, J.M., Cormier, G., Fougère, A.J., Dillenseger, J.L.: Sensors fusion for head tracking using particle filter in a context of falls detection. In: 1st International Conference on Advances in Signal Processing and Artificial Intelligence (ASPAI'2019) (2019)
53. Han, J., Shao, L., Xu, D., Shotton, J.: Enhanced computer vision with Microsoft Kinect sensor: a review. IEEE Trans. Cybern. **43**(5), 1318–1334 (2013)
54. Hayashida, Moshnyaga, V., Hashimoto, K.: The use of thermal IR array sensor for indoor fall detection. In: IEEE International Conference on Systems, Man, and Cybernetics (2017)
55. He, K., Zhang, X., Ren, S., Sun, J.: Identity mappings in deep residual networks. In: European Conference on Computer Vision, pp. 630–645 (2016)
56. Hegger, F., Hochgeschwender, N., Kraetzschmar, G., Ploeger, P.: People detection in 3d point clouds using local surface normals. In: Robot Soccer World Cup 2012. Lecture Notes in Computer Science, vol. 7500, pp. 154–165. Springer (2013)
57. Henriquez, P., Matuszewski, B.J., Andreu-Cabedo, Y., Bastiani, L., Colantonio, S., Coppini, G., D'Acunto, M., Favilla, R., Germanese, D., Giorgi, D., et al.: Mirror mirror on the wall... an unobtrusive intelligent multisensory mirror for well-being status self-assessment and visualization. IEEE Trans. Multimed. **19**(7), 1467–1481 (2017)
58. Ikemura, S., Fujiyoshi, H.: Real-time human detection using relational depth similarity features. In: Proceedings of the Asian Conference on Computer Vision, pp. 25–38 (2011)
59. Jeong, Y., Yoon, K., Joung, K.: Probabilistic method to determine human subjects for low-resolution thermal imaging sensor. In: Proceedings of the 2014 IEEE Sensors Applications Symposium (SAS), pp. 97–102 (2014)
60. Jevremovic, A., Aleksic, S., Veinovic, M., Colonna, L.: Data security in AAL. In: Salah, A.A., Colonna, L., Florez-Revuelta, F. (eds.) Privacy-Aware Monitoring for Assisted Living. Springer, Cham (2025)
61. Kelly, P., O'Connor, N., Smeaton, A.: Robust pedestrian detection and tracking in crowded scenes. Image Vis. Comput. **27**(10), 1445–1458 (2009)
62. Kessous, L., Castellano, G., Caridakis, G.: Multimodal emotion recognition in speech-based interaction using facial expression, body gesture and acoustic analysis. J. Multimodal User Interfaces **3**, 33–48 (2010)
63. Khan, F., Ghaffar, A., Khan, N., Cho, S.: An overview of signal processing techniques for remote health monitoring using impulse radio UWB transceiver. Sensors **20**, 2479 (2020)
64. Khan, F., Leem, S., Cho, S.: Hand-based gesture recognition for vehicular applications using IR-UWB radar. Sensors **17** (2017)
65. Khoshelham, K., Elberink, S.: Accuracy and resolution of Kinect depth data for indoor mapping applications. Sensors **12**(2), 1437–1454 (2012)
66. Kniaz, V., Knyaz, V., Hladuvka, J., Kropatsch, W., Mizginov, V.: ThermalGAN: multimodal color-to-thermal image translation for person re-identification in multispectral dataset. In: European Conference on Computer Vision (2018)
67. Kolotouros, N., Pavlakos, G., Black, M., Daniilidis, K.: Learning to reconstruct 3d human pose and shape via model-fitting in the loop. In: Proceedings of the IEEE/CVF International Conference on Computer Vision, pp. 2252–2261 (2019)
68. Kota, J., Papandreou-Suppappola, A.: Joint design of transmit waveforms for object tracking in coexisting multimodal sensing systems. Sensors **19**, 1753 (2019)

69. LeCun, Y., Bengio, Y., Hinton, G.: Deep learning. Nature **521**, 436–444 (2015)
70. Leem, S., Khan, F., Cho, S.: Detecting mid-air gestures for digit writing with radio sensors and a CNN. IEEE Trans. Instrum. Meas. **69**(4), 1066–1081 (2020)
71. Li, C., Lin, J., Boric-Lubecke, O., Lubecke, V., Host-Madsen, A., Park, B.K.: Development of non-contact physiological motion sensor on CMOS chip and its potential applications. In: 2007 7th International Conference on ASIC, pp. 1022–1027 (2007)
72. Loper, M., Mahmood, N., Romero, J., Pons-Moll, G., Black, M.: SMPL: a skinned multi-person linear model. ACM Trans. Graph. (TOG) **34**(6), 1–16 (2015)
73. Lumetzberger, J., Ballester, I., Kampel, M.: Fall detection. In: Salah, A.A., Colonna, L., Florez-Revuelta, F. (eds.) Privacy-Aware Monitoring for Assisted Living. Springer, Cham (2025)
74. Lutz, C., Miguel, C., Mujirishvili, T., Perez-Vega, R., Fedosov, A.: Social and societal issues in AAL. In: Salah, A.A., Colonna, L., Florez-Revuelta, F. (eds.) Privacy-Aware Monitoring for Assisted Living. Springer, Cham (2025)
75. Maaspuro, M.: A low-resolution IR-array as a doorway occupancy counter in a smart building. Int. J. Online Biomed. Eng. (iJOE) **16** (2020)
76. Makeyev, O., Lopez-Meyer, P., Schuckers, S., Besio, W., Sazonov, E.: Automatic food intake detection based on swallowing sounds. Biomed. Signal Process. Control **7**(6), 649–656 (2012)
77. Marques, G.: Ambient assisted living and internet of things. In: Harnessing the Internet of Everything (IoE) for Accelerated Innovation Opportunities, pp. 100–115 (2019)
78. Mitchell, T.: Machine Learning. McGraw Hill Series in Computer Science. McGraw-Hill, Maidenhead (1997)
79. Mohammadmoradi, H., Munir, S., Gnawali, O., Shelton, C.: Measuring people-flow through doorways using easy-to-install IR array sensors. In: Proceedings of the 13th International Conference on Distributed Computing in Sensor Systems (DCOSS), pp. 35–43. Ottawa, ON, Canada (2017)
80. Munoz, A., Augusto, J.C., Villa, A., Botía, J.A.: Design and evaluation of an ambient assisted living system based on an argumentative multi-agent system. Pers. Ubiquit. Comput. **15**, 377–387 (2011)
81. Nadee, C., Chamnongthai, K.: Ultrasonic array sensors for monitoring of human fall detection. In: Proceedings of the 12th International Conference on Electrical Engineering/Electronics, Computer, Telecommunications and Information Technology (ECTI-CON), pp. 1–4 (2015)
82. Nguyen, C., Izadi, S., Lovell, D.: Modeling Kinect sensor noise for improved 3d reconstruction and tracking. In: International Conference on 3D Imaging, Modeling, Processing, Visualization & Transmission, pp. 524–530 (2012)
83. Nguyen, T., Nebel, J., Florez-Revuelta, F.: Recognition of activities of daily living with egocentric vision: a review. Sensors **16**(1), 72 (2016)
84. Oberweger, M., Riegler, G., Wohlhart, P., Lepetit, V.: Efficiently creating 3d training data for fine hand pose estimation. In: Proceedings of the IEEE Conference on Computer Vision and Pattern Recognition, pp. 4957–4965 (2016)
85. Pan, S., Wang, N., Qian, Y., Velibeyoglu, I., Noh, H., Zhang, P.: In-door person identification through footstep induced structural vibration. In: Proceedings of the 16th International Workshop on Mobile Computing Systems and Applications (HotMobile), pp. 81–86 (2015)
86. Planinc, R., Chaaraoui, A., Kampel, M., Florez-Revuelta, F.: Computer vision for active and assisted living. In: Florez-Revuelta, F., Chaaraoui, A.A. (eds.) Active and Assisted Living: Technologies and Applications. The Institution of Engineering and Technology (2016)
87. Plizzari, C., Goletto, G., Furnari, A., Bansal, S., Ragusa, F., Farinella, G.M., Damen, D., Tommasi, T.: An outlook into the future of egocentric vision. Int. J. Comput. Vis. 1–57 (2024)
88. Portet, F., Caffiau, S., Ringeval, F., Vacher, M., Bonnefond, N., Rossato, S., Lecouteux, B., Desot, T.: Context-aware voice-based interaction in smart home-vocadom@ a4h corpus collection and empirical assessment of its usefulness. In: 2019 IEEE International Conference on Dependable, Autonomic and Secure Computing, International Conference on Pervasive Intelligence and Computing, International Conference on Cloud and Big Data Computing, International Conference on Cyber Science and Technology Congress (DASC/PiCom/CBDCom/CyberSciTech), pp. 811–818. IEEE (2019)

89. Pramerdorfer, C., Strohmayer, J., Kampel, M.: SDT: a synthetic multi-modal dataset for person detection and pose classification. In: 2020 IEEE International Conference on Image Processing (ICIP), pp. 1611–1615 (2020)
90. Principi, E., Droghini, D., Squartini, S., Olivetti, P., Piazza, F.: Acoustic cues from the floor: a new approach for fall classification. Expert Syst. Appl. **60**, 51–61 (2016)
91. Päßler, S., Fischer, W.J.: Food intake monitoring: automated chew event detection in chewing sounds. IEEE J. Biomed. Health Inform. **18**(1), 278–289 (2014)
92. Qifan, Y., Hao, T., Xuebing, Z., Yin, L., Sanfeng, Z.: Dolphin: ultrasonic-based gesture recognition on smartphone platform. In: Proceedings of the IEEE 17th International Conference on Computational Science and Engineering, pp. 1461–1468 (2014)
93. Quero, J., Burns, M., Razzaq, M., Nugent, C., Espinilla, M.: Detection of falls from non-invasive thermal vision sensors using convolutional neural networks. In: Multidisciplinary Digital Publishing Institute Proceedings, vol. 2 (2018)
94. Qureshi, M., Qureshi, K., Jeon, G., et al.: Deep learning-based ambient assisted living for self-management of cardiovascular conditions. Neural Comput. Appl. (2021)
95. Rahman, A., Lubecke, V., Boric-Lubecke, O., Prins, J., Sakamoto, T.: Doppler radar techniques for accurate respiration characterisation and subject identification. IEEE J. Emerging Select. Top. Circuits Syst. **8**(2), 350–359 (2018)
96. Rashidi, P., Mihailidis, A.: A survey on ambient-assisted living tools for older adults. IEEE J. Biomed. Health Inform. **17**(3), 579–590 (2012)
97. Rodrigues, J.J., Segundo, D., Junqueira, H.A., Sabino, M.H., Prince, R.M., Al-Muhtadi, J., De Albuquerque, V.: Enabling technologies for the internet of health things. IEEE Access **6**, 13129–13141 (2018)
98. Rogez, G., Weinzaepfel, P., Schmid, C.: LCR-Net++: multi-person 2d and 3d pose detection in natural images. IEEE Trans. Pattern Anal. Mach. Intell. **42**(5), 1146–1161 (2019)
99. Rong, Y., Shiratori, T., Joo, H.: Frankmocap: a monocular 3d whole-body pose estimation system via regression and integration. In: Proceedings of the IEEE/CVF International Conference on Computer Vision, pp. 1749–1759 (2021)
100. Salah, A.A., Iren, D., Kaya, H.: Affective computing in active assisted living. In: Salah, A.A., Colonna, L., Florez-Revuelta, F. (eds.) Privacy-Aware Monitoring for Assisted Living. Springer, Cham (2025)
101. Santofimia, M.J., del Toro, X., Bolaños, C., Dorado, J., Colantonio, S.: A smart mirror to your health: personalized virtual coaching for active and healthy ageing. In: Salah, A.A., Colonna, L., Florez-Revuelta, F. (eds.) Privacy-Aware Monitoring for Assisted Living. Springer, Cham (2025)
102. Sazonov, E., Schuckers, S., Lopez-Meyer, P., Makeyev, O., et al.: Non-invasive monitoring of chewing and swallowing for objective quantification of ingestive behavior. Physiol. Meas. **29**, 525 (2008)
103. Shotton, J., Fitzgibbon, A., Cook, M., Sharp, T., Finocchio, M., Moore, R., Kipman, A., Blake, A.: Real-time human pose recognition in parts from single depth images. In: Proceedings of the Conference on Computer Vision and Pattern Recognition (CVPR), pp. 1297–1304. IEEE, Colorado Springs, USA (2011)
104. Singh, S., Aksanli, B.: Non-intrusive presence detection and position tracking for multiple people using low-resolution thermal sensors. J. Sens. Actuator Netw. **8**(40) (2019)
105. Sixsmith, A.: An evaluation of an intelligent home monitoring system. J. Telemed. Telecare **6**, 63–72 (2000)
106. Sixsmith, A.: New technologies to support independent living and quality of life for people with dementia. Alzheimer's Care Today **7**(3), 194–202 (2006)
107. Spasova, V., Iliev, I., Petrova, G.: Privacy preserving fall detection based on simple human silhouette extraction and a linear support vector machine. Int. J. Bioautom. **20**(2), 237–252 (2016)
108. Spinello, L., Arras, K.: People detection in RGB-D data. In: Proceedings of the International Conference on Intelligent Robots and Systems, pp. 3838–3843 (2011)

109. Spinsante, S., Stara, V., Felici, E., Montanini, L., Raffaeli, L., Rossi, L., Gambi, E.: The human factor in the design of successful ambient assisted living technologies. In: Ambient Assisted Living and Enhanced Living Environments, pp. 61–89. Elsevier (2017)
110. Spremolla, I., Antunes, M., Aouada, D., Ottersten, B.: RGB-D and thermal sensor fusion—application in person tracking. In: Proceedings of VISAPP, pp. 612–619 (2016)
111. Szeliski, R.: Computer Vision: Algorithms and Applications. Springer (2021)
112. Tan, L., Jiang, J.: Digital Signal Processing. Academic Press (2018)
113. Tao, L., Volonakis, T., Tan, B., Jing, Y., Chetty, K., Smith, M.: Home activity monitoring using low resolution infrared sensor array (2018)
114. Tellioglu, H.: Integrating ethics by design and co-design principles in the development of ambient assisted living technologies. In: Salah, A.A., Colonna, L., Florez-Revuelta, F. (eds.) Privacy-Aware Monitoring for Assisted Living. Springer, Cham (2025)
115. Trofimova, A., Masciadri, A., Veronese, F., Salice, F.: Indoor human detection based on thermal array sensor data and adaptive background estimation. J. Comput. Commun. **5**, 16–28 (2017)
116. Vacher, M., Aman, F., Rossato, S., Portet, F.: Development of automatic speech recognition techniques for elderly home support: applications and challenges. In: Zhou, J., Salvendy, G. (eds.) Human Aspects of IT for the Aged Population. Design for Everyday Life (ITAP). Lecture Notes in Computer Science, vol. 9194. Springer (2015)
117. Vacher, M., Bouakaz, S., Chaumon, M.E., Aman, F., Khan, R., et al.: The CIRDO corpus: comprehensive audio/video database of domestic falls of elderly people. In: Proceedings of the Tenth International Conference on Language Resources and Evaluation (LREC"16), pp. 1389–1396. Portorož, Slovenia (2016)
118. Vacher, M., Portet, F., Fleury, A., Noury, N.: Development of audio sensing technology for ambient assisted living: applications and challenges. Int. J. E-Health Med. Commun. (IJEHMC) **82**(1), 35–54 (2011)
119. Wu, S., Yu, S., Chen, W.: An attempt to pedestrian detection in depth images. In: Proceedings of the Chinese Conference on Intelligent Visual Surveillance, pp. 97–100 (2011)
120. Xenakidis, C.N., Hadjiantonis, A.M., Milis, G.M.: Assistive technologies for people with dementia. In: Handbook of Research on Innovations in the Diagnosis and Treatment of Dementia, pp. 269–289. IGI Global (2015)
121. Xiao, Y., Lin, X.: Fall detection using low-resolution thermal sensor. Technical report, Tech Report No. ECE-2019-03 (2019)
122. Zdravevski, E., Lameski, P.: Machine learning for AAL. In: Salah, A.A., Colonna, L., Florez-Revuelta, F. (eds.) Privacy-Aware Monitoring for Assisted Living. Springer, Cham (2025)
123. Zdravevski, E., Lameski, P., Trajkovik, V., Kulakov, A., Chorbev, I., Goleva, R., Pombo, N., Garcia, N.: Improving activity recognition accuracy in ambient-assisted living systems by automated feature engineering. IEEE Access **5**, 5262–5280 (2017). https://doi.org/10.1109/ACCESS.2017.2684913
124. Zhang, S.: High-speed 3d shape measurement with structured light methods: a review. Opt. Lasers Eng. **106**, 119–131 (2018)

Open Access This chapter is licensed under the terms of the Creative Commons Attribution 4.0 International License (http://creativecommons.org/licenses/by/4.0/), which permits use, sharing, adaptation, distribution and reproduction in any medium or format, as long as you give appropriate credit to the original author(s) and the source, provide a link to the Creative Commons license and indicate if changes were made.

The images or other third party material in this chapter are included in the chapter's Creative Commons license, unless indicated otherwise in a credit line to the material. If material is not included in the chapter's Creative Commons license and your intended use is not permitted by statutory regulation or exceeds the permitted use, you will need to obtain permission directly from the copyright holder.

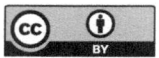

Chapter 2
Machine Learning for Active Assisted Living: Core Concepts, Challenges, and Solutions

Eftim Zdravevski and Petre Lameski

Abstract This chapter explains the process of Machine Learning (ML). First, we explain the concept of ML, what makes machines able to learn, and how they are doing it by introducing the reader to the basic underlying concept and, after that, giving the terminology and an overview of the entire ML process and life cycle. Then, we introduce ML into the Active Assisted Living (AAL) concept by defining where in AAL we can leverage the state-of-the-art concepts introduced by ML to improve the AAL applications and give users additional benefits. We will explore briefly all the problems and tasks in AAL that leverage ML. At the end of this chapter, we will give an overview of some privacy and security considerations related to ML. This chapter defines ML as a general process applicable to a wide range of AAL problems.

Keywords Active Assisted Living (AAL) · Machine learning · Action recognition · Anomaly detection · Class imbalance

2.1 Introduction to Machine Learning

ML is a transformative technology in numerous fields, demonstrating particular promise in AAL applications. This chapter describes how ML, a branch of artificial intelligence, enhances AAL systems. ML involves algorithms and models that enable computers to learn and perform specific tasks without or with minimal human intervention. Instead, these systems develop their capabilities by identifying patterns in data. During the training phase, an ML model learns from a dataset. It is a

---

E. Zdravevski (✉) · P. Lameski
Faculty of Computer Science and Engineering, Ss Cyril and Methodius University in Skopje, Skopje, North Macedonia
e-mail: eftim.zdravevski@finki.ukim.mk

P. Lameski
e-mail: petre.lameski@finki.ukim.mk

mathematical model that encapsulates the relationships within such data. Trained models can predict or make decisions based on new data it has never seen before, a process known as inference.

ML is a term that represents a set of methods enabling machines or computers to learn. Like human learning, it involves sensory input, memory, and appropriate response from the machine. Learning can be supervised, where a teacher guides the process, or unsupervised, where the data are not labeled and the algorithm tries to find groups, patterns and clusters to model the properties of the data. It can also be driven by reward and punishment, as in reinforcement learning, or used to detect abnormal behavior patterns, as in anomaly detection.

The 'knowledge' or memory the machines have is called a model. The model is a set of parameters and variables with a certain structure used in a certain function. This function transfers the input parameters or sensory inputs to a decision, a prediction, or another specific result.

So, how does the machine learn? Learning is the process of optimization where we select the best type of model and try to optimize the values of the model parameters so that we have as accurate a representation of the data as possible. The accuracy of the representation should be as high as possible, and as a consequence, the error in the estimation should be as low as possible.

The learning process is essentially about selecting the model and adjusting the model parameters to minimize the error between the actual values and those calculated using the model. There are various methods to achieve this.

2.2 Machine Learning Fundamentals

We will first define the general terms used in ML and then give an overview of several specific types of learning and some approaches.

2.2.1 Datasets

Training ML models requires learning samples, which are derived from the data at our disposal. These data are typically organized into datasets, which can be generated through sensor readings, user inputs or other sources. Additionally, datasets can be assembled from a variety of external sources, including web scraping, document parsing, and the extraction of information from images, videos, or audio files. Each individual measurement, paired with its corresponding outcome, is treated as a single sample within the dataset. Very often, the datasets are represented in tabular format, where each sample represents a row (or record).

2.2.1.1 Data Types

When analyzing and processing data, it's essential to recognize that data come in various forms, each with its own characteristics and use cases. Understanding these different types allows for more effective data management, analysis, and application in various fields. The data, depending on its nature and structure, can be classified into several categories. There are multiple ways that the data can be categorized. One is based on the way the data are saved:

- Structured
  - Categorical (i.e., nominal) data (e.g., Gender, Marital Status, Category, etc.)
  - Numerical data (e.g., Age, Height, Width, Temperature, etc.)
- Unstructured (Text, Images, Audio, Video)
- Semi-structured data (JSON, XML, HTML, etc.)

Another way to categorize the data is based on the sources and what they represent:

- Time series data (data with timestamps associated with it)
- Sensor data (data from sensor devices)
- Geo-spatial data (data from locations of objects)
- Transactional data (data from sales, transfers, purchases)
- Behavioral data (data from click-streams, user interaction)

When a dataset includes more than one type of data, it is referred to as a multimodal dataset. Multimodal datasets are increasingly common in real-world applications, where data from different sources and in various formats need to be integrated and analyzed together. For example, in a healthcare application, a multimodal dataset might include numerical data from patient vital signs, categorical data from diagnoses, textual data from doctor's notes, and image data from medical scans.

2.2.1.2 Variables

Each sample in the dataset is often described by variables. If the dataset was represented in tabular format, where samples are rows, columns can correspond to variables. There are usually the following types of variables:

- **Independent Variables**: These are the variables used as inputs for the machine to perform calculations. In ML, data mining, machine vision, and statistics, independent variables are often referred to by multiple terms, including features, attributes, signals, predictors, characteristics, and descriptors.
- **Dependent Variables**: Also known as response variables, target variables, or outcome variables, these are the variables that we aim to predict or explain. The values of the dependent variables are determined by the independent variables (or features) within the model.

In some cases, like in unsupervised learning, dependent variables may not be defined. In those scenarios, the focus is typically on identifying patterns or structures (e.g., clusters) rather than predicting an outcome based on inputs. Additionally, a variable can be both dependent and independent in some cases, such as depression level or amount of sleep if we use ML for predictive scenarios (using past depression level as an independent variable and future depression level as the dependent variable.

2.2.1.3 Model Development Datasets

In addition to the division between independent and dependent variables, it is necessary to split the dataset into different groups. These groups serve distinct purposes in the model development process:

- **Training Set**: This portion of the dataset is used to build or train the model.
- **Validation Set**: This set is used for tuning the model's hyperparameters and helps prevent overfitting by providing an additional dataset to evaluate the model's performance during training without directly impacting the model's learning process.
- **Test Set**: This part of the dataset is reserved for evaluating the final performance of the model. It is used to estimate the model's accuracy. Sometimes, it is also called a 'holdout' set. This set should not be used for model and parameter selection. This means that no performance measures should be evaluated on this set until the final model structure is selected and its parameters are fully determined.

There are no strict rules regarding the exact percentage of the dataset that should be allocated to each set. However, a common practice is to allocate 60–80% of the data to the training set, 10–20% to the validation set, and 10–20% to the test set. In class-imbalanced situations, stratified sampling is typically used to ensure that each of these sets receives examples from each class proportionally.

One can also use other validation techniques beyond the traditional train-validation-test split. One standard method is cross-validation, where the dataset is divided into multiple subsets, and the model is trained and validated multiple times, each time using a different subset as the validation set and the remaining data as the training set. This process helps provide a more robust estimate of the model's performance. Another method is leave-one-out cross-validation (LOOCV), where the model is trained on all but one data point, and the excluded point is used for validation; this is repeated for each data point in the dataset. For time-series data, it is often recommended to split the dataset along the time dimension. This approach involves using the oldest samples for training and the newest samples for testing, or vice versa, depending on the specific requirements of the analysis. For patient data, when training a general model, another approach that can be used is leave-one-subject-out.

Generating a high-quality dataset that enables ML algorithms to effectively solve their intended tasks is a challenging endeavor. Data typically does not come in a format suitable for direct use in training an ML model, necessitating an additional step called preprocessing. The data in its initially collected form is referred to as **raw data**. Raw data may present several issues, such as:

- Missing values (where some samples lack certain measurements),
- Duplicate data (where the same samples are entered multiple times),
- Inconsistent representations (e.g., initials instead of full names, varying addresses for the same location),
- Different data formats (e.g., various representations of gender),
- Erroneous entries or incorrect data types (e.g., a string instead of a numeric value, or 36°C recorded as "36" instead of the actual temperature value).

Various methods can address the issues arising from these and other factors compromising data quality. For instances of missing data, imputation methods can be employed to address the gap [67]. Common techniques include imputation using the mean, median, or mode; in time series data, backward or forward fill; and more advanced methods like regression imputation, k-nearest neighbor imputation, or interpolation.

Another important aspect to consider is the representativeness of the data. If the dataset does not include a sufficient number of cases for a certain group, it may introduce bias toward the majority group, which raises practical issues when the ML model is applied in real-world scenarios. Preprocessing can also involve sampling techniques to mitigate this bias.

Additionally, numeric variables may have varying scales. Such differences in scale can cause problems during the optimization process in ML. To address this, we normalize or standardize the data, often by scaling all values to a range between 0 and 1, or −1 and 1. Another approach is to normalize by subtracting the mean and dividing by the standard deviation. Normalization and standardization are performed using the training set mean and standard deviation. These values are stored and later used for normalization and standardization of the test samples.

Depending on the specific ML task and the data quality, additional preprocessing steps may be necessary, such as data imputation, text preprocessing, outlier detection and removal, etc. The performance of an ML algorithm often depends heavily on these steps, and better preprocessing leads to easier learning problems.

2.2.1.4 Overfitting

Overfitting occurs when a machine learning model becomes too complex and learns not only the underlying patterns in the training data but also the noise and irrelevant details. This leads to poor generalization on unseen data. In AAL systems, for example in activity recognition, overfitting can be a significant issue. For example, let us consider a model trained to recognize human activities like walking, running, or sitting using sensor data from wearable devices. If the model is overfit, it may learn specific patterns related to the exact individuals, sensor placements, or even environmental noise present in the training data, rather than generalizing to the broader activity patterns. As a result, when the model is tested on new individuals or in different environments, its performance may drop significantly because it is too specialized to the training conditions. Regularization techniques and using more generalized features can help mitigate overfitting in such cases, ensuring the model focuses on the core patterns of the activities rather than noise.

2.2.2 Types of ML

Here, we briefly define the most common types of ML algorithms. For more precise definitions with more examples, we refer the readers to Alpaydin et al. [4].

2.2.2.1 Supervised Learning

Supervised learning is used when there are data samples for which we know the outcome. These data samples are called labeled data. In supervised learning, the algorithms learn a model or function that maps inputs to outputs, enabling the model to predict outcomes for new, unseen data. In AAL context, supervised learning is often used to recognize activities, detect falls, or monitor health conditions by analyzing sensor data.

For example, in an AAL system designed to monitor older adult residents, a supervised learning model could be trained to classify daily activities, such as walking, sitting, or sleeping, using data from wearable sensors. The model learns to associate specific sensor readings with corresponding activities based on labeled training data. A usual step before the training is the feature generation from the sensor data. Features are generated by transforming the sensor readings data using various mathematical transformations. In this case, instead of the sensor reading space, the ML model optimization problem is performed in the feature space. Once trained, it can accurately predict the current activity of a resident, enabling the system to provide assistance or raise alarms if necessary.

Support Vector Machines (SVM) [69] are frequently used in AAL systems for activity recognition [14]. SVMs work by finding the optimal boundary that separates different classes of activities, such as walking, sitting, or lying down, based on sensor data. This algorithm is particularly effective when the data are complex and not easily separable, as it can create non-linear boundaries using kernel functions.

Decision Trees [38] are another popular choice in AAL applications. These algorithms operate by splitting the data into subsets based on the value of input features, forming a tree-like structure. Each branch represents a decision rule, and each leaf node represents an outcome. Decision trees are intuitive and easy to interpret, making them ideal for detecting specific events like falls or irregular movements, where clear decision paths are necessary. Multiple decision trees can be combined in a single ML model. Random Forests [12] is a widely used ensemble method that builds multiple decision trees and merges their results. By averaging the predictions of several trees, random forests increase accuracy and reduce the risk of overfitting.

K-Nearest Neighbors (KNN) [39] is another straightforward yet powerful algorithm often used in AAL. KNN classifies new instances based on the majority class of the nearest 'k' instances in the training data. This algorithm is particularly useful in scenarios where the system needs to recognize or classify activities in real time, as it can quickly adapt to new data without extensive retraining.

Naive Bayes [62] is a probabilistic algorithm that applies Bayes' theorem with the assumption of independence between features. Despite this seemingly strong assumption, Naive Bayes performs well in practice, especially in classification tasks where the probability of certain activities given sensor data can be effectively modeled [2].

Artificial Neural Networks (ANN) [9], particularly deep learning (DL) models [42], are increasingly being applied in AAL due to their ability to model complex patterns in large datasets. These models are particularly suited for tasks like continuous health monitoring or detecting subtle changes in behavior that might indicate the onset of health issues. Neural networks can automatically extract and learn features from raw sensor data, making them powerful tools in AAL systems. However, depending on the size and complexity of the model, it may require a very large amount of data to train.

Each of these algorithms brings unique strengths to the table, and the choice of which to use depends on the specific requirements of the AAL system. Often, multiple algorithms are combined in a hybrid approach to enhance the system's overall performance, ensuring that it can accurately monitor and assist individuals in various scenarios. As the training of the models is an optimization problem, there is no silver bullet regarding the choice of the algorithm for training as the models heavily rely on the data used.

2.2.2.2 Unsupervised Learning

In unsupervised learning the goal is to discover hidden patterns or intrinsic structures in data without the need for labeled outcomes. Unlike supervised learning, where the model is trained on labeled datasets, unsupervised learning works with unlabeled data, making it particularly useful in situations where manual labeling is impractical or impossible. In AAL, unsupervised learning is often employed for clustering, anomaly detection, and pattern recognition, contributing to the overall intelligence and adaptability of the system.

Clustering algorithms [75] are some of the most widely used unsupervised learning techniques in AAL. These algorithms group similar data points based on their features, enabling the system to identify different patterns of behavior or activity without prior knowledge of what those patterns might be. For instance, K-Means Clustering is a popular method that partitions the data into 'k' clusters, where each data point belongs to the cluster with the nearest mean. In an AAL setting, K-Means can be used to cluster sensor data to identify common daily activities, helping to establish a baseline of normal behavior for each individual. Another effective clustering method is Hierarchical Clustering, which builds a tree of clusters by iteratively merging or splitting existing clusters. Hierarchical clustering provides a more detailed insight into the data structure, allowing the system to detect subtle variations in behavior. Gaussian Mixture Models (GMM) [61], unlike K-Means Clustering, which takes into account only the Euclidean distance, also consider the covariance matrix of the clusters into account. GMMs are used in a similar way as k-means clustering and have the number of clusters as input parameter, although there are methods that can estimate this parameter [26].

Autoencoders [8], a type of neural network, are another powerful tool in unsupervised learning for AAL. Autoencoders learn to compress input data into a lower-dimensional space (encoding) and then reconstruct it (decoding) as closely as possible to the original. This process helps in identifying the underlying structure of the data. In AAL, autoencoders can be used for anomaly detection by training the model on normal behavior and then detecting deviations that the model cannot accurately reconstruct, which may signal unusual or potentially dangerous situations like falls or sudden health changes.

Isolation Forests [43] are algorithms particularly useful for anomaly detection in AAL systems. This method is based on isolating outliers by randomly partitioning the data. Data points that require fewer partitions to be isolated are considered anomalies. In an AAL context, Isolation Forests can monitor continuous data streams from various sensors, automatically identifying behaviors that deviate from the norm, such as erratic movement patterns that might indicate distress [56].

Even though, by definition, labels are not available in unsupervised learning, in practical scenarios, often the clusters or anomalies need to be understood. Therefore, it can be the case when experts label the clusters after they are discovered. In other situations, clusters could be compared and mapped to known labels. This simplifies the evaluation and comparison of unsupervised models.

These unsupervised learning algorithms are important to the development of AAL systems that can adapt to the unique needs and behaviors of individuals without requiring extensive labeled data. By automatically discovering patterns, identifying anomalies, and simplifying complex data, unsupervised learning enhances the ability of AAL systems to provide personalized, real-time assistance and improve the quality of life for those who rely on them.

2.2.2.3 Semi-supervised Learning

Semi-supervised learning [68] is a powerful ML approach that leverages both labeled and unlabeled data to improve model performance. In real-world applications like AAL systems, labeled data can be scarce and expensive to obtain, while unlabeled data are often abundant.

Applying semi-supervised learning in AAL systems enables the development of more accurate and adaptable systems with reduced reliance on labeled data. For instance, an AAL system might start with a small set of labeled data representing activities or health conditions (e.g., walking, sitting, or a potential fall). Still, as it collects new unlabeled sensor data, it can automatically label it, and improve its accuracy over time [65].

Related concepts within this framework include one-shot [64] and few-shot learning, where a model is trained to recognize new patterns from just one or a few examples. These approaches are beneficial in AAL systems, where collecting large amounts of labeled data for every possible activity or health condition may be impractical. For example, an AAL system could use a pretrained network and apply few-shot learning to learn users' gestures [23].

Several common methods are used in semi-supervised learning, each offering specific advantages to AAL systems. With self-training [65], the model initially trained on labeled data are used to label the unlabeled data, gradually expanding the training set. This method is simple yet effective for improving model accuracy in AAL applications, such as activity recognition.

Another approach is co-training [51], which uses two models trained on different feature sets of the data. Each model labels the unlabeled data, and these new labels are then used to train the other model. Co-training is beneficial in AAL systems where multiple sensor types (e.g., motion sensors and wearables) provide different perspectives on the same activities.

Methods like Variational Autoencoders (VAEs) and Generative Adversarial Networks (GANs) can generate synthetic data that resembles the real data, thus augmenting the training set. This approach can be helpful in AAL for creating more diverse training scenarios, helping the system to better handle variability in user behavior. In addition, using synthetic data generation techniques like VAEs and GANs can also simulate digital twins of real-world systems, providing a virtual environment for testing and optimizing algorithms without the need for real-world data collection. This is especially practical when acquiring large, diverse datasets, which is challenging or expensive, allowing the model to generalize better and improve its robustness to unseen situations.

2.2.2.4 Reinforcement Learning

Reinforcement Learning (RL) is a ML paradigm where an agent learns to make decisions by interacting with an environment, perceives information about its current state and takes actions [71]. Conversely, the environment provides a reward signal (positive or negative), and the agent aims to maximize the expected cumulative reward over the period of interaction. The policy of an agent defines how the agent selects its actions based on the available information. A policy can be either deterministic or stochastic and either stationary or history-dependent. In [71] authors provide a comprehensive collection of survey articles covering key areas in reinforcement learning, including partially observable environments, hierarchical task decomposition, and relational knowledge representation. This book can serve as an essential resource for readers interested in the fundamentals in reinforcement learning. Similarly, in Arulkumaran et al. [6] are described central algorithms in deep reinforcement learning (deep RL), including the deep Q-network (DQN), trust region policy optimization (TRPO), and the asynchronous advantage actor critic algorithm, which lead to more robust and faster learning in RL.

In the context of AAL, a common use of RL is in sign-language recognition. For example, authors in [82] propose integrating a transformer model with RL to improve continuous sign language recognition by directly optimizing non-differentiable metrics like word error rate.

2.2.2.5 Anomaly Detection

Anomaly detection in AAL systems is essential for early identification of potentially dangerous situations, enabling timely interventions that can prevent accidents or provide assistance when needed. By continuously learning and adapting to the individual's behavior, these systems offer a personalized and proactive approach to enhancing safety and independence in assisted living environments. Consider an AAL system that continuously monitors a person's movements and health-related metrics through sensors embedded in their environment and wearable devices. Over time, the system learns the individual's typical patterns of behavior, such as walking speed, gait, and daily routines. This learned model serves as a baseline for normal behavior. As the person goes about their daily activities, the AAL system continuously compares real-time sensor data against the established model of normal behavior. If the system detects a considerable deviation from expected patterns—such as an abrupt, rapid movement followed by an extended period of inactivity, which might indicate a fall—it flags this as an anomaly. This detection can then trigger various alerting mechanisms, such as notifying caregivers or activating emergency protocols.

Even though anomaly detection improves safety and independence in AAL environments, it also presents challenges, particularly concerning false positives. False alarms can occur when the system misinterprets harmless deviations from routine behavior as dangerous situations. For instance, if an individual changes their daily schedule or engages in atypical physical activity, the system might mistakenly identify this as a risk, leading to unnecessary interventions and potential stress for both the person and caregivers. Striking a balance between convenience and safety is still a challenge. On the one hand, systems must be sensitive enough to detect real dangers. On the other hand, they need to be robust against normal variations in behavior to avoid overwhelming users with false alerts. Achieving this balance requires fine-tuning detection thresholds and incorporating context-aware processing to better discern genuine emergencies from benign anomalies.

Common algorithms used include statistical methods like Z-Score Analysis and Gaussian Mixture Models (GMM), ML approaches such as One-Class SVM and Isolation Forest, and deep learning techniques like Autoencoders [53]. These algorithms help detect anomalies such as sudden falls by comparing real-time sensor data against learned models of normal behavior. Anomaly detection is also vital in the context of open set learning, where the system must handle new, unseen data that does not fit within the predefined categories. The new scenarios will be interpreted as potential outliers or anomalies in such cases. The challenge here is that these new scenarios may not necessarily indicate danger; they could simply represent natural changes in the person's lifestyle or environment. Despite that, AAL systems can gradually adapt to new scenarios, even if an anomaly is treated as a dangerous event. Sometimes, being alarmed about an anomaly could be a preferred option compared to a misclassification of the event in one of the actions of a closed set. In practical scenarios, experts might even analyze the anomalies, cluster them via unsupervised learning, and even assign labels to them if there are distinct patterns, that can result in another iteration of re-training a (semi-)supervised model. So, ultimately, anomaly detection can contribute to maintaining users' safety and well-being in dynamic environments.

2.2.2.6 Transfer Learning

Transfer learning in activity recognition typically involves leveraging a pre-trained model on a similar or related task and fine-tuning it for a specific target activity recognition task. This approach enables the system to learn a more generalized representation of human activities, enhancing its capability to accurately recognize both common and uncommon activities within the home environment [13].

An exemplary scenario of transfer learning for activity recognition is the following. A model pre-trained on a large dataset of common physical activities (like walking, running, and sitting) using wearable sensor data are adapted to recognize new, more complex activities (such as biking or climbing stairs) with limited data. The earlier layers of the pre-trained model (e.g., a CNN or RNN), which capture general motion patterns, are kept frozen, while only the final layers are fine-tuned using the smaller dataset for the new activities [70]. This approach reduces training time, improves generalization, and allows efficient use of scarce labeled data for the target task.

In the context of AAL, transfer learning is particularly beneficial for adapting models to recognize subtle variations in activities, such as changes in gait or the performance of routine tasks. Another practical application of transfer learning in AAL systems is the ability to tune models trained in controlled settings to real-life environments where the people's behavior and specifics might be different.

2.2.3 Evaluation Metrics

To evaluate the performance of a classification model, several measures and metrics are commonly used. The terms metrics and measures are terms that are sometimes used interchangeably, but they can have distinct meanings depending on the context. A measure is a general term for a quantity that can be observed or calculated from the data (in the list below, it would be TP, TN, FP, FN). A metric is typically derived from one or more measures and is used to assess how well a model performs in a specific task, so they are useful for comparison, evaluation, and optimization of models.

Some of the listed metrics are usable for binary-classification problems (where there are only two classes), but in the context of AAL, it is much more common to have multiple classes, requiring metrics that can evaluate the performance of the models accordingly. Here we list the most important metrics, and for a comprehensive list of metrics, we refer the readers to Alpaydin et al. [4].

2.2.3.1 Binary Classification

Below are listed the most common metrics for binary classification problems:

- **True Positives (TP)**: The number of instances correctly classified as positive.
- **True Negatives (TN)**: The number of instances correctly classified as negative.
- **False Positives (FP)**: The number of instances incorrectly classified as positive. An example would be the total number of cases when a normal movement was misclassified as a fall.
- **False Negatives (FN)**: The number of instances incorrectly classified as negative. An example of this would be falls misclassified as regular movements. Typically, the impact of false negatives is far greater than that of false positives. In the earlier example, a fall incorrectly classified as a normal situation can have fatal consequences for the person. On the other hand, a routine activity misclassified as a fall could be annoying (e.g., a caregiver is alarmed) but not as critical.
- **Confusion Matrix**: A table that summarizes the performance of a classification model by displaying the counts of TP, TN, FP, and FN.
- **Accuracy**: The proportion of correctly classified instances among all instances. It is calculated as:
$$\text{Accuracy} = \frac{TP + TN}{TP + TN + FP + FN}$$
- **Balanced Accuracy**: The average of recall obtained on each class, useful in cases of class imbalance, which is common in AAL. It is calculated as:
$$\text{Balanced Accuracy} = \frac{1}{2}\left(\frac{TP}{TP + FN} + \frac{TN}{TN + FP}\right)$$
- **Precision**: The proportion of true positives among all positive predictions. It is defined as:
$$\text{Precision} = \frac{TP}{TP + FP}$$
- **Recall (Sensitivity)**: The proportion of true positives among all actual positive instances. It is defined as:
$$\text{Recall} = \frac{TP}{TP + FN}$$
- **Weighted Error Rate (WER)**: Is a variation of the standard error rate, where different types of errors are assigned different weights, as explained when defining

FP and FN. In simple error rate calculations, all errors are treated equally, but in many real-world applications, one might want to penalize certain errors more heavily than others. WER is calculated as:

$$\text{WER} = \frac{w_{\text{FP}} \times \text{FP} + w_{\text{FN}} \times \text{FN}}{w_{\text{FP}} \times (\text{FP} + \text{TN}) + w_{\text{FN}} \times (\text{TP} + \text{FN})}$$

where w_{FP} and w_{FN} are the weights assigned to false positives (FP) and false negatives (FN), respectively.

- **Cost Matrix**: It defines the cost associated with different types of classification errors and is defined as:

$$\text{Cost Matrix} = \begin{pmatrix} 0 & C(\text{False Negative}) \\ C(\text{False Positive}) & 0 \end{pmatrix}$$

where C(False Positive) is the cost of FP, and C(False Negative) is the cost of FN. Similarly to WER, this metric aims to address the case when not all errors are equal.

- **F1 Score**: The harmonic mean of precision and recall, providing a balance between the two. It is calculated as:

$$\text{F1 Score} = \frac{2 \times \text{Precision} \times \text{Recall}}{\text{Precision} + \text{Recall}}$$

- **Area Under the ROC Curve (AUC-ROC)**: AUC-ROC measures the ability of the model to distinguish between normal and anomalous points across different threshold settings. The ROC curve plots the true positive rate (sensitivity) against the false positive rate (1-specificity).
- **Area Under the Precision-Recall Curve (AUC-PR)**: Similar to AUC-ROC, but more informative in cases of class imbalance, AUC-PR plots precision versus recall.
- **Binary cross-entropy**:, which compares the predicted probabilities with the actual class labels, penalizing the model more when the predicted probability for the correct class is low. It is designed to handle probability distributions, making it ideal for classification where the output of the model is a probability distribution over the classes. For binary classification, it is defined as:

$$\mathscr{L}_{\text{Binary}} = -\frac{1}{n} \sum_{i=1}^{n} \left[y_i \log(\hat{y}_i) + (1 - y_i) \log(1 - \hat{y}_i) \right].$$

2.2.3.2 Multi-class Classification

In multi-class classification, the most commonly used measures are:

- **Confusion Matrix**: A square matrix of size $n \times n$ (where n is the number of classes), with rows representing the actual classes and columns representing the predicted classes. The diagonal elements represent true positives for each class, while off-diagonal elements represent misclassifications.
- **Accuracy**: The proportion of correctly classified instances across all classes. It is computed as:

$$\text{Accuracy} = \frac{\sum_{i=1}^{n} \text{TP}_i}{\sum_{i=1}^{n} \text{TP}_i + \sum_{i \neq j} \text{CM}_{ij}}$$

where TP_i is the number of true positives for class i, and CM_{ij} is the confusion matrix element for actual class i and predicted class j.
- **Precision**: The precision for each class i is defined as:

$$\text{Precision}_i = \frac{\text{TP}_i}{\text{TP}_i + \text{FP}_i}$$

where FP_i is the number of false positives for class i. The overall precision can be computed using macro-average or weighted-average across classes.
- **Recall (Sensitivity)**: The recall for each class i is defined as:

$$\text{Recall}_i = \frac{\text{TP}_i}{\text{TP}_i + \text{FN}_i}$$

where FN_i is the number of false negatives for class i. Like precision, recall can be averaged across classes.
- **F1 Score**: The F1 score for each class i is the harmonic mean of precision and recall:

$$\text{F1 Score}_i = \frac{2 \times \text{Precision}_i \times \text{Recall}_i}{\text{Precision}_i + \text{Recall}_i}$$

The overall F1 score can also be calculated using macro-average or weighted-average.
- **Macro-Averaging**: Calculates the metric independently for each class and then takes the average, treating all classes equally:

$$\text{Macro-Metric} = \frac{1}{n} \sum_{i=1}^{n} \text{Metric}_i$$

- **Weighted-Averaging**: Averages the metric for each class, weighted by the number of training instances in each class:

$$\text{Weighted-Metric} = \frac{\sum_{i=1}^{n} w_i \times \text{Metric}_i}{\sum_{i=1}^{n} w_i}$$

where w_i is the number of training instances in class i. Obviously, this could be challenging if the class distribution of the test and training dataset are different.
- **Multi-class cross-entropy** is defined as:

$$\mathscr{L}_{\text{Multi-class}} = -\frac{1}{n} \sum_{i=1}^{n} \sum_{k=1}^{K} y_{i,k} \log(\hat{y}_{i,k}).$$

2.2.3.3 Unsupervised Learning

In clustering, anomaly detection and other unsupervised learning tasks, evaluation metrics differ from those used in supervised learning. Common metrics include:

- **Adjusted Rand Index (ARI)**: Measures the similarity between the predicted clusters and the ground truth labels, adjusted for chance. It ranges from −1 to 1, where 1 indicates perfect clustering, 0 indicates random labeling, and negative values indicate worse-than-random labeling:

$$\text{ARI} = \frac{\text{RI} - \text{Expected RI}}{\text{Max RI} - \text{Expected RI}}$$

where RI is the Rand Index. If there are no available ground truth labels, even in the training process, then this metric is not appropriate for unsupervised learning.
- **Silhouette Score**: Assesses how similar each point is to its own cluster compared to other clusters. The score ranges from −1 to 1, where 1 indicates well-separated clusters, 0 indicates overlapping clusters, and negative values indicate points assigned to the wrong cluster:

$$\text{Silhouette Score} = \frac{b - a}{\max(a, b)}$$

where a is the average intra-cluster distance and b is the average distance between the data point and all the points in the nearest neighboring cluster (i.e., the cluster that is not its own, but is closest to it).

- **Purity**: Measures the extent to which each cluster contains data points from primarily one class. It is calculated by assigning each cluster to the class that is most frequent in the cluster, and then counting the number of correctly assigned points:

$$\text{Purity} = \frac{1}{n} \sum_{k} \max_{j} |c_k \cap l_j|$$

where c_k is the set of points in cluster k, and l_j is the set of points in class j.

2.2.4 Model Monitoring

After a model is trained, it must be integrated into an application tailored to the specific problem it aims to solve. Typically, this involves using the model to make decisions, predictions, or classifications on new, unseen data. In AAL systems, integration of ML systems with alerting and monitoring systems is required so that appropriate actions can be taken immediately. Model maintenance is also necessary once the model is deployed. It involves continuously monitoring performance and retraining the model with new data to maintain its accuracy and relevance. Over time, models can become outdated due to issues like data drift, concept drift, or feature drift, where the distribution of data or features changes [10]. Addressing these drifts requires specific coping mechanisms and performance monitoring. Additionally, maintenance includes standard software upkeep, ensuring that the underlying infrastructure and supporting software remain functional and secure. Bayram et al. [10] provides a good overview on performance-aware drift detectors, covering solutions for detecting data and concept drift, as well as methods for detecting model degradation.

2.3 ML and AAL Systems

In the context of AAL, ML applications focus on personalization, safety, and efficiency. These systems process data from various wearables or sensors and devices embedded in the living environment to learn residents' daily patterns and needs and provide continuous and unobtrusive assistance. The integration of ML in AAL helps analyze complex data streams automatically, contributing to the autonomy, independence, and safety of the older adults and disabled people [33].

In AAL systems, activity recognition allows for the monitoring and understanding of physical activity, detecting changes in daily patterns that may signify health issues, and identifying emergencies, such as falls or abnormal vital signs [21]. ML models analyze behavior patterns to detect early signs of dementia, Alzheimer's, or other cognitive impairments [32]. The detection of falls (see Chap. 5 in this volume [35]) represents a pivotal aspect of emergency monitoring, employing a combination of accelerometers, gyroscopes, and visual sensors to provide real-time alerts.

Furthermore, AAL systems ensure the safety and security of the living environment by monitoring the status of doors and windows and alerting caregivers or security services to any unusual activities that could indicate potential security breaches or safety issues. Sleep patterns are tracked through wearables and bed sensors, offering data for health monitoring purposes [18]. The detection of food intake and analyzing eating and drinking habits, facilitated by wrist-worn sensors and environmental monitoring, provides valuable insights into the nutritional intake and hydration levels of the older adults [49].

In the healthcare setting, ML can be seen as a sophisticated tool that assists in diagnosing diseases, predicting patient outcomes, and managing treatment plans more efficiently [31]. In the domain of health-related activities, AAL systems assist in medication management through smart dispensers and sensors that confirm the intake of prescribed drugs. Similarly, ML systems could optimize and personalize medication schedules, monitor adherence, and predict potential adverse reactions [46]. They also support physical therapy by ensuring exercises are performed correctly, thus aiding in rehabilitation and recovery processes [44].

According to Gajarawala and Pelkowski [27], telehealth or telemedicine has transformed healthcare delivery by improving access to care and reducing the necessity for in-person visits. This is beneficial in the context of AAL. Health monitoring systems have rapidly evolved during the past two decades and can potentially change how healthcare is delivered [7]. Nowadays, Internet of Things (IoT) technologies and ML are applied together in AAL settings [34, 37]. IoT is an assistant in healthcare and is extremely important in broad scopes of medicinal services observing applications. In hospital settings, AAL systems can identify and reduce false alarms to avoid alarm fatigue of medical personnel [40].

2.4 ML Challenges Specific to AAL Systems

2.4.1 Closed Set Versus Open Set Action Recognition

Open set versus closed set action recognition refers to two different scenarios in the context of recognizing actions from sensory or visual data. These scenarios deal with the challenges of generalizing the recognition models to unseen or new actions.

In closed set action recognition, the system is trained and tested on the same set of actions. The system only encounters a fixed number of action categories during both training and testing. The primary challenge here is to develop models that can accurately distinguish between these known actions. The most common example is when a model is trained to recognize actions like walking, running, and jumping, and then tested on these same actions. In real-world recognition and classification tasks, it is often impractical to gather training samples that encompass all possible classes due to various constraints. Furthermore, it is also challenging to develop models that can effectively recognize novel or rare activities that were not encountered during training [16].

Consequently, a more realistic scenario is open set recognition (OSR), where the training data represents only a subset of the possible classes, and the system may encounter novel, previously unseen classes during testing. The system is trained on a limited set of known actions but needs to identify whether a new action belongs to one of the known classes or is something completely new. The major challenge is that the model must not only recognize known actions but also detect and appropriately handle unknown actions. For example, a model trained to recognize walking, running, and jumping but tested on a video containing a new action like falling.

In Geng et al. [28], the authors present a comprehensive review of existing OSR techniques in general but also mention activity recognition in the context of AAL. It addresses key aspects such as definitions, model representations, datasets, evaluation methods, and algorithm comparisons. Additionally, it explores the connections between OSR and related tasks like zero-shot, one-shot (few-shot) learning, and classification with a reject option. The review also extends to open-world recognition, an evolution of OSR.

2.4.1.1 Challenges

Open set action recognition presents several significant challenges that must be addressed for the development of robust and effective systems. First, the system must demonstrate the ability to generalize beyond the known categories, effectively managing the risk of overfitting to the training data. A crucial aspect of this generalization is the system's capacity to identify when an observed action does not belong to any of the known classes. One way to address this is by well-calibrated thresholds that can accurately distinguish between known and unknown actions.

2.4.1.2 Potential Solutions

Out-of-distribution detection is a crucial technique in open set action recognition [76]. It involves training models to identify when an input does not belong to any of the known classes. A common method used for this purpose is softmax thresholding, where the confidence scores from the softmax output are analyzed to determine whether an action is unknown [76]. More advanced techniques have also been developed, such as using generative models like Variational Autoencoders (VAEs) [57] or Generative Adversarial Networks (GANs) [63, 77]. These models can model the distribution of known actions, enabling the identification of out-of-distribution samples.

In addition to these techniques, open set neural networks have been specifically designed to address the challenges of open set recognition [29]. These networks modify the loss function during training to penalize both misclassifications and incorrect confidence in unknown classes. An example of this approach involves combining traditional classification loss with an additional term that encourages low confidence for unknown actions, thus improving the model's ability to recognize when an action does not belong to any known class.

Handling new or unseen actions in open-set action recognition requires several strategies to improve model robustness. One approach is to maintain a rich "other" or "garbage" class during training, allowing the model to generalize better and handle actions outside the known classes. This prevents overfitting and reduces false positives by ensuring the model can classify unfamiliar actions into a non-specific category [28, 77]. Additionally, maintaining strong contextual features helps filter out irrelevant detections, further reducing the likelihood of false positives. Incorporating multiple modalities, such as combining visual, audio, and sensor data, enhances detection accuracy by cross-verifying signals from different sources [59]. Temporal filters are also a viable solution, as they help fill in gaps from non-detections and eliminate too-short, spurious detections, improving temporal consistency [60]. Finally, integrating data quality assessments enhances the system's confidence in its predictions by factoring in the quality and reliability of the incoming data, leading to more accurate classification.

Another approach in this domain is the use of hybrid models, which combine traditional classification models with anomaly detection models [54]. In this setup, the classifier first attempts to recognize the action. If the model is uncertain, an anomaly detector steps in to determine if the action is unknown. This method proves particularly effective in scenarios with limited training data or when there is a high likelihood of encountering numerous unknown actions.

Few-shot learning and meta-learning are also practical techniques in open set action recognition [19]. These approaches focus on making models more adaptable to new classes with minimal examples. Few-shot learning, for instance, enables a model to quickly learn a new action category from only a few examples, while meta-learning trains the model to be more adaptable to learning new tasks. These techniques enhance the model's ability to generalize to unknown actions by improving its adaptability. Few-shot learning can be sensitive to data quality of the few provided examples, can struggle with class imbalance, and often requires extensive pretraining. Similarly, meta-learning, while powerful, is computationally complex, may overfit to specific tasks on which it was trained, and relies on a diverse set of training tasks for effective generalization.

2.4.2 Action Spotting Problem

Action spotting is a common task within the field of activity recognition which involves identifying specific actions or events within continuous data streams generated by various sensors, including motion detectors, cameras, and wearable devices. In AAL systems, action spotting is important for detecting activities or incidents, such as falls, unusual behavior patterns, or other events that may require immediate intervention. Unlike general activity recognition, which typically classifies entire sequences of data into specific categories like walking or sitting, action spotting focuses on pinpointing the exact moment when a particular action or event occurs. It is also important when counting certain activities, measuring their duration statistics, or labeling them accurately.

The challenge of action spotting lies in several factors unique to AAL contexts. First, the continuous flow of information makes it difficult to isolate and identify specific actions accurately. Moreover, the actions that need to be spotted can be subtle and vary significantly between individuals, adding another layer of complexity to the problem. The necessity for real-time processing further complicates the task, demanding efficient algorithms and robust models.

Recent advances in deep learning have provided promising solutions to the challenges of action spotting. Deep learning models, particularly those utilizing convolutional neural networks (CNNs) and recurrent neural networks (RNNs), have demonstrated the capability to learn complex features from raw data [74]. As mentioned in Subsect. 2.2.2.6, transfer learning has been instrumental in enhancing these models' performance.

Temporal modeling techniques, such as temporal convolutional networks (TCNs) [41] and long short-term memory (LSTM) networks, have also played a crucial role in action spotting [5]. These techniques enable the modeling of the temporal dynamics of actions, allowing the system to accurately recognize the start and end points of actions within continuous data streams [41]. The sliding window approach is a commonly used method in this domain, where the continuous data stream is divided into overlapping segments [81]. Each segment is independently analyzed to detect whether the target action occurs within that window. A challenge here is to tune the window size, considering that different actions can have different duration. In such scenarios, several different models can be used, each trained with different window sizes and making them focused on recognizing activities with particular expected duration. Alternatively, the length of the window size can be dynamic [52].

Attention mechanisms have been integrated into deep learning models to further enhance the accuracy of action spotting. These mechanisms allow the models to focus on specific parts of the data stream that are more likely to contain the action of interest. By weighting the importance of different data segments, attention mechanisms help to more accurately identify the relevant action, thus reducing false positives and improving overall detection performance [78]. Their drawbacks are increased computational complexity, risk of overfitting, and challenges in interpretability. They may also be sensitive to noise, require large datasets, and sometimes add unnecessary complexity without significant performance gains in simpler tasks. Therefore, for each specific application a careful analysis is required to balance their advantages and disadvantages.

Hybrid approaches that combine deep learning with traditional signal processing techniques have also been explored. For instance, initial preprocessing steps might involve filtering out noise or irrelevant data, making it easier for the deep learning model to focus on the essential aspects of the data. This combination of methods has been shown to improve both the accuracy and efficiency of action spotting in AAL systems [3]. However, with filtering there is always a risk of removing valid data points and filtering methods and their suitability depends on the data modalities.

2.4.3 Class Imbalance

In the context of AAL, not all actions or health-related events occur with equal frequency. For instance, typical daily activities such as walking, sitting, or eating are performed multiple times throughout the day. In contrast, actions like falling or exhibiting symptoms of a health condition, such as a sudden loss of balance or a heart arrhythmia, are relatively rare. This often results in the model being biased towards the majority class, leading to overfitting. Consequently, the model may perform poorly in detecting or predicting rare but important events. In the context of AAL, a high false positive rate can lead to unnecessary interventions, causing distress or discomfort to the user. However, a high false negative rate, which can result in missed detections of important events, poses a significant threat to the user's health and safety. For instance, a fall detection system that frequently generates false alarms may cause the user to lose trust in the system, while failing to detect an actual fall can lead to severe injury.

Class distributions are often inherently skewed in real-world scenarios, leading to imbalanced classification problems. Despite this, many datasets used in the development of ML models for AAL are artificially balanced, often by oversampling minority classes, undersampling majority classes, or using the synthetic minority over-sampling (SMOTE) technique [15].

2.4.3.1 Strategies to Address Class Imbalance

Addressing class imbalance in AAL requires a combination of strategies, as covered in much more detail in Japkowicz and Stephen [30].

Simple Balancing

With oversampling, the minority class gets more representation, the model becomes better at learning from the minority class data during training. This reduces the chance of the model getting biased toward the majority class. Oversampling can lead to overfitting on the minority class, especially if the same instances are repeated (in simple oversampling). This is because the model might become too focused on a few examples of the minority class.

Undersampling allows the model to focus on both classes more equally by reducing the number of majority class samples. However, undersampling can lead to underfitting the majority class, as it discards potentially useful information about the majority class.

Data Augmentation

There are methods like the Synthetic Minority Over-sampling Technique (SMOTE) [15] that can be used to create synthetic samples for the minority class and help balance the dataset, improving model performance on rare events. Originally, SMOTE is most effective with continuous or discrete numeric features because it generates new samples by interpolating between feature values. However, with extensions like SMOTE-NC and SMOTE-ENC (SMOTE—Encoded Nominal and Continuous) [47] it can be applied to categorical (nominal) data, by first converting nominal attributes to numeric.

If the imbalance is mild, simpler techniques like undersampling or class weighting may suffice. SMOTE can be more effective if there is a significant imbalance between the classes (e.g., 90:10 or worse). SMOTE is more effective when the minority class has enough instances to calculate meaningful synthetic points. If the minority class is extremely small, generating synthetic points may not yield a good result. In such cases, hybrid approaches like SMOTE-ENN [48] might be more effective. Likewise, SMOTE can struggle with high-dimensional datasets due to the curse of dimensionality. In such cases, it can be used in a combination with feature engineering and dimensionality reduction techniques.

Cost-Sensitive Learning

In class imbalance scenarios, the typical goal of minimizing overall error often leads to poor performance for the minority class, since the classifier can achieve high accuracy by simply predicting the majority class. Cost-sensitive learning addresses this by assigning different weights or penalties to misclassifications, encouraging the model to pay more attention to the minority class. In Mienye and Sun [45] a performance analysis of cost-sensitive learning methods with application to imbalanced medical data was performed, covering in more detail the following approaches.

One approach to cost-sensitive learning is to utilize metrics like AUC-ROC, F1-score, Weighted Error Rate, Cost matrix, and balanced or weighted accuracy during classifier training and hyperparameter tuning.

Alternatively, classifiers can adjust their decision thresholds to favor the class with the higher cost of misclassification. For instance, a classifier might lower the threshold for predicting the minority class (e.g., a fall) to reduce the number of false negatives (since falls might have a higher cost).

Another approach is to assign weights to training examples such that errors on minority class examples are penalized more heavily. Many cost-sensitive classifiers do this by multiplying the loss function by a weight factor for each example based on its class and minority class examples get a higher weight, while majority class examples get a lower weight. This approach ensures that the model focuses more on correctly classifying the minority class, as errors in these cases carry higher penalties.

Determining the correct cost matrix or weights can be difficult, as it requires domain-specific knowledge. Methods like considering the inverse of class ratios to set the weights are often simple, yet effective.

Anomaly Detection Techniques

Given the rarity of certain events, framing the detection of these events as an anomaly detection problem can be effective. This involves training the model primarily on majority class data (normal events) and identifying deviations from this as potential minority class events (anomalies). More about these approaches is discussed in Subsect. 2.2.2.5.

Ensemble Methods

Ensemble methods in machine learning combine the predictions of multiple models to improve accuracy, reliability, and generalization. By aggregating the strengths of different models, ensemble methods aim to minimize errors, reduce bias, and lower variance compared to individual models [80].

There are several types of ensemble methods, and they can be used in various domains, including AAL, to enhance decision-making, safety, and care quality:

- **Bagging** trains multiple models independently using random subsets of the training data (created through bootstrapping) and then averages their predictions (for regression) or uses majority voting (for classification) [11].
- **Boosting** works by sequentially training models, where each model focuses on correcting the errors made by the previous one. It gives higher weights to incorrectly classified instances to improve overall performance. The models are combined by weighting their predictions based on performance. Notable algorithms for this are XGBoost [17] and LightGMB [36].
- **Stacking** involves training multiple different models (not necessarily of the same type) and combining them with a meta-model (a model that learns how to best combine the outputs of the base models). The meta-model makes the final prediction based on the base models' outputs. For example, in Zdravevski et al. [79] authors stack Support Vector Machine (SVM) and Random Forest algorithms to improve recognition of complex human activities.

2.4.3.2 Practical Trade-Offs

Addressing class imbalance in AAL systems requires careful consideration of the practical trade-offs between accuracy, privacy, and convenience. High accuracy in detecting rare but critical events often necessitates extensive data collection, which can raise significant privacy concerns, for example, if audio or video data are to be collected. Meanwhile, prioritizing convenience through less intrusive monitoring may compromise the system's ability to detect these rare events accurately. The challenge lies in designing systems that can effectively manage class imbalance—ensuring rare but crucial events are detected without overwhelming users with false alarms—while balancing the need for privacy and ease of use. Achieving this balance demands a user-centric approach (i.e., the system will require user testing for convenience, usability perception, etc.), adaptive monitoring strategies, and the application of advanced techniques like anomaly detection and synthetic data generation, all aimed at creating a system that is both reliable and respectful of user needs.

In summary, with these methods for addressing class imbalance, the training performance of the minority class often improves, which is often the more important class (e.g., a fall). However, balancing the dataset might not always result in better overall test performance if oversampling leads to overfitting or undersampling removes too much data. This potential performance drop can also be acceptable if the metric is focused on recall (specificity), which favors the positive class, even if the overall accuracy is reduced.

2.4.4 Personalization of AAL Systems

Personalization is an important aspect of AAL systems, as it ensures that the technology is tailored to the specific needs, preferences, and habits of the individual inhabitants of the AAL space. Personalization involves user adaptation and modeling, where the system continuously learns and adapts to the unique patterns of the user's daily activities, health conditions, and behavioral changes. By building a detailed user profile, the system can provide more accurate and relevant support, such as reminders for medication, customized emergency responses, or adjustments in environmental controls like lighting and temperature.

Approaches like Ferrari et al. [24, 25] show that personalization in human activity recognition can be applied practically, while offering substantial benefits for end-users. Similarly, in Sztyler and Stuckenschmidt [66] authors show a method for online personalization of cross-subjects activity recognition models with wearable devices. Additionally, ML has been successfully applied in personalizing fall detection systems, such as Ngu et al. [50].

However, this level of personalization raises privacy concerns, as it requires the collection and processing of extensive personal data. The system must strike a balance between gathering enough information to provide meaningful assistance and maintaining the user's privacy. Techniques such as differential privacy, federated learning, and local data processing can help mitigate privacy risks by ensuring that sensitive information is anonymized or processed locally without being transmitted to central servers [22]. Differential privacy is a technique that adds controlled noise to data or computations to protect individual information while allowing useful insights from aggregate data. Federated Learning in AAL enables the training of machine learning models across distributed devices, like resident monitoring systems, while keeping most of the data localized to each device, enhancing privacy and security [22].

2.4.5 Dealing with Extra People in the Environment

AAL systems must also be capable of distinguishing between the primary inhabitant and other individuals who might enter the AAL space, such as caregivers, visitors, or service providers. The presence of extra people can complicate the system's ability to accurately monitor and assist the primary user. For instance, the system might incorrectly attribute the actions or behaviors of a visitor to the primary user, leading to incorrect conclusions or triggering unnecessary alerts.

To address this challenge, AAL systems need to incorporate sensing and recognition technologies that can differentiate between different individuals based on physical characteristics (such as face recognition), movement patterns like gait recognition, or the use of wearable devices. Additionally, the system should be able to adapt to varying levels of interaction with these extra individuals, such as temporarily ignoring data from a visitor or adjusting the monitoring intensity when a caregiver is present. Some approaches utilize WiFi signal characteristics to identify extra people in the environment [1]. Other approaches for activity recognition of multiple individuals utilize 3d point cloud sequences [72].

Incorporating such capabilities adds complexity to the system design but is essential for maintaining accuracy and reliability in environments where multiple people may be present. Monitoring extra people might lead to inadvertent data collection about individuals who have not consented to being part of the AAL system. Therefore, it also necessitates clear protocols and user controls to ensure that privacy is maintained, such as enabling the primary user to easily adjust monitoring settings when guests are present or ensuring that data related to extra individuals is handled in compliance with privacy regulations.

2.4.6 Multimodality of AAL Data

A promising direction in activity recognition and fall detection is the use of multimodal systems [58]. These systems combine multiple types of sensors and data sources. Combining multiple modalities in machine learning involves three main approaches [83]. In early fusion, data from different modalities are combined at the input level (e.g., concatenating features from text, audio, and images). Next, in late fusion, each modality is processed separately, and their outputs are combined at the decision level (e.g., combining predictions from audio and video models). There is also intermediate or hybrid fusion, where modality-specific features are first extracted and then integrated at a mid-layer before the final prediction (e.g., merging text and image features after independent processing). Additionally, cross-modal learning uses one modality to predict or enhance another. Each method captures multimodal relationships at different stages of processing.

In Zhao et al. [83] also the challenges in multi-modal learning are discussed. Different modalities like audio, video, and text may need to be aligned and synchronized in time or space. Data heterogeneity arises as different modalities have varied structures, making integration difficult. Missing or incomplete modalities can complicate learning when one modality's data are unavailable. Additionally, noise and modality-specific errors can propagate through the model. Other concerns include scalability and computational complexity, as multimodal models are resource-intensive, and issues related to bias and fairness, where one modality may introduce unintended biases. Lastly, interpretability and explainability are also challenging, as multimodal models can become unclear and harder to explain.

Multimodal fall detection approaches are used to gain higher precision and more robustness. In the work presented in Xefteris et al. [73], the authors propose a multimodal fall detection system based on wearable sensors, ambient sensors and vision devices. They also use long short-term memory networks (LSTM) and convolutional neural networks (CNN) for the analysis.

Audio-based approaches for AAL are reviewed in Despotovic et al. [20], and the authors identify several trends. Namely, physiological monitoring, emotion recognition in the context of AAL, human activity recognition, fall detection, and food intake monitoring could leverage audio sensors. Human activities can also be recognized by audio fingerprinting of noises in the environment [55].

2.5 Conclusion

In this chapter, we explored the core concepts of machine learning (ML) and its application to Active Assisted Living (AAL) systems, highlighting the fundamental aspects and unique challenges such systems pose. We began with an introduction to ML fundamentals. First we introduced the typical data types and variables used for modeling. Further, we introduced the common challenges, such as overfitting. The chapter then continues with an overview of the different types of ML techniques, including supervised, unsupervised, semi-supervised, reinforcement learning, and transfer learning. While discussing this, we covered certain specifics and actual use-cases of these types of ML in AAL. The discussion also included the most widely used evaluation measures and metrics for assessing the performance of ML models across binary and multi-class classification, as well as unsupervised learning tasks.

Our focus then shifted to the application of ML in AAL systems, where we emphasized specific challenges in this domain. These challenge include open and closed set action recognition, the action spotting problem, and class imbalance issues. We reviewed potential strategies for overcoming these challenges, such as addressing class imbalance through various techniques and discussing the practical trade-offs inherent to these solutions. The chapter also examined the complexities of personalizing AAL systems, managing scenarios with extra people in the environment, or when processing and fusing multimodal data.

ML is a very dynamic field where new approaches are being introduced daily and is one of the fastest-growing fields in science and technology. Although we have covered the basics in this chapter and introduced the typical ML application development workflow, the reader needs to refer to the newest literature available to obtain the latest developments in ML and the current state-of-the-art algorithms, especially in the AAL domain.

Acknowledgements This publication is based upon work from COST Action GoodBrother—Network on Privacy-Aware Audio- and Video-Based Applications for Active and Assisted Living (CA19121), supported by COST (European Cooperation in Science and Technology). This work was partially financed by the Faculty of Computer Science and Engineering at the Ss. Cyril and Methodius University in Skojpe, Macedonia.

References

1. Abuhoureyah, F., Sim, K.S., Chiew Wong, Y.: Multi-user human activity recognition through adaptive location-independent WiFi signal characteristics. IEEE Access **12**, 112,008–112,024 (2024). https://doi.org/10.1109/ACCESS.2024.3438871
2. Addepalli, N., Pabolu, R.K., Chennuru, S.G., Vissampalli, V.L., Madhumati, G.: Conversion of American sign language to text using deep learning for feature extraction and Naive Bayes for classification. In: 2023 IEEE 8th International Conference for Convergence in Technology (I2CT), pp. 1–5. IEEE (2023)
3. Ahmed, M.F., He, G., Wang, S.: Trifusion Hybrid Model for Human Activity Recognition. Signal, Image and Video Processing, pp. 1–8 (2024)
4. Alpaydin, E.: Introduction to Machine Learning, 4th edn. MIT Press (2020)
5. Alwassel, H., Heilbron, F.C., Ghanem, B.: Action search: spotting actions in videos and its application to temporal action localization. In: Proceedings of the European Conference on Computer Vision (ECCV), pp. 251–266 (2018)
6. Arulkumaran, K., Deisenroth, M.P., Brundage, M., Bharath, A.A.: Deep reinforcement learning: a brief survey. IEEE Signal Process. Mag. **34**(6), 26–38 (2017). https://doi.org/10.1109/MSP.2017.2743240
7. Baig, M.M., Gholamhosseini, H.: Smart health monitoring systems: an overview of design and modeling. J. Med. Syst. **37**, 1–14 (2013)
8. Baldi, P.: Autoencoders, unsupervised learning, and deep architectures. In: Proceedings of ICML Workshop on Unsupervised and Transfer Learning, pp. 37–49. JMLR Workshop and Conference Proceedings (2012)
9. Basheer, I.A., Hajmeer, M.: Artificial neural networks: fundamentals, computing, design, and application. J. Microbiol. Methods **43**(1), 3–31 (2000)
10. Bayram, F., Ahmed, B.S., Kassler, A.: From concept drift to model degradation: an overview on performance-aware drift detectors. Knowl.-Based Syst. **245**, 108,632 (2022)
11. Breiman, L.: Bagging predictors. Mach. Learn. **24**, 123–140 (1996)
12. Breiman, L.: Random forests. Mach. Learn. **45**(1), 5–32 (2001)
13. Chakraborty, S., Mondal, R., Singh, P.K., Sarkar, R., Bhattacharjee, D.: Transfer learning with fine tuning for human action recognition from still images. Multimedia Tools Appl. **80**, 20547–20578 (2021)
14. Chathuramali, K.M., Rodrigo, R.: Faster human activity recognition with SVM. In: International Conference on Advances in ICT for Emerging Regions (ICTer2012), pp. 197–203. IEEE (2012)
15. Chawla, N.V., Bowyer, K.W., Hall, L.O., Kegelmeyer, W.P.: Smote: synthetic minority oversampling technique. J. Artif. Intell. Res. **16**, 321–357 (2002)
16. Chen, K., Zhang, D., Yao, L., Guo, B., Yu, Z., Liu, Y.: Deep learning for sensor-based human activity recognition: overview, challenges, and opportunities. ACM Comput. Surv. (CSUR) **54**(4), 1–40 (2021)

17. Chen, T., Guestrin, C.: Xgboost: a scalable tree boosting system. In: Proceedings of the 22nd ACM SIGKDD International Conference on Knowledge Discovery and Data Mining, pp. 785–794 (2016)
18. Chen, Z., Lin, M., Chen, F., Lane, N.D., Cardone, G., Wang, R., Li, T., Chen, Y., Choudhury, T., Campbell, A.T.: Unobtrusive sleep monitoring using smartphones. In: 2013 7th International Conference on Pervasive Computing Technologies for Healthcare and Workshops, pp. 145–152. IEEE (2013)
19. Coskun, H., Zia, M.Z., Tekin, B., Bogo, F., Navab, N., Tombari, F., Sawhney, H.S.: Domain-specific priors and meta learning for few-shot first-person action recognition. IEEE Trans. Pattern Anal. Mach. Intell. **45**(6), 6659–6673 (2021)
20. Despotovic, V., Pocta, P., Zgank, A.: Audio-based active and assisted living: a review of selected applications and future trends. Comput. Biol. Med. **149**, 106,027 (2022)
21. Dhiman, C., Vishwakarma, D.K.: A review of state-of-the-art techniques for abnormal human activity recognition. Eng. Appl. Artif. Intell. **77**, 21–45 (2019)
22. El Ouadrhiri, A., Abdelhadi, A.: Differential privacy for deep and federated learning: a survey. IEEE Access **10**, 22359–22380 (2022)
23. Elbahri, M., Taleb, N., Ardjoun, S.A.E.M., Zouaoui, C.M.A.: Few-shot learning with pre-trained layers integration applied to hand gesture recognition for people with disabilities. Appl. Comput. Sci. (1895-3735) **20**(2) (2024)
24. Ferrari, A., Micucci, D., Mobilio, M., Napoletano, P.: On the personalization of classification models for human activity recognition. IEEE Access **8**, 32066–32079 (2020)
25. Ferrari, A., Micucci, D., Mobilio, M., Napoletano, P.: Deep learning and model personalization in sensor-based human activity recognition. J. Reliab. Intell. Environ. **9**(1), 27–39 (2023)
26. Figueiredo, M., Jain, A.K.: Unsupervised learning of finite mixture models. IEEE Trans. Pattern Anal. Mach. Intell. **24**(3), 381–396 (2002)
27. Gajarawala, S.N., Pelkowski, J.N.: Telehealth benefits and barriers. J. Nurse Pract. **17**(2), 218–221 (2021)
28. Geng, C., Huang, S.J., Chen, S.: Recent advances in open set recognition: a survey. IEEE Trans. Pattern Anal.Mach. Intell. **43**(10), 3614–3631 (2021). https://doi.org/10.1109/TPAMI.2020.2981604
29. Hassen, M., Chan, P.K.: Learning a neural-network-based representation for open set recognition. In: Proceedings of the 2020 SIAM International Conference on Data Mining, pp. 154–162. SIAM (2020)
30. Japkowicz, N., Stephen, S.: The class imbalance problem: a systematic study. Intell. Data Anal. **6**(5), 429–449 (2002)
31. Javaid, M., Haleem, A., Singh, R.P., Suman, R., Rab, S.: Significance of machine learning in healthcare: features, pillars and applications. Int. J. Intell. Netw. **3**, 58–73 (2022)
32. Javeed, A., Dallora, A.L., Berglund, J.S., Ali, A., Ali, L., Anderberg, P.: Machine learning for dementia prediction: a systematic review and future research directions. J. Med. Syst. **47**(1), 17 (2023)
33. Jovanovic, M., Mitrov, G., Zdravevski, E., Lameski, P., Colantonio, S., Kampel, M., Tellioglu, H., Florez-Revuelta, F.: Ambient assisted living: scoping review of artificial intelligence models, domains, technology, and concerns. J. Med. Internet Res. **24**(11), e36,553 (2022)
34. Kadhim, K.T., Alsahlany, A.M., Wadi, S.M., Kadhum, H.T.: An overview of patient's health status monitoring system based on Internet of Things (IoT). Wirel. Pers. Commun. **114**(3), 2235–2262 (2020)
35. Lumetzberger, J., Ballester, I., Kampel, M.: Fall detection. In: Salah, A.A., Colonna, L., Florez-Revuelta, F. (eds.) Privacy-Aware Monitoring for Assisted Living. Springer, Cham (2025)
36. Ke, G., Meng, Q., Finley, T., Wang, T., Chen, W., Ma, W., Ye, Q., Liu, T.Y.: LightGBM: a highly efficient gradient boosting decision tree. Adv. Neural Inform. Process. Syst. **30** (2017)
37. Kishor, A., Chakraborty, C.: Artificial intelligence and Internet of Things based healthcare 4.0 monitoring system. Wirel. Pers. Commun. **127**(2), 1615–1631 (2022)
38. Kotsiantis, S.B.: Decision trees: a recent overview. Artif. Intell. Rev. **39**, 261–283 (2013)

39. Laaksonen, J., Oja, E.: Classification with learning k-nearest neighbors. In: Proceedings of International Conference on Neural Networks (ICNN'96), vol. 3, pp. 1480–1483. IEEE (1996)
40. Lameski, P., Zdravevski, E., Koceski, S., Kulakov, A., Trajkovik, V.: Suppression of intensive care unit false alarms based on the arterial blood pressure signal. IEEE Access **5**, 5829–5836 (2017). https://doi.org/10.1109/ACCESS.2017.2690380
41. Lea, C., Flynn, M.D., Vidal, R., Reiter, A., Hager, G.D.: Temporal convolutional networks for action segmentation and detection. In: Proceedings of the IEEE Conference on Computer Vision and Pattern Recognition, pp. 156–165 (2017)
42. LeCun, Y., Bengio, Y., Hinton, G.: Deep learning. Nature **521**(7553), 436–444 (2015)
43. Liu, F.T., Ting, K.M., Zhou, Z.H.: Isolation forest. In: 2008 eighth IEEE International Conference on Data Mining, pp. 413–422. IEEE (2008)
44. Liu, L., Wang, S., Peng, Y., Huang, Z., Liu, M., Hu, B.: Mining intricate temporal rules for recognizing complex activities of daily living under uncertainty. Pattern Recogn. **60**, 1015–1028 (2016). https://doi.org/10.1016/j.patcog.2016.07.024
45. Mienye, I.D., Sun, Y.: Performance analysis of cost-sensitive learning methods with application to imbalanced medical data. Inform. Med. Unlocked **25**, 100,690 (2021)
46. Motulsky, A., Nikiema, J.N., Bosson-Rieutort, D.: Artificial intelligence and medication management. In: Multiple Perspectives on Artificial Intelligence in Healthcare: Opportunities and Challenges, pp. 91–101. Springer (2021)
47. Mukherjee, M., Khushi, M.: Smote-ENC: a novel smote-based method to generate synthetic data for nominal and continuous features. Appl. Syst. Innov. **4**(1), 18 (2021)
48. Muntasir Nishat, M., Faisal, F., Jahan Ratul, I., Al-Monsur, A., Ar-Rafi, A.M., Nasrullah, S.M., Reza, M.T., Khan, M.R.H.: A comprehensive investigation of the performances of different machine learning classifiers with Smote-ENN oversampling technique and hyperparameter optimization for imbalanced heart failure dataset. Sci. Program. **2022**(1), 3649,406 (2022)
49. Neves, P.A., Simões, J., Costa, R., Pimenta, L., Gonalves, N.J., Albuquerque, C., Cunha, C., Zdravevski, E., Lameski, P., Garcia, N.M., Pires, I.M.: Thought on food: a systematic review of current approaches and challenges for food intake detection. Sensors **22**(17) (2022). DOI https://doi.org/10.3390/s22176443, https://www.mdpi.com/1424-8220/22/17/6443
50. Ngu, A.H., Metsis, V., Coyne, S., Chung, B., Pai, R., Chang, J.: Personalized fall detection system. In: 2020 IEEE International Conference on Pervasive Computing and Communications Workshops (PerCom Workshops), pp. 1–7. IEEE (2020)
51. Nigam, K., Ghani, R.: Analyzing the effectiveness and applicability of co-training. In: Proceedings of the ninth international conference on Information and knowledge management, pp. 86–93 (2000)
52. Ortiz Laguna, J., Olaya, A.G., Borrajo, D.: A dynamic sliding window approach for activity recognition. In: User Modeling, Adaption and Personalization: 19th International Conference, UMAP 2011, Girona, Spain, July 11–15, 2011. Proceedings 19, pp. 219–230. Springer (2011)
53. Parada Otte, F.J., Rosales Saurer, B., Stork, W.: Unsupervised learning in ambient assisted living for pattern and anomaly detection: a survey. In: Evolving Ambient Intelligence: AmI 2013 Workshops, Dublin, Ireland, December 3-5, 2013. Revised Selected Papers 4, pp. 44–53. Springer (2013)
54. Perera, P., Patel, V.M.: Deep transfer learning for multiple class novelty detection. In: Proceedings of the IEEE/CVF Conference on Computer Vision and Pattern Recognition, pp. 11,544–11,552 (2019)
55. Pires, I.M., Santos, R., Pombo, N., Garcia, N.M., Flórez-Revuelta, F., Spinsante, S., Goleva, R., Zdravevski, E.: Recognition of activities of daily living based on environmental analyses using audio fingerprinting techniques: a systematic review. Sensors **18**(1) (2018). DOI https://doi.org/10.3390/s18010160. URL https://www.mdpi.com/1424-8220/18/1/160
56. Prenkaj, B., Aragona, D., Flaborea, A., Galasso, F., Gravina, S., Podo, L., Reda, E., Velardi, P.: A self-supervised algorithm to detect signs of social isolation in the elderly from daily activity sequences. Artif. Intell. Med. **135**, 102,454 (2023)
57. Ran, X., Xu, M., Mei, L., Xu, Q., Liu, Q.: Detecting out-of-distribution samples via variational auto-encoder with reliable uncertainty estimation. Neural Netw. **145**, 199–208 (2022)

58. Ranieri, C.M., MacLeod, S., Dragone, M., Vargas, P.A., Romero, R.: Activity recognition for ambient assisted living with videos, inertial units and ambient sensors. Sensors **21**(3), 768 (2021)
59. Ren, Z., Zhang, Q., Gao, X., Hao, P., Cheng, J.: Multi-modality learning for human action recognition. Multimedia Tools and Applications **80**(11), 16185–16203 (2021)
60. Reyes-Ortiz, J.L., Oneto, L., Ghio, A., Samá, A., Anguita, D., Parra, X.: Human activity recognition on smartphones with awareness of basic activities and postural transitions. In: Artificial Neural Networks and Machine Learning–ICANN 2014: 24th International Conference on Artificial Neural Networks, Hamburg, Germany, September 15–19, 2014. Proceedings 24, pp. 177–184. Springer (2014)
61. Reynolds, D.A., et al.: Gaussian mixture models. Encyclopedia of biometrics, **741**(659–663) (2009)
62. Rish, I., et al.: An empirical study of the Naive Bayes classifier. In: IJCAI 2001 Workshop on Empirical Methods in Artificial Intelligence, vol. 3, pp. 41–46 (2001)
63. Sabuhi, M., Zhou, M., Bezemer, C.P., Musilek, P.: Applications of generative adversarial networks in anomaly detection: a systematic literature review. IEEE Access **9**, 161,003–161,029 (2021)
64. Shaban, A., Bansal, S., Liu, Z., Essa, I., Boots, B.: One-shot learning for semantic segmentation (2017). arXiv preprint arXiv:1709.03410
65. Stikic, M., Van Laerhoven, K., Schiele, B.: Exploring semi-supervised and active learning for activity recognition. In: 2008 12th IEEE International Symposium on Wearable Computers, pp. 81–88. IEEE (2008)
66. Sztyler, T., Stuckenschmidt, H.: Online personalization of cross-subjects based activity recognition models on wearable devices. In: 2017 IEEE International Conference on Pervasive Computing and Communications (PerCom), pp. 180–189. IEEE (2017)
67. Van Buuren, S.: Flexible Imputation of Missing Data. CRC Press (2018)
68. Van Engelen, J.E., Hoos, H.H.: A survey on semi-supervised learning. Mach. Learn. **109**(2), 373–440 (2020)
69. Vapnik, V.: The Nature of Statistical Learning Theory. Springer Science & Business Media (2013)
70. Wang, J., Zheng, V.W., Chen, Y., Huang, M.: Deep transfer learning for cross-domain activity recognition. In: Proceedings of the 3rd International Conference on Crowd Science and Engineering, pp. 1–8 (2018)
71. Wiering, M.A., Van Otterlo, M. (eds.): Reinforcement learning: state-of-the-art. In: Adaptation, Learning, and Optimization, vol. 12. Springer, Berlin, Heidelberg (2012). https://doi.org/10.1007/978-3-642-27645-3
72. Wu, Z., Cao, Z., Yu, X., Zhu, J., Song, C., Xu, Z.: A novel multiperson activity recognition algorithm based on point clouds measured by millimeter-wave MIMO radar. IEEE Sens. J. **23**(17), 19509–19523 (2023)
73. Xefteris, V.R., Tsanousa, A., Meditskos, G., Vrochidis, S., Kompatsiaris, I.: Performance, challenges, and limitations in multimodal fall detection systems: a review. IEEE Sens. J. **21**(17), 18398–18409 (2021). https://doi.org/10.1109/JSEN.2021.3090454
74. Xia, K., Huang, J., Wang, H.: LSTM-CNN architecture for human activity recognition. IEEE Access **8**, 56855–56866 (2020)
75. Xu, R., Wunsch, D.: Survey of clustering algorithms. IEEE Trans. Neural Netw. **16**(3), 645–678 (2005)
76. Yang, J., Zhou, K., Li, Y., Liu, Z.: Generalized out-of-distribution detection: a survey. Int. J. Comput. Vis. 1–28 (2024)
77. Yang, Y., Hou, C., Lang, Y., Guan, D., Huang, D., Xu, J.: Open-set human activity recognition based on micro-doppler signatures. Pattern Recogn. **85**, 60–69 (2019). https://doi.org/10.1016/j.patcog.2018.07.030, https://www.sciencedirect.com/science/article/pii/S003132031830270X
78. Ye, X., Kevin, I., Wang, K.: Deep generative domain adaptation with temporal relation attention mechanism for cross-user activity recognition. Pattern Recogn. 110811 (2024)

79. Zdravevski, E., Lameski, P., Mingov, R., Kulakov, A., Gjorgjevikj, D.: Robust histogram-based feature engineering of time series data. In: 2015 Federated Conference on Computer Science and Information Systems (FedCSIS), pp. 381–388. IEEE (2015)
80. Zdravevski, E., Lameski, P., Trajkovik, V., Kulakov, A., Chorbev, I., Goleva, R., Pombo, N., Garcia, N.: Improving activity recognition accuracy in ambient-assisted living systems by automated feature engineering. IEEE Access **5**, 5262–5280 (2017). https://doi.org/10.1109/ACCESS.2017.2684913
81. Zdravevski, E., Risteska Stojkoska, B., Standl, M., Schulz, H.: Automatic machine-learning based identification of jogging periods from accelerometer measurements of adolescents under field conditions. PLOS One **12**(9), 1–28 (2017). https://doi.org/10.1371/journal.pone.0184216
82. Zhang, Z., Pu, J., Zhuang, L., Zhou, W., Li, H.: Continuous sign language recognition via reinforcement learning. In: 2019 IEEE International Conference on Image Processing (ICIP), pp. 285–289 (2019). https://doi.org/10.1109/ICIP.2019.8802972
83. Zhao, T., Zhang, L., Ma, Y., Cheng, L.: A survey on safe multi-modal learning systems. In: Proceedings of the 30th ACM SIGKDD Conference on Knowledge Discovery and Data Mining, pp. 6655–6665 (2024)

Open Access This chapter is licensed under the terms of the Creative Commons Attribution 4.0 International License (http://creativecommons.org/licenses/by/4.0/), which permits use, sharing, adaptation, distribution and reproduction in any medium or format, as long as you give appropriate credit to the original author(s) and the source, provide a link to the Creative Commons license and indicate if changes were made.

The images or other third party material in this chapter are included in the chapter's Creative Commons license, unless indicated otherwise in a credit line to the material. If material is not included in the chapter's Creative Commons license and your intended use is not permitted by statutory regulation or exceeds the permitted use, you will need to obtain permission directly from the copyright holder.

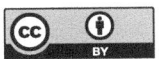

Chapter 3
Privacy Preservation in Audio and Video

Tom Bäckström, Siddharth Ravi, and Francisco Florez-Revuelta

Abstract Audio and video sensors are useful in Active Assisted Living (AAL) systems as they provide a rich source of information in well-known formats and since such sensors are readily available. This, however, also means that audio and video sensors will record a wide range of private information. Misusing this private information can have far-reaching consequences, including extortion, theft, and harassment. This chapter provides an overview of privacy issues in video and audio from the perspective of AAL systems and the most important protections for privacy.

Keywords Active assisted living (AAL) · Privacy · Privacy preservation · Machine learning · Image and video processing · Audio processing

3.1 Introduction

Active Assisted Living (AAL) systems represent a significant advancement in using information and communication technologies to enhance the quality of life for older adults and individuals with disabilities. These systems, encompassing a diverse range of environments from homes to public spaces, integrate an array of sensors—worn by users or installed in the environment—to monitor and interact with the individual's status and surroundings. This enables the provision of personalized and advanced healthcare services, which are increasingly important in our aging society.

T. Bäckström (✉)
Department of Information and Communications Engineering, University of Aalto, Aalto, Finland
e-mail: tom.backstrom@aalto.fi

S. Ravi
University of Alicante, Alicante, Spain
e-mail: siddharth.ravi@ua.es

F. Florez-Revuelta
Department of Computing Technology, University of Alicante, Alicante, Spain
e-mail: francisco.florez@ua.es

In recent years, audio- and video-based devices have significantly evolved, offering enhanced processing power, improved quality, wireless data transmission, and greater integration with Internet of Things (IoT) systems. In the context of AAL, cameras and microphones provide a more intelligent means of monitoring and assistance, supporting activities like gait analysis, fall detection, rehabilitation, and social communication. These technologies enable a more natural way to observe and describe events, actions, and interactions. Recent advances in computer vision and speech analytics have transformed these devices into smart systems capable of analyzing behaviors and providing real-time feedback.

However, these technological advancements also introduce significant challenges, primarily concerning privacy and ethical considerations. Traditionally, video surveillance has been widely used in public spaces for security purposes, but its extension into private spaces like homes, especially within the context of AAL, raises substantial privacy concerns. There are also concerns that smart speakers may be recording conversations without users' consent. The key concerns involve the potential for misuse of data, constant monitoring, and the infringement upon individuals' rights to privacy.

The need for privacy preservation in AAL systems cannot be overlooked. As intelligent monitoring systems become more prevalent in both public and private spheres, they pose a threat to individual privacy rights. If privacy-aware smart systems, including both cameras and audio devices, can be appropriately implemented, they could enable the use of video and audio monitoring in private settings like homes or care facilities, previously unthinkable due to ethical and privacy issues, with the potential to improve the quality of life and support the independence of individuals needing long-term care, while still addressing privacy concerns.

3.2 Privacy Issues in Audio and Video

Auditory and visual inputs are, for humans, important sources for gathering information about their surroundings. In addition, sounds and images, in general, and speech in particular, are also the main methods of communication among people. Practically all private communication is thus conveyed through sounds and images. In addition to communication, sounds, and images of people's activities and their surroundings carry a plethora of private information beyond intentional communication. For example, speech signals contain information about emotions, health, personal relationships, etc. (see Table 3.1).

Threats to privacy in AAL scenarios can cause a wide variety of problems and damage (see Table 3.2). Notably, such threats include material damage such as economic damage, social threats such as public humiliation, and loss of dignity and psychological threats both from psychological violence (e.g. harassment) as well as through the *fear* of loss of privacy.

Table 3.1 Categories of information about the patient, in audio and video signals, as well as an example of their potential relevance for the caretaker(s) in an AAL scenario. Observe that the relevance of categories may vary from scenario to scenario and should be cataloged in an impact assessment

Category	Examples	Relevance in AAL
Physiological	Health	Important
	Identity	Required
	Other characteristics and state	Known/irrelevant
Psychological	Health	Important
	Emotions	Potentially relevant
	Other characteristics and state	Private/irrelevant
Communication	To caretaker	Important
	To others (local or remote)	Private/irrelevant
Activities	Indicators of trouble (screams, sounds, and video of a person falling, unusual inactivity)	Important
	All other	Potentially relevant
Visitor(s)	Relationship character, state and history	Potentially relevant
	Visitor characteristics	Potentially relevant
Physical environment	Background sounds, interior decoration, TV programs, literature, art, lighting	Private/irrelevant
Physical setup	Reverberation, location, transmission distance, sensor type and manufacturer	Known/irrelevant

Table 3.2 Examples of threats to privacy relevant in AAL scenarios [61, 63]

Threats	Examples
Extortion, public humiliation	Romantic affairs and unusual domestic activities could be used for blackmail or made public against a user's wishes.
Theft	Audio, and video can leak passwords and other information of secure storage, enabling illegal access.
Harassment, inappropriate advances	The private activities of users could be monitored to enable harassment and for entertainment.
Fear of monitoring	Users can *fear* that they have no privacy due to continuous monitoring, causing psychological damage. It may also stifle political expression, damaging democratic societies.
Loss of dignity	Users may feel that they lose control of private aspects of their activities and information about them.

Audio and video thus contain both *private messages* as well as consequential, sensitive *side-information*, both of which warrant protection [6]. Unlike most applications where privacy must be protected, in AAL environments, where usually only one person is present (e.g., an older individual living alone), user identification is often not a major concern. The primary issues are more focused on the potential disclosure of conversations, the person's appearance (e.g., whether the person is dressed or undressed), and their behavior. Besides, in difference to most speech applications, in AAL, the primary object of interest for the monitoring system is not the communication (the private messages), but the well-being of the user. Communication, such as cries for help, can naturally be important sounds to monitor for, but we can safely assume that such cries are exceptional and most communication is in fact private. The types of information monitored in AAL can thus be roughly categorized into two particular classes:

- critical events, signifying acute dangers, such as evidence of the user falling and cries for help, that require immediate attention from the caretakers and
- long-term trends in the well-being of the users, such as movement patterns, that can give important information about the user's health.

The two types of information present very different challenges for both the design of algorithms and the daily processes of the caretakers. First, critical events require both immediate automatic identification and a rapid response from the caretaker. Second, they are in character outlier events, such that it is challenging to collect data about them in sufficient quantities for typical machine learning approaches. While we can, in theory, construct algorithms that detect outlier events, it is unclear to which extent they would catch outliers that are not critical. For example, how would the algorithm classify unusual expressions of joy, such as when winning the lottery? Such events are, by design, unusual and potentially highly private.

Long-term trends are, in this sense, easier to anonymize since algorithms can, for example, take long-term averages, thus removing information about private events. Moreover, analysis of long-term trends can use more computing power since the results are typically not urgent.

While the level of objective privacy is a prerequisite for a good AAL system, one should also consider how users *subjectively perceive* such monitoring systems. Clearly, a system that is perceived as threatening a user's privacy will not be perceived favorably by the users. Such subjective experience of privacy is closely linked to the level of *trust* that the user has towards the system [38, 62]. From a psychological perspective, people have a need for privacy [52], and lacking privacy, low levels of trust, and betrayal can, in turn, cause psychological trauma and issues like shock, loss, grief, morbid preoccupation, damaged self-esteem, self-doubting, and anger [58].

Optimizing the level of subjective experience of privacy is a task of user-experience design [62]. The central goal in such design is that the subjective experience should reflect the actual, objective level of privacy. Communicating a higher level of privacy than the true level would be deceptive and unethical and is known as a *dark design pattern* [77]. The reverse, understating the privacy level would unnecessarily undermine users' trust in the system and is thus also undesirable.

Privacy-preserving techniques can be categorised into three main types: limiting the audio/visual field and reach, secure computations, and attribute and feature protection. The first category involves methods that prevent the capture or transmission of sensitive data through software or hardware solutions. The second, secure computation, allows multiple parties to collaboratively compute a function without revealing their inputs or the function itself, ensuring privacy during processing. The third category, attribute and feature protection, involves modifying sensitive data to conceal private information.

In applying these privacy-preserving techniques, it is important to consider the inherent privacy-utility trade-off. While limiting the audio/visual field and reach can effectively protect sensitive information, it may also remove valuable data needed for accurate monitoring and intervention in AAL applications. Similarly, secure computation methods, although ensuring privacy during data processing, may introduce additional computational overhead, potentially affecting the system's real-time performance. Attribute and feature protection, such as anonymization or obfuscation, can mask private information but may also degrade data quality, impairing the system's ability to provide reliable outcomes. Thus, one should carefully balance privacy preservation with data utility, ensuring that privacy is protected without significantly compromising the system's effectiveness in delivering AAL services.

3.3 Privacy Preservation in Audio

Protecting privacy for acoustic signals is special in at least three ways. First, acoustic signals travel indiscriminately from the source in all directions of the acoustic space. Any listener or sensor in that space, even behind a corner, can thus eavesdrop on signals. In fact, human listeners can have difficulty in *ignoring* auditory cues [45] such that they can eavesdrop involuntarily. Second, audio, in general, and speech, in particular, are central modalities in human communication such that we can expect that audio signals contain much of our private communication [6]. Third, the hardware required, i.e. microphones, are cheap and useful for a wide range of tasks. Many devices will thus need microphones for their intended functionalities, potentially exposing private sounds in the same acoustic environment.

The intended tasks, also known as *trusted tasks*, in the context of AAL and in recording audio signals can include, for example, detection of screams [31], fall detection [44], and detection of unusual audio events [37]. The data-minimization principle, stated, for example, in the General Data Protection Regulation (GDPR) [23], requires that service providers minimize processing, storing, and transmission of all data, not explicitly required for that intended functionality. Privacy-preserving audio processing is thus primarily focused on removing or obfuscating any sounds from a signal that is not required for those intended functionalities. A secondary approach is to limit access to signals such that they may be used only for authorized purposes.

Methods of privacy-preserving processing can be categorized according to whether they operate in the acoustic space or within the computing devices and whether they prevent access to, obfuscate, or remove private information. In particular, early work on privacy focused on computationally modifying audio signals such that private information becomes difficult to access [12, 42] (see Sect. 3.3.1). Recently, a dominant approach has been to attempt to remove private information with information bottlenecks [26, 72] and disentanglement methods [4, 11, 64, 76] (see Sect. 3.3.2). In parallel, cryptography offers methods that prevent the extraction of private information while still allowing trusted processing tasks [30, 66–68, 83, 86] (see Sect. 3.3.3). These are all computational methods. In the acoustic space, with beamforming, we can extract sounds focusing only on the target and ignore other private sound sources [74], or in reverse, reproduce audio such that only users in a target location receive an intelligible signal at a "sound zone" [75] (see Sect. 3.3.4). In addition, often, privacy can be improved by improving the performance of the methods used in the trusted task (see Sect. 3.3.5).

3.3.1 Obfuscation in Speech and Audio

Much of generic privacy-preserving methodologies, like those of differential privacy [19], rely on obfuscation through added noise to preserve privacy. For speech and audio, however, this presents a problem. Adding noise to a speech or audio signal will distort the desired signal as much as its private parts, thus reducing utility as much as privacy is improved. The issue is that we should operate on the level of descriptions of the content rather than raw data. For example, we may replace identifying words such as names or even regenerate sentences with language models, such that meaning is preserved but the exact grammatical form is modified [30]. This is applicable where the abstraction level of the private information is in the language and grammar. However, the specifics of the scenario are decisive; Removing or replacing words or parts of audio implies the processing of private information. Such processing requires that we trust the processing service or device and, most importantly, that such processing is legally justified.

Much of the desired data sought from speech and audio exists on a lower abstraction level, such as the voice itself, including para- and extralinguistic information. By paralinguistic information, we refer to non-verbal communication, such as speech style, and by extralinguistic information, to voice characteristics that do not have a communicative purpose, such as the audible state of health [20]. Higher-abstraction level information, like the text, is encoded into and with the voice. We would thus like to obfuscate the higher-level information without corrupting the lower-level information. An approach, invented independently multiple times, is to cut the audio signal into smaller segments and randomize the ordering of those segments [12, 42]. By randomizing the ordering of speech segments, we effectively protect privacy by anonymizing the text and any other content dependent on its temporal structure. Any short-time features of the audio will, however, be preserved, thus retaining utility.

Observe that temporal randomization works only if the number of segments is large. Audio and speech, in general, contain plenty of information that has large variability but is slowly changing over time, such as the fundamental frequency (the pitch) of a speech signal. Matching up segments where the fundamental frequency is continuous over the border can significantly reduce the number of possible combinations of segments. The mixed-up segments could thus potentially be recombined and private information reconstructed if the number of frames with similar fundamentals is sufficiently small. Features of speech and audio signals that could potentially be matched in this way include the fundamental frequency, loudness, distance to the microphone, hoarseness, vocal tract shape, etc. It is thus useful to consider if the higher-level information could be removed entirely rather than just obfuscated.

3.3.2 Information Isolation

To protect privacy, we can isolate and extract only the target information from a signal and exclude everything else. Formally, this means that from the isolated data channel, we can extract the target information with sufficient accuracy, but simultaneously, we make sure that this channel does not give any indication about other private information. In other words, even if we try to predict a private attribute from the protected channel, our estimate of the private attribute will not improve.

Such isolation of information can be achieved mainly through two alternative approaches. First, with an *information bottleneck*, we can limit the information rate of the target data so low that nothing other than the target data can pass through [72]. We thus need to ensure that the accuracy of the target data is retained while reducing the information rate so that utility is not lost. By information rate, we refer to the number of bits per unit of time. Second, we can use an *adversarial approach* to train a data-driven model such that utility is maximized but simultaneously such that a simulated attacker cannot extract any private information from the protected channel. Adversarial learning is thus based on two competing machine learning models; one trained for the desired task and the other, the adversarial model, to extract such private information from the desired output that we want to protect. By balancing the desired and adversarial models, we can design a model that minimizes the private information in the desired output while retaining the utility of the desired functionality.

The structure of neural networks using information bottlenecks is illustrated in Fig. 3.1. The bottleneck is embedded in a structure known as an *autoencoder*, where a neural network with an encoder, bottleneck, and decoder is trained with unsupervised learning to model the desired features of a signal [14, 18, 76]. To protect privacy with such structures, it is central that the bottleneck is quantized since the information rate passing through the bottleneck is dependent on the accuracy of quantization. The information rate passing through the bottleneck should, moreover, correspond to the information rate of the desired data. By limiting the information rate to match the rate of the desired data, we can ensure that no private information can pass through.

The alternative approach, illustrated in Fig. 3.2, is to use an *adversarial* model to simulate an attacker and train the network to exclude private information from the output [46, 53, 80]. Training of the models then requires two opposing targets. The

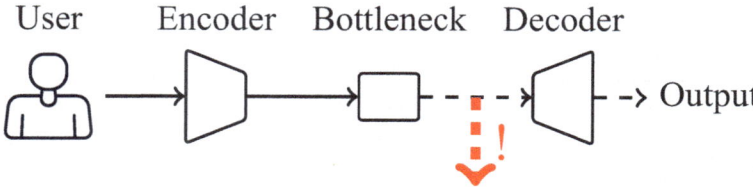

Fig. 3.1 Privacy-preserving audio analysis through information isolation with an *information bottleneck* within an autoencoder structure. The protected data flows are indicated by dashed lines and the point of attack by the red, thick arrow and exclamation mark

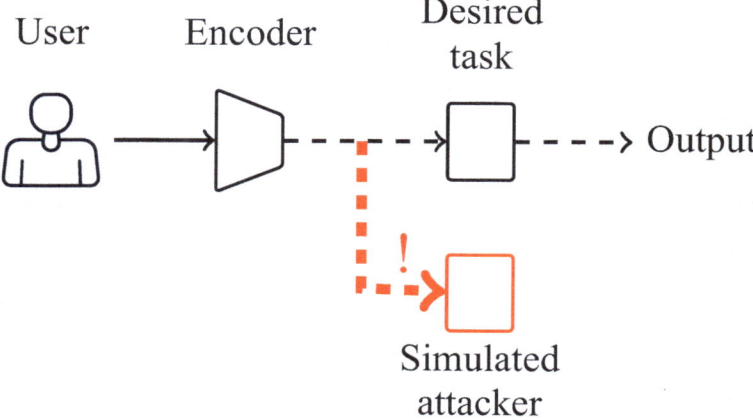

Fig. 3.2 Privacy-preserving speech analysis through information isolation with an *adversarial* approach. The desired task is authorized to extract some information, while the simulated attacker (drawn with red, thick line) is attempting to extract some other private information. Privacy is protected by training the encoder to exclude all private information. Protected data flows are illustrated by dashed lines

desired functionality of the network is trained such that the accuracy of the desired output is maximized and the accuracy of the simulated attacker (i.e., the adversarial model) is minimized. Simultaneously, the adversarial model is trained to *maximize* the accuracy of the private information extracted. The encoder must thus learn to preserve the desired output while excluding other private information.

Adversarial learning thus provides a straightforward way of protecting privacy, and its training simultaneously gives empirical evidence of the extent of protection. It does, however, not ensure protection against future, improved, or larger adversarial models or other categories of private information that were not considered during training. For example, if a model is trained to exclude linguistic content from a speech signal, it does not ensure that emotions would be also excluded. Moreover, the training of adversarial models requires data where private information is labelled. Such data is both expensive to collect and inherently sensitive since it contains labelled private

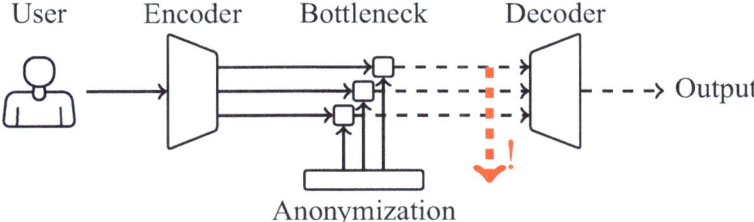

Fig. 3.3 Privacy-preserving speech processing through *disentanglement*, where categories of audio information are isolated into independent streams of information and where the level of anonymization can be individually chosen for each category. The point of attack is indicated by the red, thick arrow and exclamation mark

information. On the other hand, to give provable protection, training neural networks using information bottlenecks requires prior knowledge of the information rate of the desired output. This is not always easy to come by. The training process of information bottlenecks also does not inherently give any empirical evidence of the extent of protections, but adversarial models have to be constructed separately to verify the protections.

Both information bottlenecks and adversarial training can isolate a single category of information. Typical applications of speech and audio, however, involve multiple categories of private information, such as linguistic content, emotions, and health attributes. In an approach known as *disentanglement* (Fig. 3.3), we can then construct multiple channels, each trained with information bottlenecks or adversarial training, to separately isolate each category of information [4, 11, 64, 76]. When all categories are isolated, we can pick and choose which ones to anonymize or preserve, depending on the application or situation. For example, if we detect the linguistic exclamation "Help!", we can then enable an analysis of emotions and speech style, to determine whether it was a scream or a part of normal conversation.

3.3.3 Cryptography in Audio

It is widely accepted common praxis to use encryption to protect all transmission channels potentially accessible by outsiders. This provides sufficient protection to the security of the transmission channel. However, the receiver will, in this scenario, have the key to open the encrypted communication, and any private information contained in the transmission will then be exposed to the recipient. We thus need ways of protecting data from intrusions by the intended recipient.

Homomorphic encryption is a category of cryptographic methods where a user can encrypt messages such that a recipient can perform operations on the encrypted message and return an encrypted response so only the original user can decrypt the response. This enables the user to offload computationally complex tasks, such as speech recognition, to a server without exposing private information [68, 86]. Alternatively, *zero-knowledge* approaches have been proposed to allow the recipient to extract some information without revealing anything else [1]. With such methods, two or more agents can perform operations on private data jointly, such that any one agent gains access to data from the others only in encrypted form, they jointly perform operations on the encrypted data, and at the end, only the output of the processing is available in unencrypted form.

The primary issues with such methods are their computational complexity and transmission requirements. Operations in the encrypted domain must be approximated by piecewise linear operations, introducing an exponential increase in the overall complexity. The sizes of the transmitted encrypted messages are also an order of magnitude larger than those of the corresponding messages without encryption. These issues have kept homomorphic encryption beyond the practical applications. Work on secure multiparty computations and deep polynomial networks have recently reduced both issues [66, 67, 83].

3.3.4 Interventions in the Acoustic Space

Recall that acoustic signals travel indiscriminately in all directions from the source, such that any microphone can pick up any sound source in the same acoustic space. Any private sound sources can thus be picked up together with the intended source. For example, suppose the target user of an AAL scenario has a visitor, and the target user has given informed consent, but the visitor has not. Both the visitor's and the target user's voices will then be picked up, thus exposing any private information of the visitor. Conversely, if the AAL system outputs sound to the user, then any visitor will hear the sounds, irrespective of whether the sounds are private or not.

On the receiver/pick-up side, there is a long tradition of researching the task of extracting a target sound or target speaker from a mixture of sounds and speakers [8, 74]. If we can extract and isolate only the target sound source, then all the other sound sources would be protected. This task is known as *sound source separation*. The most straightforward scenario is where we have multiple microphones available, such as a linear array of microphones, so we can use wave propagation's physical properties to differentiate between sources. For example, sources in different directions will arrive at different times to the individual microphones. Such time differences can be used to isolate the desired sound source in an approach known as *beamforming*. A central problem in beamforming is that, in practical scenarios, sound sources will move in the acoustic space. Hence, we must track their location over time and identify the desired source. Such tracking of acoustic sources is an independent research problem of its own [24].

However, even with a single microphone, we can use the fact that sound sources are typically separated in time and frequency; different sounds appear at different times and at different frequencies. By identifying which portions of a time-frequency representation belong to which sound source, we can isolate individual sound sources and thus protect the privacy of other sound sources. The problem of identifying and tracking sources, however, remains.

A practical AAL system can also include notifications to the user, such as reminders to take medications. Such notifications can contain private information that is also revealed to other occupants of and visitors to the home. As an inverse of beamforming, with an approach known as *sound zones*, it is possible to play sounds such that they are intelligible only at a specific location in the acoustic space and unintelligible elsewhere [75]. This protects the user's privacy by anonymizing the content of a message, though other listeners can hear that there is "a message". Like in beamforming, the system requires knowledge of the location of the desired recipient and it must thus track the location of the user. As usual, such tracking however extracts private information from the user, thus potentially exposing the user's privacy in a new way.

3.3.5 Improving the Performance of the Trusted Task

Consider the practical scenario of detecting screams; the trusted task is to label audio signals as screams and non-screams. We can *a priori* assume that screams are rare (unless there is a baby in the house), but it is very important to positively identify every scream since that is the primary functionality of the whole system, and false negatives can have a serious impact on the well-being of the user. A conservative approach to tuning the scream detector would then be to trigger positive identifications of screams easily. As the detector will invariably make some errors, this means that it will more often suffer from false positives, where non-screams are identified as screams. The caretaker team must react to every detected scream and check whether the user has a problem, thereby intruding on the private sphere of the user. The sensitive trigger of the scream detector thus increases the number and likelihood of intrusions on the users' privacy.

By improving the performance of the scream detector, we can thus reduce the number of false positives without increasing the number of false negatives. In other words, such improvements reduce the number of times the detector incorrectly identifies a scream, thus improving privacy while simultaneously detecting screams as well as before, thus maintaining (or even improving) the utility of the system.

This is a common pattern in many systems, where inaccuracies of the trusted task lead to accidental intrusions into the users' privacy (c.f [41]). Interestingly, while privacy and utility are often seen as opponents on a Pareto-optimal performance limit, where improving one necessarily leads to the degradation of the other, by improving the accuracy of the trusted task, it may be possible to improve both privacy *and* utility.

3.4 Privacy Preservation in Video

Following the surveys by Padilla-López et al. [50] and Ravi et al. [59], visual privacy preservation methods can be categorised into intervention methods, blind vision, secure processing, data hiding, and visual obfuscation (Fig. 3.4).

3.4.1 Intervention Methods

Intervention methods are techniques that disrupt the data collection phase to prevent unauthorized visual data capture. These methods fit into those techniques, limiting the visual field and reach. Perez et al. [54] categorize these methods into *sensor saturation*, *broadcasting commands*, and *context-based approaches*.

Sensor saturation involves overwhelming a device's sensor with signals beyond its processing capability. This category includes physical devices like webcam covers, also known as privacy stickers, which manually block camera lenses and vary in design and adhesive quality [7, 33]. Notable systems like the BlindSpot [51], and anti-paparazzi devices described by Harvey and Knight [27] use light pulses to corrupt or overexpose captured images. The LiShield system by Zhu et al. [85] employs smart LEDs that emit modulated light waveforms designed to interfere with camera sensors without affecting human vision. Devices like the PinePhone [57] incorporate hardware 'kill switches' to physically disable cameras as a form of sensor saturation.

Broadcasting commands involves sending signals to deactivate or alter camera operations within a vicinity, such as Hewlett-Packard's camera that blurs faces upon receiving specific commands [56]. However, these methods rely on the user's consent, limiting their effectiveness.

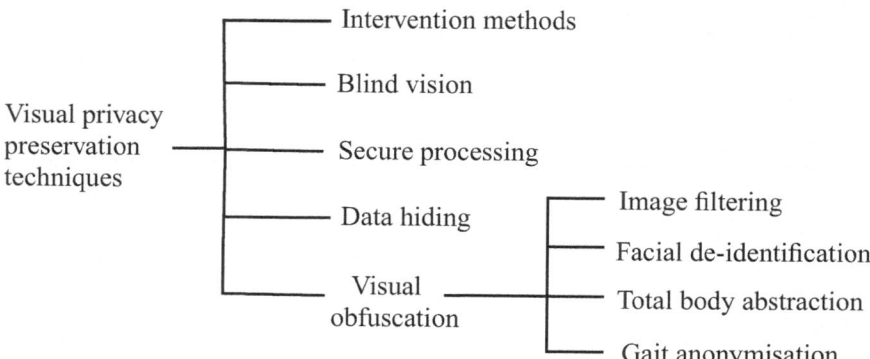

Fig. 3.4 A taxonomy of visual privacy preservation techniques for AAL (adapted from [59])

Context-based approaches leverage environmental data to control data collection. The *Virtual Walls* framework by Kapadia et al. [34] uses Global Positioning System (GPS) data to disable device sensors based on location, providing control over digital footprints. Despite their potential, these methods have not been widely adopted in commercial devices.

3.4.2 Blind Vision

Blind vision involves processing images and videos anonymously using secure multi-party computation (SMC) techniques, a subfield of cryptography that protects both the algorithms and the data. SMC ensures that neither party learns about the other's inputs or processes. This method supports privacy-sensitive applications, allowing tasks like face detection, image segmentation, and object tracking to be performed without disclosing underlying data or algorithms.

Avidan and Butman [5] introduced a secure face detection algorithm using SMC to ensure the privacy of both the images and the detection model. The goal is to perform face detection on sensitive image data without either party learning unnecessary information about the other. This is achieved using cryptographic techniques like oblivious transfer, which allows one party to choose an element from another party's dataset without revealing the choice, and secure dot product, which enables two parties to compute the dot product of their vectors without revealing the actual values. While this approach ensures strong privacy, it is computationally expensive. To speed up face detection, Histogram of Oriented Gradients (HoG) is employed to encode detection windows by computing image gradients, while scrambling the pixel order to obscure the original image. Additionally, fake HoGs are introduced to further protect privacy. This method allows quick filtering of detection windows, accelerating the process while still preserving some privacy, although some information about the original image may be exposed.

Erkin et al. [22] proposed a system for secure face recognition that protects both biometric data and the results of the recognition process. It addresses a two-party problem, where one party holds a face image and the other maintains a database of facial templates. The system ensures that neither party learns sensitive information about the other while jointly executing a face recognition algorithm to determine if the image matches any in the database. Using SMC techniques and cryptographic methods, the image data remains encrypted throughout the process. The party with the image only learns whether a match is found, while the party with the database keeps its contents private. The protocol ensures that the server performing the matching has no access to the input image or the recognition result. Despite the computational complexity involved in these cryptographic operations, the system runs efficiently on standard hardware, offering strong privacy protection without significant performance trade-offs.

3.4.3 Secure Processing

Secure processing methods facilitate the privacy-respectful handling of visual information and are distinguished from Secure Multi-party Computation (SMC). These methods ensure privacy in a unidirectional sense: databases may be publicly accessible, but the queries and their results are confidential. Notable examples include private content-based image retrieval (PCBIR) algorithms that ensure query privacy [60], and phase-only correlation techniques that maintain the privacy of images in a template database by transforming and scrambling them in the frequency domain [32].

These methods also include techniques that omit unnecessary visual information to preserve privacy. Using depth or thermal sensors restricts data to non-identifiable metrics such as the number of people or their activities, protecting sensitive details like facial identity or location [29]. Visual anonymisation strategies create anonymised silhouettes for action recognition, allowing the observation of motion without revealing identities [3]. Privacy can also be implicitly preserved by simplifying images to basic elements, which significantly reduces identifiable features [48].

Additionally, secret sharing schemes within secure processing involve splitting images into parts that contain no meaningful information individually, yet allow for private processing across distributed nodes [73]. Homomorphic encryption is another relevant technique, enabling operations on encrypted data to perform tasks without compromising privacy [9, 81].

3.4.4 Data Hiding

Data hiding techniques used in visual privacy protection might involve embedding the original video inside a privacy-protected version or extracting and encrypting specific objects from a video, then embedding them back into the video in a way that ensures privacy yet allows for later extraction and usage. These methods, which include steganography, digital watermarking, and fingerprinting, modify privacy-sensitive regions in images while maintaining the ability to recover the original content. Steganography secures a secret message within a cover message, often a video frame, using a key for later retrieval [55]. Digital watermarking embeds visible or hidden ownership marks, like logos or serial numbers, to detect copyright violations and manage license agreements [17].

Watermarking techniques also serve in privacy protection by embedding sensitive attributes of an original video into an obfuscated version, such as hiding real faces in video frames replaced with generated faces [82]. This often uses quantisation index modulation for data hiding, which can be reversible or non-reversible. Reversible methods restore the original video without loss, while non-reversible methods increase hiding capacity but prevent full restoration [49, 79].

PECAM [78] is a recent versatile method that incorporates data-hiding techniques to enable both reversible and irreversible privacy-preserving transformations of images. This method allows for dual modalities; it can either restore the original image completely or make the changes permanent, depending on the required application. Other redaction methods also employ data hiding to enable future retrieval of the original information when necessary, using techniques that develop reversible methods [13].

3.4.5 Visual Obfuscation

Visual obfuscation or redaction methods aim to protect visual privacy by making privacy-sensitive elements in images perceptually different from their originals. This approach is designed for users who need to conceal private information from those without appropriate access privileges. These techniques can be broadly categorized into five subcategories based on the visual results they produce: image filtering, facial de-identification, total body abstraction, and gait anonymisation. These methods can be either reversible, allowing the original image to be restored, for instance, by using data hiding techniques, or irreversible, where the changes are permanent.

Image filtering is a class of visual obfuscation techniques that rely on the alteration/redaction of images in a way to impart privacy to that image. These can be applied globally (to whole images), or locally (to privacy-sensitive parts of images).

The simplest forms of filtering techniques are blurring and pixelation (see Fig. 3.5). Pixelation relies on a grid of a certain size to be chosen for an image. For the regions of interest in the image, the average colour value over all the pixels within the grid is calculated and assigned to the individual pixels within the box. Blurring filters slide Gaussian kernels over images, using neighbourhood pixels to alter the values of a

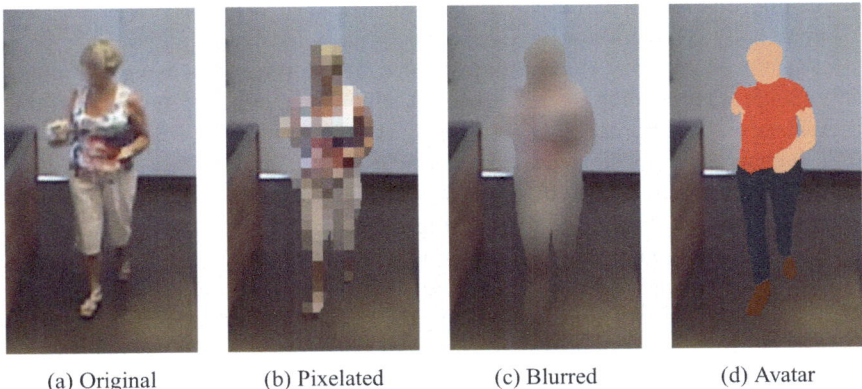

(a) Original   (b) Pixelated   (c) Blurred   (d) Avatar

Fig. 3.5 Visual privacy preservation of a person by applying different filters

central pixel. Adaptive blurring [84] is a technique that uses semantic segmentation masks to apply a scale dependent Gaussian blur selectively on privacy-sensitive areas of videos, but it may inaccurately determine blurring parameters based solely on bounding box size, leading to potential under- or over-blurring.

Other noteworthy filtering techniques include:

- Morphing and warping: These are techniques mainly used for face anonymisation. In morphing, the input face is transformed into a target face by adjusting keypoints through interpolation and intensity parameters [35]. In warping, keypoints identified by face detection are shifted based on a 'warping strength' parameter, with new intensity values determined by interpolation [36].
- False colouring: This technique converts RGB images to greyscale and map pixel intensities to pre-defined RGB values according to a chosen colour palette [15]. However, this method is vulnerable to attacks that can reverse the process if the relationship between false and original colours is determined.
- Cartooning, for instance, proposing mean shift-based approach simplifying colours and textures while preserving edge sharpness [21], or replacing privacy-sensitive objects in videos with abstract cartoon clip art [28].

Although image filtering has been widely used by the media, particularly to obscure the identity of subjects who wish to remain anonymous, simpler filtering techniques like blurring and pixelation are known not to be robust to attacks [43].

Facial de-identification methods generate artificial faces to protect identities, traditionally using k-same algorithms to blend these faces into original images [47]. Recent advancements leverage Generative Adversarial Networks (GANs) for more sophisticated de-identification, such as Sun et al.'s approach [65] that uses keypoint generation to condition an adversarial autoencoder for creating realistic inpainted faces, and Gafni et al.'s live de-identification technique for videos [25], which distances facial descriptors from a target image. Additionally, Li and Lin's Anonymous-Net [39] employs neural networks and random forests to generate de-identified faces with features that resemble real-world distributions.

Human body abstraction methods enhance privacy by replacing the entire body of a subject in an image or video with generated alternatives, often using techniques like semantic segmentation to create avatars, silhouettes, or background inpainting [16], with advanced approaches incorporating generative models [10] and 3D avatar fitting, such as the Skinned Multi-Person Linear (SMPL) model [40] and its extensions, to create realistic body replacements while addressing challenges like garment modelling and body shape variation (see Fig. 3.5d).

Gait is also an important biomarker for identifying individuals due to its unique characteristics. Gait anonymisation, a relatively new field, has evolved from traditional methods like pixelation and blurring, which often produce artificial results [2], to more advanced techniques using deep neural networks [70] and generative adversarial networks [69, 71] to create natural-looking, anonymised gaits, even for low-quality silhouettes.

3.5 Conclusion

The intersection of AAL technologies with privacy preservation techniques, as examined in this chapter, reveals both the potential benefits and challenges associated with ensuring user privacy in environments enriched with audio and visual monitoring. While AAL systems promise enhanced support and care for individuals, especially older and disabled people, their integration into private spaces raises significant concerns about privacy violations and data misuse.

One key insight is the need for a balance between privacy preservation and the utility of AAL systems. While privacy is paramount, overly restrictive privacy measures could hinder the system's ability to effectively monitor and support users, particularly in detecting critical events such as falls or medical emergencies. Therefore, privacy preservation strategies must be carefully designed to ensure that they do not compromise the primary functions of AAL systems.

Moreover, the subjective perception of privacy by users plays a crucial role in the adoption and acceptance of AAL technologies. Users' trust in these systems is heavily influenced by how well the system communicates its privacy-preserving capabilities, as well as its transparency and honesty about potential limitations. This calls for a user-centered design approach where privacy features are not just technically robust but also aligned with users' expectations and comfort levels.

The development of privacy-preserving AAL systems is a complex but important task that requires continuous advancements in both technology and ethical considerations. Future work should focus on improving the robustness of privacy techniques against emerging threats, enhancing the computational efficiency of secure processing methods, and fostering greater user trust through transparent and user-friendly privacy interfaces. The ultimate goal is to create AAL systems that not only enhance the quality of life for users but also respect and protect their fundamental rights to privacy.

Acknowledgements This publication is based upon work from COST Action GoodBrother—Network on Privacy-Aware Audio- and Video-Based Applications for Active and Assisted Living (CA19121), supported by COST (European Cooperation in Science and Technology). This work is part of the visuAAL project on Privacy-Aware and Acceptable Video-Based Technologies and Services for Active and Assisted Living (https://www.visuaal-itn.eu/). This project has received funding from the European Union's Horizon 2020 research and innovation programme under the Marie Skłodowska-Curie grant agreement No. 861091.

References

1. Adelsbach, A., Sadeghi, A.R.: Zero-knowledge watermark detection and proof of ownership. In: Information Hiding: 4th International Workshop, pp. 273–288. Springer (2001). https://doi.org/10.1007/s00530-003-0098-z
2. Agrawal, P., Narayanan, P.J.: Person de-identification in videos. IEEE Trans. Circuits Syst. Video Technol. **21**(3), 299–310 (2011). https://doi.org/10.1109/TCSVT.2011.2105551

3. Al-Obaidi, S., Al-Khafaji, H., Abhayaratne, C.: Modeling temporal visual salience for human action recognition enabled visual anonymity preservation. IEEE Access **8**, 213,806–213,824 (2020). https://doi.org/10.1109/ACCESS.2020.3039740
4. Aloufi, R., Haddadi, H., Boyle, D.: Privacy-preserving voice analysis via disentangled representations. In: Proceedings of the 2020 ACM SIGSAC Conference on Cloud Computing Security Workshop, pp. 1–14 (2020). https://doi.org/10.1145/3411495.3421355
5. Avidan, S., Butman, M.: Blind vision. In: Leonardis, A., Bischof, H., Pinz, A. (eds.) Computer Vision - ECCV 2006. Lecture Notes in Computer Science, vol. 3953, pp. 1–13. Springer, Berlin / Heidelberg (2006)
6. Bäckström, T.: Privacy in speech technology. arXiv:2305.05227 (2023). https://doi.org/10.48550/arXiv.2305.05227
7. Barangan, A.P., Cocchia, V.E., Fiske, M.S., Haddad, W.S.: Microphone and Camera Disruption Apparatus and Method (2015). US Patent 9,124,792
8. Benesty, J., Sondhi, M.M., Huang, Y., et al.: Springer Handbook of Speech Processing, vol. 1. Springer (2008). https://doi.org/10.1007/978-3-540-49127-9
9. Bian, S., Wang, T., Hiromoto, M., Shi, Y., Sato, T.: ENSEI: efficient secure inference via frequency-domain homomorphic convolution for privacy-preserving visual recognition. In: Proceedings of the IEEE/CVF Conference on Computer Vision and Pattern Recognition (CVPR) (2020). https://doi.org/10.1109/cvpr42600.2020.00942
10. Brkic, K., Sikiric, I., Hrkac, T., Kalafatic, Z.: I know that person: generative full body and face de-identification of people in images. In: IEEE Conference on Computer Vision and Pattern Recognition Workshops (CVPRW), pp. 1319–1328 (2017). https://doi.org/10.1109/CVPRW.2017.173
11. Champion, P., Larcher, A., Jouvet, D.: Are disentangled representations all you need to build speaker anonymization systems? In: Proceedings of the Interspeech, pp. 2793–2797 (2022). https://doi.org/10.21437/Interspeech.2022-10586
12. Chen, F., Adcock, J., Krishnagiri, S.: Audio privacy: reducing speech intelligibility while preserving environmental sounds. In: Proceedings of the 16th ACM International Conference on Multimedia, pp. 733–736 (2008). https://doi.org/10.1145/2699343.2699366
13. Cheung, S.C., Venkatesh, M., Paruchuri, J., Zhao, J., Nguyen, T.: Protecting and managing privacy information in video surveillance systems. In: Senior, A. (ed.) Protecting Privacy in Video Surveillance, pp. 11–33. Springer, London (2009)
14. Chorowski, J., Weiss, R.J., Bengio, S., Van Den Oord, A.: Unsupervised speech representation learning using WaveNet autoencoders. IEEE/ACM Trans. Audio, Speech, Lang. Process. **27**(12), 2041–2053 (2019). https://doi.org/10.1109/TASLP.2019.2938863
15. Çiftçi, S., Akyüz, A.O., Ebrahimi, T.: A reliable and reversible image privacy protection based on false colors. IEEE Trans. Multimed. **20**(1), 68–81 (2018). https://doi.org/10.1109/TMM.2017.2728479
16. Climent-Pérez, P., Florez-Revuelta, F.: Protection of visual privacy in videos acquired with RGB cameras for active and assisted living applications. Multimed. Tools Appl. 1–16 (2021). https://doi.org/10.1007/s11042-020-10249-1
17. Cox, I., Honsinger, C., Miller, M., Bloom, J.: Digital watermarking. J. Electron. Imaging **11**(3), 414–414 (2002)
18. Deng, J., Xu, X., Zhang, Z., Frühholz, S., Schuller, B.: Semisupervised autoencoders for speech emotion recognition. IEEE/ACM Trans. Audio, Speech, Lang. Process. **26**(1), 31–43 (2017)
19. Dwork, C.: Differential privacy: a survey of results. In: International Conference on Theory and Applications of Models of Computation, pp. 1–19. Springer (2008). https://doi.org/10.1007/978-3-540-79228-4
20. Ephratt, M.: Linguistic, paralinguistic and extralinguistic speech and silence. J. Pragmat. **43**(9), 2286–2307 (2011). https://doi.org/10.1016/j.pragma.2011.03.006
21. Erdélyi, Á., Winkler, T., Rinner, B.: Serious fun: cartooning for privacy protection. In: Proceedings of the MediaEval (2013)
22. Erkin, Z., Franz, M., Guajardo, J., Katzenbeisser, S., Lagendijk, I., Toft, T.: Privacy-preserving face recognition. In: Goldberg, I., Atallah, M. (eds.) Privacy Enhancing Technologies. Lecture Notes in Computer Science, vol. 5672, pp. 235–253. Springer, Berlin / Heidelberg (2009)

23. European Parliament: Directive 95/46/EC General Data Protection Regulation (2016). http://data.europa.eu/eli/reg/2016/679
24. Evers, C., Löllmann, H.W., Mellmann, H., Schmidt, A., Barfuss, H., Naylor, P.A., Kellermann, W.: The LOCATA challenge: acoustic source localization and tracking. IEEE/ACM Trans. Audio, Speech, Lang. Process. **28**, 1620–1643 (2020). https://doi.org/10.1109/TASLP.2020.2990485
25. Gafni, O., Wolf, L., Taigman, Y.: Live face de-identification in video. In: Proceedings of the IEEE/CVF International Conference on Computer Vision (ICCV), pp. 9378–9387 (2019). https://doi.org/10.1109/iccv.2019.00947
26. Gârbacea, C., van den Oord, A., Li, Y., Lim, F.S., Luebs, A., Vinyals, O., Walters, T.C.: Low bitrate speech coding with VQ-VAE and a WaveNet decoder. In: IEEE International Conference on Acoustics, Speech and Signal Processing (ICASSP), pp. 735–739 (2019). https://doi.org/10.1109/ICASSP.2019.8683277
27. Harvey, A., Knight, H.: Anti-Paparazzi Fashion. www.marilynmonrobot.com. Accessed on 30 June 2021 (2009)
28. Hassan, E.T., Hasan, R., Shaffer, P., Crandall, D., Kapadia, A.: Cartooning for enhanced privacy in lifelogging and streaming videos. In: Proceedings of the IEEE Conference on Computer Vision and Pattern Recognition (CVPR) Workshops (2017). https://doi.org/10.1109/cvprw.2017.175
29. Heitzinger, T., Kampel, M.: IPT: a dataset for identity preserved tracking in closed domains. In: 2020 25th International Conference on Pattern Recognition (ICPR), pp. 8228–8234 (2021). https://doi.org/10.1109/ICPR48806.2021.9412979
30. Hu, Z., Havrylov, S., Titov, I., Cohen, S.B.: Obfuscation for privacy-preserving syntactic parsing. In: Proceedings of the 16th International Conference on Parsing Technologies and the IWPT 2020 Shared Task on Parsing into Enhanced Universal Dependencies, pp. 62–72 (2020)
31. Huang, W., Chiew, T.K., Li, H., Kok, T.S., Biswas, J.: Scream detection for home applications. In: 2010 5th IEEE Conference on Industrial Electronics and Applications, pp. 2115–2120. IEEE (2010). https://doi.org/10.1109/ICIEA.2010.5515397
32. Ito, I., Kiya, H.: One-time key based phase scrambling for phase-only correlation between visually protected images. EURASIP J. Inform. Secur. **2009**, 1–11 (2009). https://doi.org/10.1155/2009/841045. Article ID: 2009:841045
33. Jonsson, K.S., Bergthorsdottir, S.H.: Webcam Privacy Shield (2016). US Patent 9,465,276
34. Kapadia, A., Henderson, T., Fielding, J.J., Kotz, D.: Virtual walls: protecting digital privacy in pervasive environments. In: LaMarca, A., Langheinrich, M., Truong K.N. (eds.) Pervasive Computing, pp. 162–179. Springer Berlin Heidelberg, Berlin, Heidelberg (2007). https://doi.org/10.1007/978-3-540-72037-9
35. Korshunov, P., Ebrahimi, T.: Using face morphing to protect privacy. In: 10th IEEE International Conference on Advanced Video and Signal Based Surveillance, pp. 208–213 (2013). https://doi.org/10.1109/AVSS.2013.6636641
36. Korshunov, P., Ebrahimi, T.: Using warping for privacy protection in video surveillance. In: 2013 18th International Conference on Digital Signal Processing (DSP), pp. 1–6 (2013). https://doi.org/10.1109/ICDSP.2013.6622791
37. Lee, Y., Han, D.K., Ko, H.: Acoustic signal based abnormal event detection in indoor environment using multiclass adaboost. IEEE Trans. Consum. Electron. **59**(3), 615–622 (2013). https://doi.org/10.1109/TCE.2013.6626247
38. Leschanowsky, A., Rech, S., Popp, B., Bäckström, T.: Evaluating privacy, security, and trust perceptions in conversational AI: a systematic review. Comput. Hum. Behav. 108344 (2024). https://doi.org/10.1016/j.chb.2024.108344
39. Li, T., Lin, L.: AnonymousNet: natural face de-identification with measurable privacy. In: Proceedings of the IEEE/CVF Conference on Computer Vision and Pattern Recognition (CVPR) Workshops (2019). https://doi.org/10.1109/cvprw.2019.00013
40. Loper, M., Mahmood, N., Romero, J., Pons-Moll, G., Black, M.J.: SMPL: a skinned multi-person linear model. ACM Trans. Graph. **34**(6) (2015). https://doi.org/10.1145/2816795.2818013

41. Lynskey, D.: Alexa, are you invading my privacy?—The dark side of our voice assistants. The Guardian (2019). https://www.theguardian.com/technology/2019/oct/09/alexa-are-you-invading-my-privacy-the-dark-side-of-our-voice-assistants
42. Maouche, M., Srivastava, B.M.L., Vauquier, N., Bellet, A., Tommasi, M., Vincent, E.: Enhancing speech privacy with slicing. In: Proceedings of the Interspeech (2022). https://hal.inria.fr/hal-03369137/
43. McPherson, R., Shokri, R., Shmatikov, V.: Defeating Image Obfuscation With Deep Learning. arXiv:1609.00408 (2016)
44. Mubashir, M., Shao, L., Seed, L.: A survey on fall detection: principles and approaches. Neurocomputing **100**, 144–152 (2013). https://doi.org/10.1016/j.neucom.2011.09.037
45. Murphy, S., Spence, C., Dalton, P.: Auditory perceptual load: a review. Hear. Res. **352**, 40–48 (2017). https://doi.org/10.1016/j.heares.2017.02.005
46. Nelus, A., Martin, R.: Gender discrimination versus speaker identification through privacy-aware adversarial feature extraction. In: 13th ITG-Symposium on Speech Communication, pp. 1–5 (2018). https://ieeexplore.ieee.org/abstract/document/8578003
47. Newton, E., Sweeney, L., Malin, B.: Preserving privacy by de-identifying face images. IEEE Trans. Knowl. Data Eng. **17**(2), 232–243 (2005)
48. Ng, P.L., Ang, L., Seng, K.P.: Privacy preserving stereoscopic vision with one-bit transform. In: 2010 3rd IEEE International Conference on Computer Science and Information Technology (ICCSIT), vol. 9, pp. 70–74 (2010)
49. Ni, Z., Shi, Y.Q., Ansari, N., Su, W.: Reversible data hiding. IEEE Trans. Circuits Syst. Video Technol. **16**(3), 354–362 (2006). https://doi.org/10.1109/tcsvt.2006.869964
50. Padilla-López, J.R., Chaaraoui, A.A., Flórez-Revuelta, F.: Visual privacy protection methods: a survey. Expert Syst. Appl. **42**(9), 4177–4195 (2015). https://doi.org/10.1016/j.eswa.2015.01.041. https://www.sciencedirect.com/science/article/pii/S0957417415000561
51. Patel, S.N., Summet, J.W., Truong, K.N.: BlindSpot: Creating Capture-Resistant Spaces, pp. 185–201. Springer, London (2009). https://doi.org/10.1007/978-1-84882-301-3
52. Pedersen, D.M.: Psychological functions of privacy. J. Environ. Psychol. **17**(2), 147–156 (1997). https://doi.org/10.1006/jevp.1997.0049
53. Perero-Codosero, J.M., Espinoza-Cuadros, F.M., Hernández-Gómez, L.A.: X-vector anonymization using autoencoders and adversarial training for preserving speech privacy. Comput. Speech Lang. 101351 (2022). https://doi.org/10.1016/j.csl.2022.101351
54. Perez, A.J., Zeadally, S., Griffith, S.: Bystanders' privacy. IT Prof. **19**(3), 61–65 (2017). https://doi.org/10.1109/MITP.2017.42
55. Petitcolas, F., Anderson, R., Kuhn, M.: Information hiding-a survey. Proc. IEEE **87**(7), 1062–1078 (1999). https://doi.org/10.1109/5.771065
56. Pilu, M.: Detector For Use With Data Encoding Pattern (2007). US Patent App. 11/491,174
57. Pine64: Pinephone. https://www.pine64.org/pinephone/. Accessed on 05 May 2021 (2021)
58. Rachman, S.: Betrayal: a psychological analysis. Behav. Res. Therapy **48**(4), 304–311 (2010). https://doi.org/10.1016/j.brat.2009.12.002
59. Ravi, S., Climent-Pérez, P., Florez-Revuelta, F.: A review on visual privacy preservation techniques for active and assisted living. Multimed. Tools Appl. **83**(5), 14715–14755 (2024)
60. Shashank, J., Kowshik, P., Srinathan, K., Jawahar, C.: Private content based image retrieval. In: 2008 IEEE Conference on Computer Vision and Pattern Recognition, pp. 1–8 (2008). https://doi.org/10.1109/CVPR.2008.4587388
61. Solove, D.J.: A taxonomy of privacy. Univ. Pa. Law Rev. **154**, 477 (2005). https://doi.org/10.2307/40041279
62. de Souza, P.C., Maciel, C.: Legal issues and user experience in ubiquitous systems from a privacy perspective. In: Human Aspects of Information Security, Privacy, and Trust: Third International Conference, HAS 2015, Held as Part of HCI International 2015, Los Angeles, CA, USA, August 2–7, 2015. Proceedings 3, pp. 449–460. Springer (2015). https://doi.org/10.1007/978-3-319-20376-8
63. Staats, K., Grov, E.K., Husebø, B.S., Tranvåg, O.: Dignity and loss of dignity: experiences of older women living with incurable cancer at home. Health Care Women Int. **41**(9), 1036–1058 (2020). https://doi.org/10.1080/07399332.2020.1797035

64. Stoidis, D., Cavallaro, A.: Protecting gender and identity with disentangled speech representations. In: Proceedings Interspeech, pp. 1699–1703 (2021). https://doi.org/10.21437/Interspeech.2021-2163
65. Sun, Q., Ma, L., Oh, S.J., Van Gool, L., Schiele, B., Fritz, M.: Natural and effective obfuscation by head inpainting. In: Proceedings of the IEEE Conference on Computer Vision and Pattern Recognition (CVPR) (2018). https://doi.org/10.1109/cvpr.2018.00530
66. Teixeira, F., Abad, A., Raj, B., Trancoso, I.: Towards end-to-end private automatic speaker recognition. In: Proceedings of the Interspeech, pp. 2798–2802 (2022). https://doi.org/10.21437/Interspeech.2022-10672
67. Teixeira, F., Abad, A., Raj, B., Trancoso, I.: Privacy-preserving automatic speaker diarization. In: International Conference on Acoustics, Speech and Signal Processing (ICASSP). IEEE (2023). https://doi.org/10.1109/ICASSP49357.2023.10096113
68. Thaine, P., Penn, G.: Extracting Mel-frequency and Bark-frequency cepstral coefficients from encrypted signals. In: Proceedings of the Interspeech, pp. 3715–3719 (2019). https://doi.org/10.21437/Interspeech.2019-1136
69. Tieu, N.D.T., Nguyen, H.H., Fang, F., Yamagishi, J., Echizen, I.: An RGB gait anonymization model for low-quality silhouettes. In: 2019 Asia-Pacific Signal and Information Processing Association Annual Summit and Conference (APSIPA ASC), pp. 1686–1693 (2019). https://doi.org/10.1109/APSIPAASC47483.2019.9023188
70. Tieu, N.D.T., Nguyen, H.H., Nguyen-Son, H.Q., Yamagishi, J., Echizen, I.: An approach for gait anonymization using deep learning. In: IEEE Workshop on Information Forensics and Security (WIFS), pp. 1–6. IEEE (2017)
71. Tieu, N.D.T., Nguyen, H.H., Nguyen-Son, H.Q., Yamagishi, J., Echizen, I.: Spatio-temporal generative adversarial network for gait anonymization. J. Inf. Secur. Appl. **46**, 307–319 (2019)
72. Tishby, N., Pereira, F.C., Bialek, W.: The information bottleneck method. https://arxiv.org/abs/physics/0004057 (2000)
73. Upmanyu, M., Namboodiri, A., Srinathan, K., Jawahar, C.: Efficient privacy preserving video surveillance. In: 2009 IEEE 12th International Conference on Computer Vision, pp. 1639–1646 (2009)
74. Vincent, E., Virtanen, T., Gannot, S.: Audio Source Separation and Speech Enhancement. Wiley (2018). https://doi.org/10.1002/9781119279860
75. Wallace, D., Cheer, J.: Combining background noise and artificial masking to achieve privacy in sound zones. Comput. Speech Lang. **72**, 101,285 (2022). https://doi.org/10.1016/j.csl.2021.101285. https://www.sciencedirect.com/science/article/pii/S0885230821000875
76. Williams, J.: Learning disentangled speech representations. Ph.D. Thesis, The University of Edinburgh (2022). https://doi.org/10.7488/era/1980
77. Willis, L.E.: Deception by design. Harvard J. Law Technol. **34**, 115 (2020). https://ssrn.com/abstract=3694575
78. Wu, H., Tian, X., Li, M., Liu, Y., Ananthanarayanan, G., Xu, F., Zhong, S.: PECAM: privacy-enhanced video streaming and analytics via securely-reversible transformation. In: Proceedings of the 27th Annual International Conference on Mobile Computing and Networking, MobiCom'21, pp. 229–241. Association for Computing Machinery, New York, NY, USA (2021). https://doi.org/10.1145/3447993.3448618
79. Yabuta, K., Kitazawa, H., Tanaka, T.: A new concept of security camera monitoring with privacy protection by masking moving objects. In: Pacific-Rim Conference on Multimedia, pp. 831–842. Springer (2005). https://doi.org/10.1007/11581772
80. Yang, C.H.H., Siniscalchi, S.M., Lee, C.H.: PATE-AAE: incorporating adversarial autoencoder into private aggregation of teacher ensembles for spoken command classification. In: Proceedings of the Interspeech, pp. 881–885 (2021). https://doi.org/10.21437/Interspeech.2021-640
81. Yonetani, R., Naresh Boddeti, V., Kitani, K.M., Sato, Y.: Privacy-preserving visual learning using doubly permuted homomorphic encryption. In: IEEE International Conference on Computer Vision (ICCV) (2017). https://doi.org/10.1109/iccv.2017.225

82. Yu, X., Babaguchi, N.: Privacy preserving: hiding a face in a face. In: Asian Conference on Computer Vision, pp. 651–661. Springer (2007). https://doi.org/10.1007/978-3-540-76390-1
83. Zhang, S.X., Gong, Y., Yu, D.: Encrypted speech recognition using deep polynomial networks. In: ICASSP 2019—2019 IEEE International Conference on Acoustics, Speech and Signal Processing (ICASSP), pp. 5691–5695 (2019). https://doi.org/10.1109/ICASSP.2019.8683721
84. Zhang, Z., Cilloni, T., Walter, C., Fleming, C.: Multi-scale, class-generic, privacy-preserving video. Electronics **10**(10) (2021). https://doi.org/10.3390/electronics10101172. https://www.mdpi.com/2079-9292/10/10/1172
85. Zhu, S., Zhang, C., Zhang, X.: Automating visual privacy protection using a smart LED. In: Proceedings of the 23rd Annual International Conference on Mobile Computing and Networking, MobiCom'17, pp. 329–342. Association for Computing Machinery, New York, NY, USA (2017). https://doi.org/10.1145/3117811.3117820
86. Zuber, M., Carpov, S., Sirdey, R.: Towards real-time hidden speaker recognition by means of fully homomorphic encryption. In: International Conference on Information and Communications Security, pp. 403–421. Springer (2020). https://doi.org/10.1007/978-3-030-61078-4

Open Access This chapter is licensed under the terms of the Creative Commons Attribution 4.0 International License (http://creativecommons.org/licenses/by/4.0/), which permits use, sharing, adaptation, distribution and reproduction in any medium or format, as long as you give appropriate credit to the original author(s) and the source, provide a link to the Creative Commons license and indicate if changes were made.

The images or other third party material in this chapter are included in the chapter's Creative Commons license, unless indicated otherwise in a credit line to the material. If material is not included in the chapter's Creative Commons license and your intended use is not permitted by statutory regulation or exceeds the permitted use, you will need to obtain permission directly from the copyright holder.

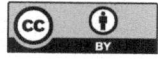

Chapter 4
Data Security in AAL

Aleksandar Jevremovic, Slavisa Aleksic, Mladen Veinovic, and Liane Colonna

Abstract Active assisted living (AAL) environments inherently collect, generate, and use large amounts of data. These environments are inherently distributed and often use external services, so data can be in different states and locations. This data is often very sensitive, and its compromise can endanger the privacy and security of users. Additionally, data unavailability can jeopardize the proper functioning of critical environment functions. This chapter presents relevant aspects of data protection. General principles, risks, approaches, and solutions for data protection are analyzed, taking into account the specificities applicable in AAL environments. The first part of the chapter provides an overview of security and data protection, along with a chapter outline. The second part offers a retrospective of the evolution of relevant information technologies, with an emphasis on two critical technologies for AAL: the Internet of Things and cloud computing. The third part outlines the relevant cryptological fundamentals of data protection. In the fourth part, a synthesis of the fundamentals, technologies, risks, and possible solutions is presented. The fifth part of the chapter expands the view on data protection from the perspective of the importance of open source and technological sovereignty. The sixth part reviews the importance of proper management of the entire lifecycle of AAL environments and their components. Finally, the last part of the chapter analyzes relevant and current legal aspects of data protection.

A. Jevremovic (✉) · M. Veinovic
Faculty of Informatics and Computing, Singidunum University, Belgrade, Serbia
e-mail: ajevremovic@ieee.org

M. Veinovic
e-mail: mveinovic@singidunum.ac.rs

S. Aleksic
Faculty of Digital Transformation, HTWK Leipzig, Leipzig, Germany
e-mail: slavisa.aleksic@htwk-leipzig.de

L. Colonna
Stockholm University, Stockholm, Sweden
e-mail: Liane.Colonna@juridicum.su.se

© The Author(s) 2025
A. A. Salah et al. (eds.), *Privacy-Aware Monitoring for Assisted Living*, Intelligent Systems Reference Library 270,
https://doi.org/10.1007/978-3-031-84158-3_4

Keywords Active assisted living (AAL) · Data protection · Cryptography · Cipher systems · Open source · Fail-secure design · Cyber resilience act (CRA)

4.1 Introduction

Principally, AAL environments operate based on sensors and actuators, connected through processing units that, by processing input data obtained from the sensors, make decisions that are forwarded to the actuators. This process today typically involves a large amount of stored or externally obtained data, and it can be executed locally or in a distributed or external environment. The data in this process are most often considered sensitive, meaning that their compromise can threaten the privacy and security of users, as well as the functionality of the environment itself. Therefore, such data must be adequately protected, regardless of whether they are in communication channels or in the memory and processing units of the components.

AAL environments can be considered among the most complex computing environments today, as they utilize almost the entire spectrum of hardware, software, and telecommunication solutions—from microcontrollers to supercomputers, from simple algorithms to artificial intelligence, general and specialized operating systems, libraries, and more. This complexity, as a prerequisite for achieving a high level of functionality, makes data protection in AAL environments particularly demanding and based on a wide range of solutions and approaches.

The three main aspects of data protection are confidentiality, integrity, and availability [13]. Confidentiality is the property that only authorized parties can access the content of the data. For example, if an unauthorized party could access current or stored content obtained from a camera or another sensor in an AAL environment, it would compromise the confidentiality aspect. User privacy is mostly based on the confidentiality of data related to them, but in certain cases, it can also be achieved through the specific data modification step of anonymization. With anonymization, the data are available to a third party, but all identifiers that could link a data point to the entity it relates to are removed beforehand.

Data integrity is the property that ensures data can be considered trusted. This encompasses two things. First, it means that it can be determined that the data have not been altered by an unauthorized party, or accidentally corrupted. For example, data emitted by a temperature sensor should not be damaged or altered, either accidentally or intentionally, by a high-intensity signal emitted by a third party. Second, integrity also means that it can be verified that the data indeed come from the claimed source. For instance, a fire alarm signal should genuinely originate from the sensor installed in the smart home, not from an attacker aiming to automatically unlock the front door. This latter characteristic is also known as authenticity and is sometimes considered a separate fundamental property [25], although it essentially falls under data integrity. Nevertheless, it fundamentally falls under integrity. Integrity protection does not imply confidentiality protection, and vice versa. For example, data from certain sensors that are not privacy-sensitive do not need to be encrypted during transmission (to avoid unnecessary battery drain), but it may be necessary to ensure their integrity is verified on the receiving end.

Finally, the third attribute of data protection—availability—precisely implies that data are accessible for use when needed. For example, an attacker can disrupt communication between sensors and actuators in AAL environments by emitting strong electromagnetic radiation, thus hindering the timely reaction of actuators. Or, by sending a large number of requests to the services used by the environment (i.e. Denial of Service attack[1]), it can prevent the timely execution of requests coming from regular components. Moreover, it is even possible for a regular provider of a specific service, on which the AAL environment relies, to suddenly withdraw from it. In real-time environments, including AAL environments, prior or subsequent availability of data and services can be entirely useless, even detrimental in terms of security or functionality.

Each of these three fundamental data protection properties involves the application of specific principles and approaches to achieve it. Cryptographic functions, described in more detail in the third section of this chapter, form the basis for protecting confidentiality and integrity. Specifically, encryption functions protect unauthorized access to data content, while asymmetric cryptography and digital signatures guarantee integrity. Additionally, cryptographic functions are used for many system functions such as secure storage of passwords or biometric data for user authentication. On the other hand, cryptography generally does not provide a direct ability to contribute to data availability, while some types of attacks on data availability, such as ransomware (where the encryption is used to prevent the owner from accessing the data, with the aim of demanding ransom), are based on cryptography.

To achieve the efficacy of cryptographic functions, their application requires deployment in an environment that is secure according to other criteria. For instance, if outdated hardware or software components with known security vulnerabilities are used, or if they contain backdoors, or if requirements for proper generation and management of cryptographic keys are not adhered to, cryptography will not be able to provide the expected results. On the other hand, cryptography can help compensate for security shortcomings at other levels - for example, data confidentiality can be preserved even in situations where the physical medium on which they are stored is physically stolen, provided they have been previously encrypted.

---

[1] https://www.ncsc.gov.uk/collection/denial-service-dos-guidance-collection, Accessed 9 September 2024.

4.2 Retrospective of Data Protection

Data protection is one of the primary goals of information security, whether it involves professional security systems (military, police, security services, etc.), business systems, private devices, or smart environments. The commonly used analogy in literature, where data are portrayed as the circulatory system of information systems, is incomplete, because data often possesses critically important attributes of confidentiality and authenticity. Society in which we currently live is often described as an "information society," [32] emphasizing its reliance on information, or data, in many essential aspects. Therefore, data protection today can be regarded as a form of safeguarding societal order and progress.

Traditionally, data protection was associated exclusively with professional security organizations, and possibly large business systems, that handled confidential and secret information. The data were mostly kept in isolated environments and transmitted through special and secure communication channels. However, the emergence and widespread use of the Internet and personal computers, along with the availability and cost-effectiveness of digital media for data storage, have led to the fact that in the last two decades of the twentieth century and beyond, small business organizations, as well as individuals, have started intensively using these technologies to achieve business or personal goals. As expected, in accordance with general principles related to value and risk, this migration of value from the physical world to the digital one implied the emergence of essentially or formally new risks. A completely new environment has been created in which an individual, for example, is compelled to develop an awareness that failing to keep a few digits related to a credit card secret is equally harmful as its physical theft, or that the presence of digital pathogens on their computer can have an equally negative impact on the quality of their life as when it comes to compromising their physical health. However, the benefits associated with the use of these new technologies outweigh the risks related to them, or at least the awareness of them, so it is estimated that by the year 2025, two-thirds of the world's population will be using computers and the Internet [26].

The beginning of the 21st century was marked by two new trends in the world of computing: cloud computing and the Internet of Things (IoT). Cloud computing re-emerged as a kind of reincarnation of mainframe computing, addressing the inadequacy of existing technologies and architectures to meet the extremely growing demands for data processing driven by the expansion and evolution of the Internet. Key characteristics of this approach to computing include on-demand self-service, broad network access, resource pooling, rapid elasticity, and measured service [22].

The three basic service models in the cloud environment are Infrastructure as a Service (IaaS), Platform as a Service (PaaS), and Software as a Service (SaaS). From a deployment aspect, typical cloud models are private cloud, community cloud, public cloud, and hybrid cloud [22]. This relatively wide range of options across different dimensions has made cloud computing services attractive for developing services for AAL (Active Assisted Living) environments. For example, relocating server functions (whose on-site implementation is impractical for various reasons

4 Data Security in AAL

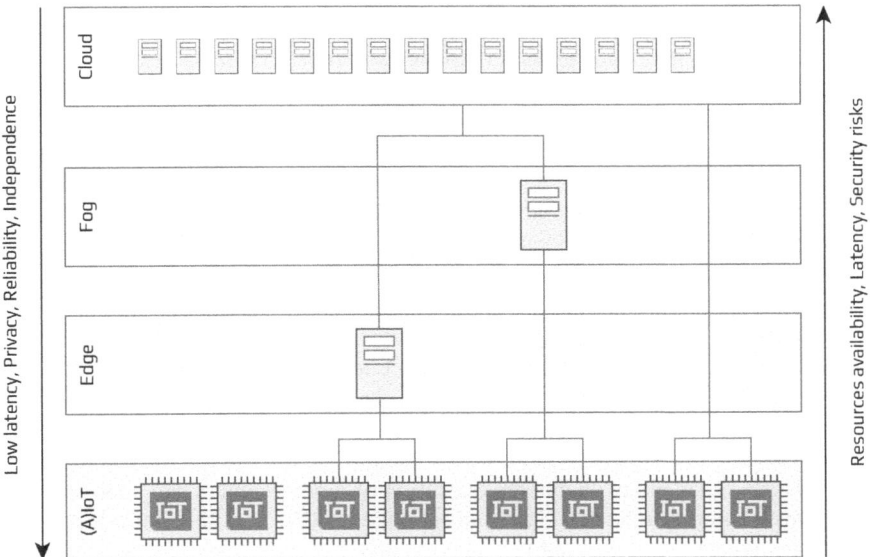

Fig. 4.1 Some high end IoT devices (primarily artificial intelligence of things, AIoT) process data locally, while others use the service of remote servers (edge/fog/cloud) which have significant processing and memory resources. Local processing and processing at the edge/fog layer imply greater data security, given their reduced movement and retention in the user's ownership

such as oversized and overly expensive devices, inadequate environmental conditions, difficult updates, etc.) to a cloud environment offers the possibility of significantly reducing costs, increasing availability, providing sophisticated and computationally demanding functions, and fostering more dynamic development, among other benefits.

Another important characteristic of using the cloud is the facilitated inter-process communication between different devices, which is a common requirement in AAL environments. For these reasons, the vast majority of all ready-made devices for smart homes and environments inherently base their functionality on using manufacturers' cloud services. The services for interacting with and configuring these devices are generally so user-friendly that users are often unaware that the communication between their smartphone and a nearby IoT device is mediated by a cloud environment located on the other side of the world (Fig. 4.1).

Advances in the development of computer hardware—primarily in terms of lower costs, smaller sizes, and increased processing and memory resources—have enabled the explosion of the second trend, the Internet of Things [10].[2] The primary characteristic of this approach to computing is embedding data processing and communication capabilities through local networks and the Internet into devices in the end-user environment. In this way, the direct interaction of users with computer

---

[2] https://aws.amazon.com/what-is/iot, Accessed 26 September 2024.

services, whether local or distributed, is reduced (e.g. various sensors or actuators that lack any user-interface related components, but are controlled exclusively via network). The benefit of using them is achieved through automated influence on the environment and greater convenience in using the devices themselves. Alongside the reduced interactivity with the user comes a decrease in user's awareness of their technological complexity and background activities, and even of their existence in the environment. A crucial characteristic of IoT devices is rigorous dimensioning, i.e., adapting the hardware and software capabilities of the devices to their planned functionality. This is particularly important for achieving an affordable device price and usage in battery-powered scenarios, but it can be a limitation in terms of improving the functional and security features of the devices. Finally, the lack of a direct user interface implies the need for automated device maintenance and software updates on them.

More recently, the IoT concept in some domains has been replaced by the Artificial Intelligence of Things (AIoT), where the hardware-software stack and device potentials are enhanced to enable the execution of more complex and sophisticated algorithms, primarily related to artificial intelligence [9]. This shift introduces significant potentials for improving the functionality and usability of devices. From a security perspective, the existence of more significant computing resources enables local data processing, autonomy in operation, and a reduced need to exchange sensitive data with other local or remote nodes. Additionally, the enhanced computational potential allows for the application of more advanced encryption to protect stored or exchanged data. On the other hand, a more complex technological stack introduces additional challenges and risks in terms of maintaining the system secure and resilient to potential software and configuration errors [34]. For example, the latest versions of the Linux kernel—the most commonly used operating system on AIoT devices—contains over 60 thousand files with 1.7 billion lines of code.[3] Operating system distributions installed on these devices may contain thousands of software packages with hundreds of thousands of files. It is evident that this level of complexity opens up the possibility for accidental or intentional vulnerability introduced by software authors or contributors. Some evidence of poor management of this complexity is that the vast majority of files installed on these systems are never utilized [15].

AAL environments inherently make intensive use of cloud computing and IoT services to achieve the necessary functions. From the perspective of data protection, two key issues with these approaches are the transmission of sensitive data to remote cloud environments owned by third parties, and the scattering of data across a large number of IoT devices in the local environment (which may not necessarily be physically or otherwise protected from unauthorized access). Since cloud and IoT can be seen as extreme values on the current computing spectrum, it (the spectrum) has been enriched with intermediate layers such as fog, mist, and edge computing [14], where fog computing is more complex, hierarchical, and cloud-oriented approach [12], mist computing is a lightweight and rudimentary form of fog computing, while edge computing is simpler and flatter, and closer to end (IoT) devices. In these layers, the

---

[3] The Linux Kernel Archives, available at https://kernel.org/, Accessed 25 September 2024.

main processing capacities from the cloud environment are moved closer to the user, or the point of end-use. This brings significant improvements in terms of increased availability, reduced latency, greater privacy and data security, etc., but also complicates deployment, administration, and raises the cost of establishing and using services.

4.3 Cryptological Foundations and Security Attributes of Data Protection

Cryptology (or cryptography) is a science that fundamentally enables data security, i.e. secret communication between participants (source and destination), based on the assumption that the storage media or communication channel is being eavesdropped on.[4] Secrecy remains one of the primary services of cryptology today. However, modern applications based on computer networks and the Internet have introduced additional services, such as data integrity during transmission, authentication of communication parties, service availability, and non-repudiation of transaction requests (assurance that the sender of information is provided with proof of delivery and the recipient is provided with proof of the sender's identity, so neither can later deny having processed the information [33]), all of which cryptology provides comprehensive solutions for. Today, cryptology is the foundation of computer and communication technology. It is based on strict mathematical principles in areas such as number theory, computational complexity theory, and probability theory, among others. Modern cryptology is supported by mathematically precise guarantees, temporal dimensions, and available computing technology for solving complex problems.

Modern cryptology addresses many issues in computer communication systems. The most important problem remains achieving secure communication over insecure communication channels. In cryptology, a third party, representing a source of threats, is always considered—one that has access to the communication channel or physical media, and aims to compromise the security of the data and communicating parties. The goal of cryptology is to create a perfect communication channel in terms of security, accessible only to the sender and the receiver. In the real world, there are no ideal communication channels. Data transmission occurs over private or public networks, such as the Internet, which are well-standardized, precisely defined, and thus known to attackers. The primary objective of cryptology is to enable communication that has similar properties to ideal communication channels. For this purpose, appropriate cryptographic protocols are defined, which involve the selection of algorithms for encryption/decryption, key agreements, and the alignment of other cryptographic parameters. The communicating parties must know or be able to do something that the third party (attacker) does not know or cannot do.

---

[4] https://www.fortinet.com/resources/cyberglossary/eavesdropping, Accessed 9 September 2024.

There are two basic security models in cryptology: the symmetric (or secret key model) and the asymmetric (or public and private key). Modern cryptographic systems are most often combined (hybrid) to achieve complete protection, implemented at multiple levels in a layered communication architecture. Modern AAL solutions extensively use both types of encryption.

4.3.1 Symmetric Cipher Systems

The traditional and well-known case in communication protection is when the sender and receiver share a single (secret) key that the opponent does not have. This model is called the symmetric model. The key is a random string of bits. The problem of exchanging or storing cryptographic keys for symmetric cipher systems and the procedures for negotiating a secret symmetric key represent the greatest challenge in symmetric cipher systems. In all cipher systems, special attention is given to the generation and distribution of cryptographic keys, which requires organizational measures, i.e., the implementation of specific "protection policies." The success of encryption and decryption requires procedures for initialization on both the sending and receiving sides, collectively known as cryptographic synchronization. The secrecy of symmetric cipher systems is based on the secrecy of the shared key for encryption and decryption. Due to high-tech hardware, operating systems, and the Internet itself, it is often concluded that only isolated computers, i.e., those not connected to public networks, are secure (Fig. 4.2).

The protocol used in symmetric systems is called the symmetric encryption scheme, denoted as (E, D). E denotes the encryption algorithm. The message the sender wishes to send is commonly called *plaintext*. The sender encrypts the plaintext by combining the key k, the encryption algorithm E, and the plaintext M. The resulting text is called *ciphertext*. D represents the decryption algorithm. The receiver

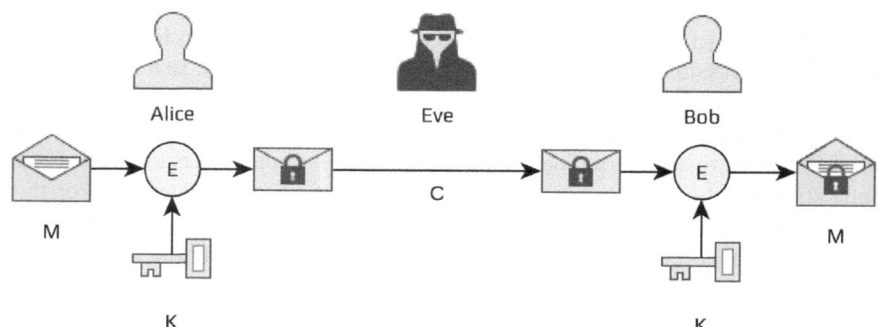

Fig. 4.2 Symmetric encryption is mainly used when it is necessary to protect the confidentiality of data during transmission or storage. The same key k is used for both encryption and decryption

applies the algorithm D with the key k to the ciphertext C. Upon successful decryption, the originally encrypted message M is obtained, i.e., the plaintext. Typically, the key is a random string of appropriate length. Encryption algorithms are standardized (DES, 3DES, AES, etc.) and generated according to strict mathematical principles.[5]

The application of symmetric cryptography is so prevalent in modern computer systems, including AAL solutions, that it is often used by default in most cases. Additionally, the performance of modern symmetric encryption algorithms is at a very high level, both in terms of the level of protection they offer and the amount of data that modern processors can encrypt and decrypt within a given time unit. Furthermore, many processors (even those with modest capabilities, used in embedded/IoT systems) have additional hardware support for faster and more energy-efficient encryption and decryption processes. This is of particular importance for AAL systems, where there is often a need to protect large amounts of data (e.g., audio and video) and to achieve high energy efficiency in the process (e.g., in battery-powered devices).

4.3.2 Asymmetric Cipher Systems

The key known only to the communicating parties and its secrecy is not the only way to maintain data secrecy or communication privacy. The asymmetric cipher system, also known as the public key model, is based on the existence of two keys: a public key and a private (secret) key. The public key is known to the public and can be published.

In asymmetric cryptography, one key is used for encryption, and the other for decryption [31]. The essence is that the encryption key can be public, while only the decryption key must remain private, or vice versa. These two keys are uniquely related. Cipher algorithms in asymmetric systems are such that successful encryption and decryption can only be achieved with the pair of keys. Decryption is not possible with the same key used for encryption. These principles eliminate one of the major problems in symmetric cipher systems related to the distribution of secret symmetric keys. Asymmetric cipher systems have properties that provide a broader set of security functions compared to symmetric cipher systems. They are typically used for efficient authentication, message integrity, non-repudiation, etc., and are rarely used for confidentiality. They are usually combined with symmetric cipher systems. For example, one application of asymmetric systems is to establish a symmetric key for encryption and decryption in a symmetric cipher system (Fig. 4.3).

Asymmetric systems are based on mathematical one-way trapdoor functions. These are functions that are easy to compute in one direction but difficult in the other (computationally or practically infeasible). The trapdoor ensures that the attacker cannot easily (directly) compute the private key from the public key. The most well-known algorithm in asymmetric cryptography, RSA, is named after its creators,

---

[5] https://www.iso.org/information-security/what-is-cryptography, Accessed 9 September 2024.

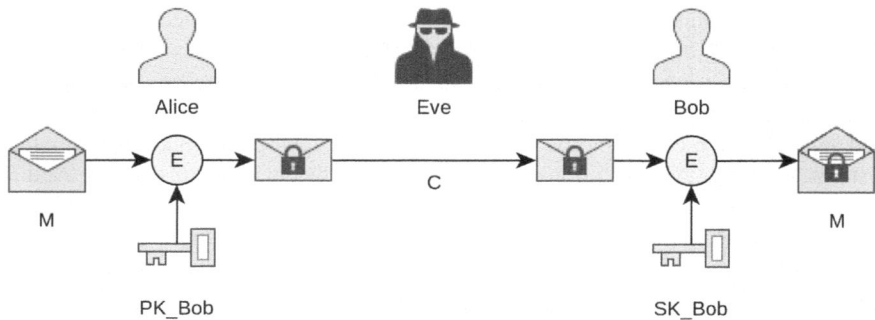

Fig. 4.3 In asymmetric encryption, a pair of keys is used—a public key and a private key. Data encrypted with the public key can only be decrypted with the private key, and vice versa

Rivest, Shamir, and Adleman [28]. It is based on the mathematically complex process of factoring the product of two large prime numbers into its factors. A problem for the widespread use of asymmetric systems, such as the RSA algorithm, is that there is no firm mathematical proof that a shorter path for factoring does not exist.

In asymmetric cipher systems, the confidentiality service is provided without the sharing of secrets. This is very important and useful in today's distributed computing environments. There is no problem with key exchange as in symmetric cipher systems. The main drawback of asymmetric systems is significantly slower operation and the application of keys that are an order of magnitude larger than those in symmetric systems. Finally, asymmetric systems in most applications assume the presence of a trusted third party, such as a certificate authority.

The application of asymmetric encryption in AAL systems, as well as in most other domains, is enormous today, as it enables protected communication between parties that do not have the ability to initially exchange keys using secure channels. In most devices within AAL systems, it is possible to embed keys during their production phase, thus enabling their mutual communication as well as communication with the manufacturer's services. However, limiting to such an approach would prevent the development of complex scenarios, the development of additional services, and the integration of devices from different manufacturers in the development of AAL solutions. That problem is resolved through the use of asymmetric cryptography. It is also important to note that asymmetric cryptography does not solve the problem of verifying the authenticity of the other party but provides a basis for such a solution in the form of digital signatures.

4.3.3 Digital Signature

A method for confirming the authenticity and integrity of a message in the asymmetric model is the digital signature, most elegantly implemented using asymmetric cipher

4   Data Security in AAL

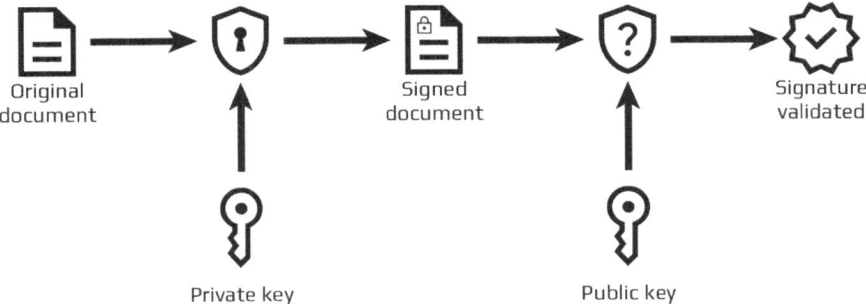

Fig. 4.4 Digital signing of documents is a specific application of asymmetric encryption, where the document's checksum (a control value for detecting errors in data, which occur during transmission, storage, handling, or intentionally) is encrypted using the private key and verified on the recipient's side using the sender's public key. This ensures the integrity of the documents

systems. In this case, the sender has their public and corresponding private (secret) key that are mutually linked. A message encrypted with the public key can only be decrypted using its pair, i.e., the private key, and vice versa. In asymmetric cipher systems, the recipient by definition knows the public key of the sender, the signing party. It is also assumed that the attacker knows the public key. When the sender wants to send a message (document), they compute a hash over it and then encrypt the hash using an asymmetric algorithm based on the private key. Upon receipt, the verification algorithm is applied, which is based on decrypting using the sender's public key. If the message is accepted (encryption and decryption over the message hash are successful), the recipient considers it authentic; if not, it is regarded as a fraud attempt. Digital signing is the basis for data integrity and participant authenticity services in communication (Fig. 4.4).

On the Internet today, only digitally signed content is trusted. Practically, nothing would function on the Internet without digital signing. To access most internet services, such as email, online banking, online shopping, etc., cryptographic computer protocols are applied. For this purpose, symmetric and asymmetric cipher systems and hash functions are used. Well-known security protocols, designed for specific purposes in the layered architecture of computer communication, include WEP, WPA, IPsec, SSL, and others.[6] The essence of these protocols is to prevent attacks such as message replay, message modification in transit, or complete communication takeover, e.g., in the case of a man-in-the-middle attack.

The use of digitally signed data is one of the foundations of security in AAL systems. Given that the components of these systems are most often automatically updated, that they intensely exchange sensitive data, etc., verifying the identity and authenticity of the other party in communication is extremely important. Otherwise,

---

[6] https://sslinsights.com/what-are-digital-signatures-in-ssl-tls, Accessed 9 September 2024.

an attacker could potentially compromise the system's security by introducing modified software or by accessing sensitive data through the mentioned communication interception.

4.3.4 Stream and Block Cipher Algorithms

Stream encryption is a method of encryption where encryption is performed bit by bit, i.e., a bit of plaintext is XORed with a bit of the key to obtain a bit of ciphertext. Absolutely secret cipher systems belong to this group. The secrecy of the ciphertext is based on the secrecy of the encryption key, which must be generated from a natural source of randomness and must possess good random properties. These systems are the best, but are impractical for use in high-bit-rate systems.[7] Therefore, practically secret symmetric stream systems are used, based on generators of pseudo-random sequences with relatively short-length keys. Generators are cryptographic algorithms characterized by good diffusion and confusion, large periods of the output generated sequence, and high nonlinear complexity that complicates cryptanalysis procedures, i.e., attacks on encrypted data. Stream cipher systems are suitable for hardware implementation and are suitable in environments with high levels of noise on the communication channel. That can be the case in AAL environments with a large number of devices using the same radio frequency range for wireless communication.

With the increase in computing power of modern systems, symmetric block cipher algorithms have been developed. The most well-known standard block cipher algorithm is AES (Advanced Encryption Algorithm), which is a NIST standard [23]. An iterative block cipher divides plaintext into fixed-length blocks and generates fixed-size ciphertext blocks. In many cases, the ciphertext is obtained from the plaintext by repeating the function F for a certain number of rounds. The function F, which depends on the output of the previous round and the key K, is known as the round function. Input parameters for each round are the key and the output from the previous round. AES is resistant to known attacks, very fast, allows for parallel design, and can be implemented on many processors, graphics cards, and smart cards. Today, AES-based encryption with 256-bit keys is considered secure encryption that cannot be broken with current computing resources within an acceptable time frame.

---

[7] AAL systems can be considered high-bit-rate systems in situations where large amounts of audio and video data are transmitted; for simple sensors—e.g., temperature, humidity, alerting, etc.—there is no need to transmit large amounts of data.

4.4 General System Architecture and Related Technologies

In computer systems, data can be found in memory units (internal or external), processing units, or on buses that connect these units or computer nodes with each other. For data located in internal memory, processing units, or mounted external memory, the term "data in use" is used. For data located on external memory that is currently not mounted, the term "data at rest" is used. For data located on buses (primarily external ones), the term "data in transit" or "data in motion" is used. All the mentioned units and buses are potentially, to a greater or lesser extent, vulnerable to accidental [35] or intentionally induced errors [16, 18, 20] during the storage, transfer, or processing of data (Fig. 4.5).

It is common for multiple copies of a single piece of data to exist simultaneously at multiple locations—for example, a file stored on external memory and its copy in the main cache memory. Or, data in main memory whose copy is transmitted through a communication channel. It is important to note that in most data removal operations (for example, releasing a variable in a running program or deleting a file from external memory), the content is not actually removed; instead, the space is only marked as free for writing new data. Only after new data is written to that memory space does the actual "destruction" of previously deleted data occur. However, even such data overwriting can be partial, meaning that some parts of the data may still remain in parts of memory blocks. Additionally, on some types of external memory, such as solid-state drives, there may be multiple versions or identical copies of the same data, as a result of complex algorithms for balanced wear of device memory cells. All of this can lead to the "leakage" of sensitive data, while also forming the basis of digital forensic investigation. The problem becomes even more complex in

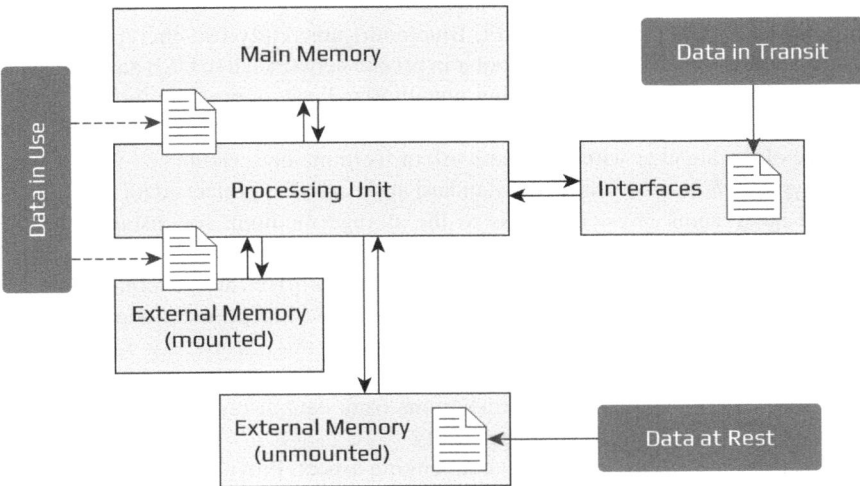

Fig. 4.5 Typical computer system architecture with possible data states

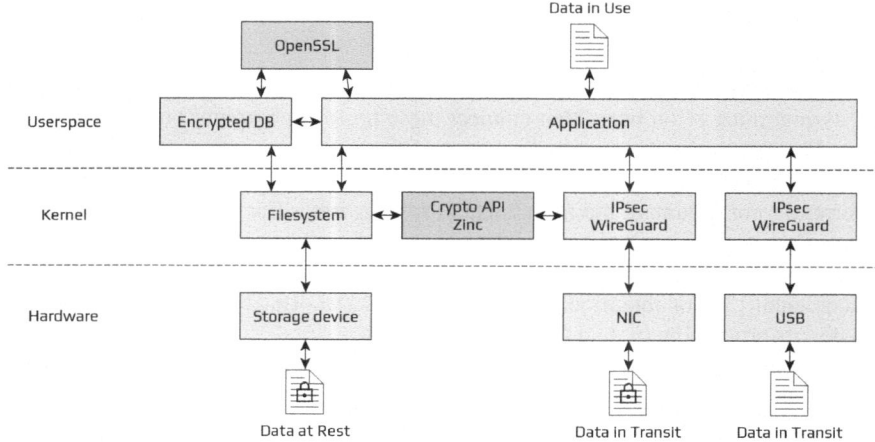

Fig. 4.6 Typical data paths through a computer system, with state changes and potential encryption points

cloud environments, where users typically lack control over which media their data will reside on, as well as physical access to them, or access at a low enough level to efficiently remove data. Efficient and precise removal of data that are no longer in use, especially from external memory media, is an important component of data protection and it is necessary to adhere to relevant recommendations [27] (Fig. 4.6).

Different approaches are used to protect data in various states and locations. Cryptography is a fundamental, but not the only method for data protection in most cases. For protecting *data-in-transit*, encryption protocols such as Virtual Private Networks (VPN), OpenSSL, IPsec, and WireGuard are commonly used. Most wireless data transmission technologies (e.g., WiFi, Bluetooth) inherently use encryption. Conversely, some wired technologies popular in private networks, like USB and Ethernet, transmit plain data by default, making unauthorized access possible through interception or electromagnetic radiation eavesdropping. This typically requires physical presence of the attacker within the network or its immediate vicinity.

Encrypting *data-at-rest* is also a standard approach that protects data if an unauthorized party gains physical access to the storage medium, for instance, in the event of a stolen laptop or hard drives from a surveillance system. Encrypted file systems or built-in encryption functions on the media drives are generally used for this kind of protection. However, there is often a misconception among users that such encryption also protects against some attacks on *data-in-use*, e.g. ransomware attacks. Once the encrypted medium is mounted and accessible through the input of a valid cryptographic key, the data transitions from data-at-rest to data-in-use, and previous protection methods no longer apply.

Protecting *data-in-use* is the most challenging aspect. Previously described solutions apply when transitioning data from "in use" to "in transit" and "at rest," and vice versa. However, to utilize and transform data, it must be "visible," meaning it cannot be encrypted. Cryptography has yet to provide ideal solutions in terms of functionality and performance in this area, although significant progress has been made over the past two decades, primarily through Fully Homomorphic Encryption, which permits computations to be performed on encrypted data without first having to decrypt it [11]. A more realistic approach to this problem involves strict control over access to the computing environment where data-in-use resides. This primarily refers to strictly controlled network access—using firewalls, up-to-date software, etc.—since physical access by attackers is usually impossible, or the data are protected by data-at-rest solutions. However, such isolation, relatively easy to implement when computing systems are physically located with the user, is practically impossible in cloud environments. Implementing unauthorized network access protection systems on cloud-based systems will yield mostly identical results concerning external attackers, but does not protect against the cloud provider. Since these providers have physical access to the machines hosting the users' virtual machines, they can access its working memory at any time, i.e., the data within it. This also potentially allows access to external memory, even if it is encrypted. There are approaches, such as confidential computing[8] or fully homomorphic encryption, that can somewhat address this issue (Fig. 4.7).

Encryption and decryption of data, to protect its confidentiality and integrity, can occur at multiple points within a system. In rare situations, it is implemented as an internal function of a specific application or service. This is often unnecessary as it significantly complicates development and maintenance, raises questions about the correct implementation of cryptographic functions, and the solution is limited to a single piece of software. Much more frequently, ready-made functions at the library level (for example, OpenSSL), the operating system kernel level (for example, Crypto API in Linux), or hardware level (for example, encryption functions built into solid state drives) are used. Multiple encryption, or encryption at multiple levels, generally does not provide any substantial benefit and unnecessarily wastes processing time. In any case, the key issue in applying cryptographic data protection relates to key storage and management. If an unauthorized party gains access to encrypted data (e.g., theft of hard drives or interception of network traffic), access to the decrypted content depends on the ability to access the decryption keys. If the key is of poor quality (e.g., low complexity or short bit length), it can be discovered in a reasonable time through dictionary attacks or brute force. Otherwise, the attacker's only option is to obtain a copy of the required key. If this copy is stored in an unprotected location (for example, in a file on an unencrypted partition of a stolen disk), the entire principle of encryption protection is compromised. Therefore, keys must be stored in a protected location, separate from the encrypted data. This can be quite demanding for users (especially for those who do not possess advanced technical knowledge, which mainly includes older people as the default users of AAL solutions) and almost unfeasible in cloud environments. It should be noted that the correct application of cryptographic functions and key management requires specific developer expertise,

---

[8] https://cloud.google.com/security/products/confidential-computing, Accessed 9 September 2024.

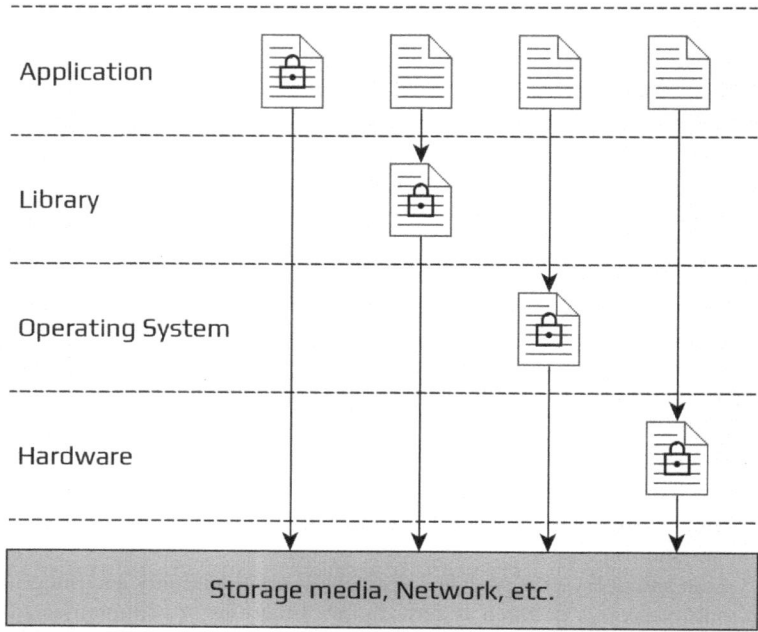

Fig. 4.7 When translating data-in-use to data-at-rest or data-in-transit, encryption/decryption can be performed at the application/library, kernel, or hardware level

which is often lacking even in solutions from large companies.[9] Data in AAL environments is often sensitive in terms of privacy/security, so their protection through proper encryption use is by default required. Additionally, since this data often consists of large audio and video files, when designing AAL solutions, it is necessary to consider the load on users created by proper key management, as well as the load on processing units introduced by the data encryption/decryption process.

4.5 Technological Sovereignty and the Significance of Open Source

All previous considerations are based on the assumption that the manufacturers of the hardware and software components used in AAL/IoT environments have no hidden intentions, meaning that their solutions do not contain intentional flaws that could be exploited for unauthorized access to data or other resources on the systems using these components. In other words, assuming that the components used have only the

---

[9] https://www.schneier.com/blog/archives/2022/08/hyundai-uses-example-keys-for-encryption-system.html, Accessed 9 September 2024.

functionalities clearly stated in their specifications, and that they are integrated into the system in the recommended manner and in accordance with best practices, the only source of vulnerabilities can be unintentional developer errors. To manage such vulnerabilities, a typical model of problem detection, patch issuance, and system updating is used, so the period of system vulnerability is considered the time during which a 0-day exploit[10]—a kind of a cyberattack that takes advantage of a currently unknown or unaddressed security flaw in the computer system—can be utilized, i.e., the period from the discovery of the vulnerability to the issuance and application of the patch. This assumption of the absence of hidden intentions by manufacturers is most often taken as a fact and is not further examined.

Another assumption, significant for the security of data and the AAL/IoT environments themselves, is that the creators of hardware and software components are thoroughly familiar with all the details of their operation and that reliable, high-quality subcomponents were used in their implementation (with which the creators are also thoroughly familiar). This requirement is significant because the quality of the components affects not only the reliability and functionality of the solution but also the security of sensitive data. For this assumption to be accurate, the creators of all components must, in addition to the previously mentioned lack of hidden intentions, possess all the necessary resources and knowledge required to create a high-quality product. A good illustration of the importance of the described principle can be the recent CrowdStrike incident,[11] where the use of closed software caused millions of computer systems and users to be disabled in one day, as a result of an error in one of the components.

Unfortunately, there is ample evidence and practical examples that these assumptions are largely unfounded. Modern computer systems are rife with intentionally or unintentionally included errors that can lead to critical functional or security issues.

Many services today are offered to users for free, with the operational costs and profits being achieved through the direct or indirect sale of data collected during use.[12] This is particularly pronounced and difficult to control with online services implemented as SaaS.[13] Moreover, some closed operating systems or user devices now have built-in functions to display ads to users based on the collected data.[14] Hardware devices are not spared from this problems.[15] Even some data protection solutions are suspected to have backdoors installed.[16] Some devices become unusable

---

[10] https://www.ibm.com/topics/zero-day, Accessed 9 September 2024.

[11] https://edition.cnn.com/2024/07/19/tech/crowdstrike-update-global-outage-explainer/index.html, Accessed 9 September 2024.

[12] https://humenglish.com/technology/slack-under-fire-for-using-user-data/, Accessed 9 September 2024.

[13] https://www.gnu.org/philosophy/who-does-that-server-really-serve.en.html, Accessed 9 September 2024.

[14] https://www.cnet.com/news/privacy/superfish-torments-lenovo-owners-with-more-than-adware/, Accessed 9 September 2024.

[15] https://arstechnica.com/information-technology/2017/06/internet-cameras-expose-private-video-feeds-and-remote-controls/, Accessed 9 September 2024.

[16] https://theintercept.com/2015/12/28/recently-bought-a-windows-computer-microsoft-probably-has-your-encryption-key/, Accessed 9 September 2024.

if the Internet connection goes down,[17] or if not supported anymore, including devices that are critical for their users, like bionic eyes[18] or other implants.[19]

One approach often used by users to protect themselves from undocumented functionalities in the solutions they use is to replace the original software (or firmware) with unofficial equivalents. For example, on specialized Internet forums, one can find complete instructions on how to replace the firmware on devices from popular smart home solution manufacturers with copies that claim to be free of backdoors, and that do not use the manufacturer's cloud services, but rather a local one provided by the user. However, there are many drawbacks to this approach. First, very few users have the necessary technical knowledge to replace the firmware and install the required alternative environment. Additionally, the quality of the unofficial firmware being installed is highly questionable, and it often contains new backdoors and other flaws. Furthermore, this kind of replacement frequently results in the loss of compatibility with other devices and services from the manufacturer. The same applies to support, regarding future firmware updates and assistance in resolving issues. Finally, such replacement may also be illegal, contradicting the end-user agreement that the user has accepted.

An extreme approach to solving these problems would involve achieving technological sovereignty through the independent development of all critical hardware and software components, as well as providing critical services via a private cloud. However, this approach, although it appears to be an attractive solution, is due to its extremely high cost, lack of skilled personnel, the time required for implementation, and other factors, a privilege only for the most technologically advanced countries and their agencies, as well as companies that are technological giants.

A crucial (though not sufficient) condition for trusting a component is that all details of its operation are accessible to the user. Open source embodies this characteristic, and today, key software components of modern computing, such as GNU/Linux and the entire spectrum of user software, are available in this form. However, this alone is not sufficient. It is necessary for all components of the system to meet this transparency requirement to evaluate the security of the entire system. If even one component in the system, whether hardware or software, does not fulfill this requirement, the security of the entire system is questionable. Unfortunately, open source hardware is quite rare today, and often manufacturers of AAL solutions use a large number of closed components.

At this point, it is worth noting that IPsec—de facto standard for encrypting data transmitted in IP-based networks—as well as Crypto API—the default resource for

---

[17] https://www.theguardian.com/business/2023/nov/10/optus-went-down-and-the-smart-lights-came-on-and-then-marayke-was-stranded-in-bed, Accessed 9 September 2024.

[18] https://futurism.com/neoscope/bionic-eye-implants-expire, Accessed 9 September 2024.

[19] https://www.healthcareitnews.com/news/medical-device-vendor-disables-internet-updates-over-hacking-risk-fda-alerts, Accessed 9 September 2024.

cryptographic functions in the Linux kernel—in 2018 received remarkable alternatives in the form of the WireGuard VPN solution and the Zinc cryptographic API [8]. The primary reason for introducing these new solutions lies in simplifying the codebase to make the security level offered by the solution verifiable. For comparison, the complete implementation of WireGuard in the Linux kernel contains fewer than 4,000 lines of code, while that number exceeds 400,000 in the case of IPsec and over 600,000 in the case of OpenSSL. It is clear that such complexity leaves ample room for accidental or intentional introduction of errors (e.g. malicious code in the upstream archive files[20]), which can be critical for data security.

4.6 Considerations About the Life Cycle of AAL Solutions

AAL technologies have the potential to improve the independence and well-being of individuals at home and to enhance the actual and perceived safety. This can be achieved by smart home elements for efficient monitoring and supporting individuals in their home environment. In this context, the key technologies are activity and behavior recognition (see Chap. 7 in this volume [1]), accident prevention such as detecting falls (Chapter 5 [21]) and recognizing frailty (Chapter 6 [4]), monitoring vital signs and other health parameters (Chapter 8 [5], this volume), support for food and medicine intake and in any daily activities (Chapters 7 and 10 [1, 29]). Thus, AAL technologies integrate functionalities that are safe-critical, and, consequently, safety is an important characteristic of AAL systems. In particular, this means that a failure of the system must not lead to any impairment of the user. In other words, the main objective of AAL systems is to improve the well-being and physical and mental health of an individual and not negatively influence it [7].

The safety of an AAL system can be analyzed according to different aspects depending on devices and sensors used, system's structure, involved parties and stakeholders, but also on the quality and safety of data acquisition, processing and storage. One can distinguish between several types of user safety [24]:

- Medical safety: Realized by monitoring of medical parameters,
- Fast safety: Fast assistance in emergencies (for example fall detection or other accidents and their prevention),
- Safety of daily living: Related to the use of technical devices and household aids,
- Structuring safety: For example reminding on appointments, intake of food or medicine,
- Felt or perceived safety: Feeling that the person in need of care is not alone.

An important goal of any AAL system and application is to increase the safety by implementing adequate measures. For example, on the one hand, monitoring applications should implement a high level of data security and safety, as well as

---

[20] CVE-2024-3094, available from MITRE, https://cve.mitre.org/cgi-bin/cvename.cgi?name=CVE-2024-3094, Accessed 26 September 2024.

modern authentication methods to access the data. On the other hand, applications for emergency detection and prevention should pay more attention to a fast, adequate and effective processing of data, especially regarding speed, accuracy, reasoning, and technical quality.

The lifecycle of each product used in AAL systems, as well as the system itself, can be categorized according to [19] into three stages: (1) beginning of life (BoL), (2) middle of life (MoL), and (3) end of life (EoL). The starting point of the lifecycle is the BoL stage, in which the product or system is designed, tested and manufactured. This stage is the stage that mostly influences the characteristics of the product in all dimensions such as performance, price, energy-efficiency, security, and safety dimensions. Once the product or a system enters the market and is installed at the customer's premises, the operational phase starts. All these steps, including the marketing, sales, installation, operation, and services, are a part of the MoL stage. Finally, after years of operation, the product or a system enters the EoL stage, which can be reached because of a number of reasons such as failure, need for an upgrade, discontinuation, safety problems, and so on. Accordingly, the system or a part of it can be refurbished, recycled, or disposed of.

4.6.1 Fail-Secure Design

A prerequisite for a working and safe AAL system is its ability to provide a high tolerance to possible errors and faults [30]. Even small faults may lead to an incorrect working or a failure of the entire system. In the worst case, failure of a single component may result in a catastrophic system failure, which can lead to a risk of harm or injury to a person. For safety-critical AAL systems, fault-tolerant design and implementation should follow the so-called fault hypothesis [17]. The goal of a fault hypothesis is to clearly indicate different types of faults to be tolerated by the system and define their units, as well as to identify the fault-containment regions (FCRs). The fault-containment regions are defined such that it is ensured that they only can fail independently. Additionally, for every FCR, failure rates and failure modes are to be determined. In case of AAL solutions, the system should be divided according to geographical, structural or technological means. For example, different rooms or buildings could be associated with different FCRs or mobile devices and wearables such as smartphones, smart watches could belong to one FCR, and permanently installed devices such as surveillance cameras, microphones, or smart mirrors, to another one. Another possibility is to separate sensors, communication infrastructure, and processing and storage equipment into different FCRs. Thus, the identification of FCRs is crucial for a fail-tolerant design.

In order to achieve a fault-tolerant system, a fault hypothesis should be precisely defined at an early stage of the design process. A fault hypothesis indicates the error types that have to be tolerated by the system [17]. These errors are referred to as normal faults, while faults that are not considered by the fault hypothesis are called

4 Data Security in AAL

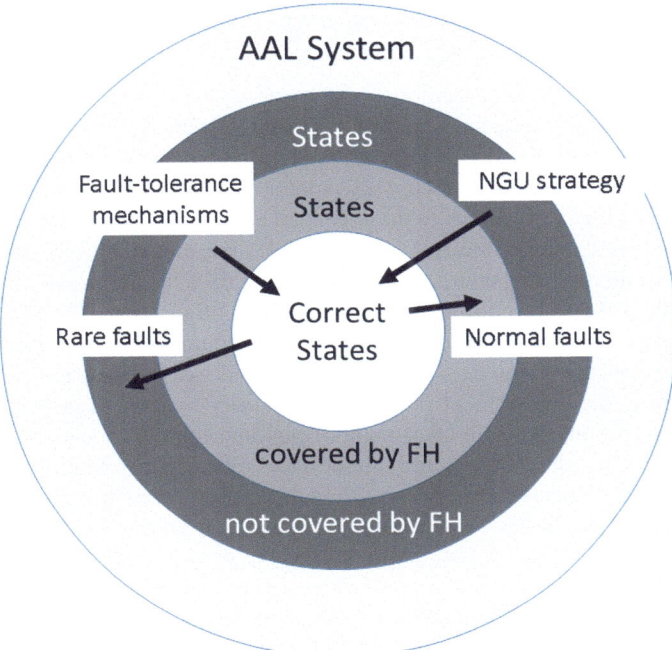

Fig. 4.8 Fault-related state space of fault-tolerant systems (FH: Fault Hypothesis, NGU: Never Give Up), adapted from [17]

"rare faults". In this way, two fault domains are created in the state space that are named as "states covered by fault hypothesis" and "states not covered by the fault hypothesis," respectively (see Fig. 4.8).

Additionally, the failure modes of independent FCRs and their associated failure rates must be determined. This means that failures are clearly assigned to FCRs and a particular failure can only affect the state of a particular FCR. All other faults that are outside the scope of the fault hypothesis need to be treated by the "never give up" (NGU) strategy. The NGU strategy could, for instance, provide a restart of an entire system in case of simultaneous occurrence of several faults in more than one FCR.

In some applications, in addition to a high level of fault-tolerance, it might be desirable to provide a fail-secure design as an additional level of safety. A fail-secure or fail-safe system is designed to protect the user and their property, e.g. by protecting the user's life and personal data from damage. In some failure states, it can be required to run the system at a reduced performance level or even to initiate a controlled shut down or a graceful exit in order to prevent any people injuries or damage to data. In such a case, it is often said that the system is "failing well".

4.6.2 Safe Disposal of Worn-Out and Obsolete Components

Since AAL systems usually comprise different sensors, processing and storage devices, communication and networking equipment, as well as software applications, the entire life cycle of all system components has to be considered when designing and operating the system. The three stages mentioned earlier are shown in Fig. 4.9. The mapping of lifecycle phases to these general stages is shown in the second line of the figure. For example, the BoL stage includes the manufacturing and deploying phases, while MoL is the largest stage that comprises the entire operation phase together with system's monitoring, updates, and reconfiguration. The third stage is the EoL stage, in which a change of the owner or decommissioning can happen.

Possible security measures are indicated in the boxes below each phase [36]. Already during the development process, the Security by Design principle should be followed. That means individual components and the entire system should be developed such that they already provide best-possible security features. Thus, the development phase results in secure-by-default products, which are secure to use "out of the box" with little or no customization and no need for upgrades, extension or complex configuration. Additionally, during the manufacturing process, physical security measures and installation of all necessary certificates are indicated. By installing certificates on devices during the manufacturing process, device identities are created that can be used for authentication in the operational phase.

During the operation phase, particular attention should be paid to the preservation of both local and end-to-end security. Within the entire MoL stage, an efficient monitoring of the entire system should be used to detect, identify, and resist any attack that could compromise the security of the system or influence the privacy and trust of users. The measures include implementation of intrusion detection systems, key/certificates, software updates, and change of configuration.

Once the system reaches the end-of-life (EoL) stage or is being sold to another owner, all sensitive information such as secret or personal data should be effectively erased or overwritten from the devices. Should a device be selected for decommissioning or recycling, all memory components need to be taken out from the device and manipulated accordingly so that they become unreadable.

4.7 Legal Aspects of Data Security

Data security in the European Union (EU) is governed by a broad legal framework designed to protect personal data and ensure cybersecurity. These laws include, for example, the General Data Protection Regulation (GDPR),[21] the

---

[21] Regulation (EU) 2016/679 on the protection of natural persons with regard to the processing of personal data and on the free movement of such data (2016) OJ L 119 ('GDPR').

4 Data Security in AAL

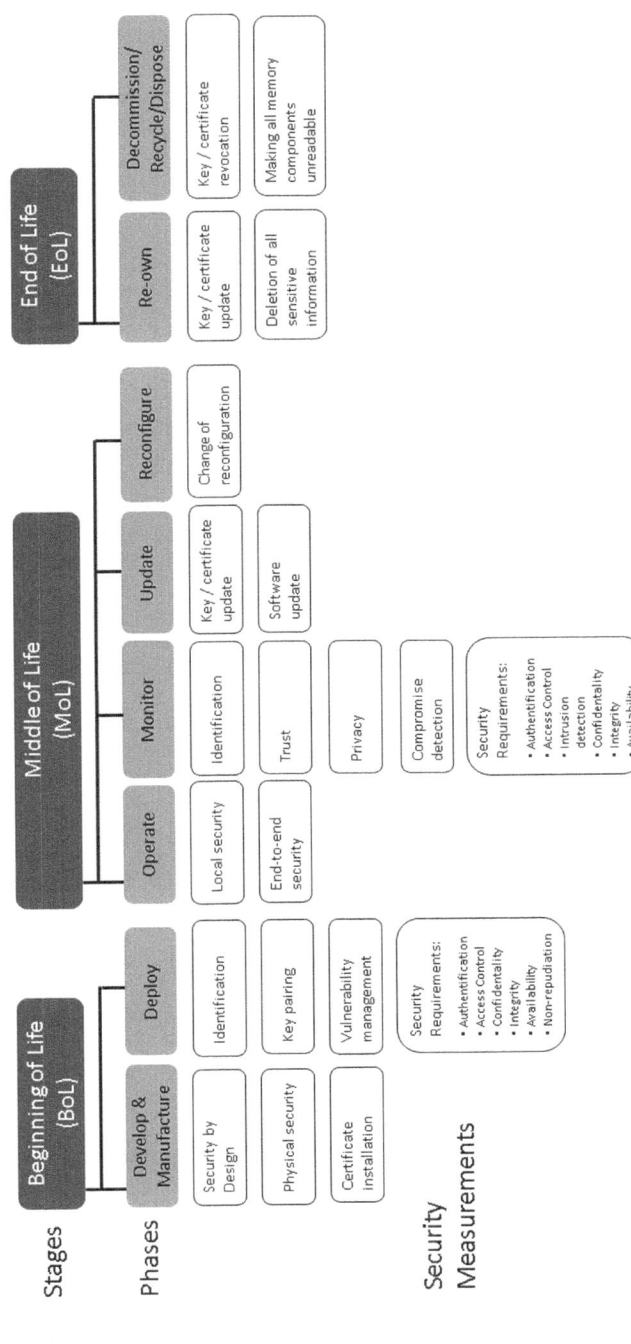

Fig. 4.9 Systems lifecycle and related security issues, adapted from [36]

Cybersecurity Act,[22] NIS 2 Directive,[23] Digital Operation Resilience Act (DORA)[24] as well as the AI Act[25] and the Cyber Resilience Act (CRA).[26] This section will focus on the CRA because it imposes stringent regulatory requirements on Products with Digital Elements (PDEs),[27] signaling an end to the "wild west" era of cybersecurity for the IoT/AioT.[28] It describes three major components of this regulatory framework which include Security by Design, vulnerability reporting, and the use of Software Bill of Materials (SBOMs).

---

[22] Regulation (EU) 2019/881 of 17 April 2019 on ENISA (the European Union Agency for Cybersecurity) and on information and communications technology cybersecurity certification and repealing Regulation (EU) No 526/2013 (Cybersecurity Act) OJ L 151.

[23] Directive (EU) 2022/2555 of 14 December 2022 on measures for a high common level of cybersecurity across the Union, amending Regulation (EU) No 910/2014 and Directive (EU) 2018/1972, and repealing Directive (EU) 2016/1148 ('NIS2'), OJ L 333. Member States have until October 2024 to transpose NIS2 into national law (Article 41).

[24] Regulation (EU) 2022/2554 of the European Parliament and of the Council of 14 December 2022 on digital operational resilience for the financial sector and amending Regulations (EC) No 1060/2009, (EU) No 648/2012, (EU) No 600/2014, (EU) No 909/2014 and (EU) 2016/1011 (DORA) OJ L 333.

[25] Regulation (EU) 2024/1689 of the European Parliament and of the Council of 13 June 2024 laying down harmonised rules on artificial intelligence and amending Regulations (EC) No 300/2008, (EU) No 167/2013, (EU) No 168/2013, (EU) 2018/858, (EU) 2018/1139 and (EU) 2019/2144 and Directives 2014/90/EU, (EU) 2016/797 and (EU) 2020/1828 (AI Act) OJ L 1689. (see also European Parliament legislative resolution of 12 March 2024 on the proposal for a regulation of the European Parliament and of the Council on horizontal cybersecurity requirements for products with digital elements and amending Regulation (EU) 2019/1020 (COM(2022)0454 – C9-0308/2022 – 2022/0272(COD)), available at https://www.europarl.europa.eu/doceo/document/TA-9-2024-0130_EN.html.

[26] Proposal for a Regulation of the European Parliament and of the Council on horizontal cybersecurity requirements for products with digital elements and amending Regulation (EU) 2019/1020, COM (2022) 454 final (CRA proposal), available at https://eur-lex.europa.eu/legal-content/EN/TXT/HTML/?uri=CELEX:52022PC0454.

[27] CRA Article 3(1)(explaining "product with digital elements" means any software or hardware product and its remote data processing solutions, including software or hardware components to be placed on the market separately.").

[28] Article 3(1) of the CRA defines PDE as "a software or hardware product and its remote data processing solutions, including software or hardware components being placed on the market separately." Annex III sets forth an explicit list of important PDEs which includes, for example, identity management systems, password managers and smart home products with security functionalities, including smart door locks, security cameras, baby monitoring systems and alarm systems. Basically, every device or software that winds up in the hands of the consumer are covered by the law, at least insofar as they are not already regulated by other legal frameworks such as Medical Device Regulation.

4.7.1 Security by Design

Security by Design is the backbone of the CRA, requiring that manufacturers adopt strategies from the very outset of system development to minimize security risks and limit vulnerabilities. According to Annex I, Section I, PDEs need to be built in a way that comply with the essential requirements from the very outset of their design and development and throughout the entire lifecycle of the product.[29] Importantly, the requirement to implement Security by Design imposed by the CRA exists as a hard law principle with respect to non-personal data, thus, extending the existing requirement to implement Security by Design where personal data are concerned under Article 32 of the GDPR.[30]

The CRA prescribes numerous ways to operationalize the requirement of Security by Design. These include ensuring a secure by default configuration[31] and having the ability to reset PDEs to their original state.[32] Manufacturers must have the ability to address or patch vulnerabilities through security updates.[33] There needs to be protection against unauthorized access which may be achieved through authentication or identity management systems.[34] There must also be a focus on the protection of the confidentiality of data which may, for example, be accomplished by encryption.[35] Additionally, PDEs should only process the data that is necessary for the function of that PDEs[36] and have inbuilt capacity to support data portability.[37] In the event of

---

[29] CRA, Annex I, Section I.

[30] See more generally [2].

[31] CRA, Annex I, Part I(2)(b) (PDEs shall "be made available on the market with a secure by default configuration, unless otherwise agreed between manufacturer and business user in relation to a tailor-made product with digital elements, including the possibility to reset the product to its original state.").

[32] CRA, Annex I, Part I 1(2)(m) (PDEs shall "provide the possibility for users to securely and easily remove on a permanent basis all data and settings…").

[33] CRA, Annex I, Part I 1(2)(c) (PDEs shall "ensure that vulnerabilities can be addressed through security updates, including, where applicable, through automatic security updates that are installed within an appropriate time frame enabled as a default setting, with a clear and easy-to-use opt-out mechanism, through the notification of available updates to users, and the option to temporarily postpone them.").

[34] CRA, Annex I, Part I(2)(d) (PDEs shall "ensure protection from unauthorised access by appropriate control mechanisms, including but not limited to authentication, identity or access management systems, and report on possible unauthorised access.").

[35] CRA, Annex I, Part I(2)(e) (PDEs shall "protect the confidentiality of stored, transmitted or otherwise processed data, personal or other, such as by encrypting relevant data at rest or in transit by state of the art mechanisms, and by using other technical means.").

[36] CRA, Annex I, Part I(2)(g) (PDEs shall "process only data, personal or other, that are adequate, relevant and limited to what is necessary in relation to the intended purpose of the product with digital elements (minimisation of data)").

[37] CRA, Annex I(2)(m) (PDEs shall "provide the possibility for users to securely and easily remove on a permanent basis all data and settings and, where such data can be transferred to other products or systems, ensure that this is done in a secure manner.").

a Denial of Service (DoS) attack, the PDE must be designed and manufactured in a way that users can access their basic and essential functions despite the attack.[38]

4.7.2 Vulnerability Reporting

PDEs shall be delivered without any known exploitable vulnerabilities.[39] The CRA defines an "exploitable vulnerability" as "a vulnerability that has the potential to be effectively used by an adversary under practical operational conditions."[40] Additionally, manufacturers are required to guarantee the efficient management of vulnerabilities for either the entirety of the anticipated product lifespan or a minimum of five years, whichever period is shorter, after the product's sale.[41] In other words, manufacturers cannot just put a product on the market without offering an extended support period.

The CRA further introduces rigorous vulnerability reporting, requiring detailed records for vulnerabilities found in PDEs. Manufacturers must report any actively exploited vulnerabilities or severe incidents affecting PDEs within 24 hours.[42] The legislation specifies that these reports are to be submitted to a new platform maintained by ENISA, which shall facilitate the formal sharing of these report.[43] The

---

[38] CRA, Annex I, Part I(2)(h) (PDEs shall "protect the availability of essential and basic functions, also after an incident, including through resilience and mitigation measures against denial-of-service attacks.").

[39] CRA, Annex I, Part I(2)(a) (PDEs shall "be made available on the market without known exploitable vulnerabilities"). Recital (55) of the CRA explains this as: "In order to ensure that products with digital elements are secure both at the time of their placing on the market as well as during the time the product is expected to be in use, it is necessary to lay down essential requirements for vulnerability handling and essential cybersecurity requirements relating to the properties of products with digital elements. While manufacturers should comply with all essential requirements related to vulnerability handling throughout the support period, they should determine which other essential requirements related to the product properties are relevant for the type of product with digital elements concerned. For that purpose, manufacturers should undertake an assessment of the cybersecurity risks associated with a product with digital elements to identify relevant risks and relevant essential requirements in order to make available their products with digital elements without known exploitable vulnerabilities that might have an impact on the security of those products and to appropriately apply suitable harmonised standards, common specifications or European or international standards.".

[40] CRA, Article 3(41).

[41] CRA, Article 13(8); See also CRA, Recital (61) (explaining, "The support period for which the manufacturer ensures the effective handling of vulnerabilities should be no less than five years, unless the lifetime of the product with digital elements is less than five years, in which case the manufacturer should ensure the vulnerability handling for that lifetime.".

[42] CRA, Article 14(1) (explaining, "A manufacturer shall notify any actively exploited vulnerability contained in the product with digital elements that it becomes aware of simultaneously to the CSIRT designated as coordinator…and to ENISA…").

[43] CRA, Article 14(1) and Article 16.

platform will maintain a comprehensive list of vulnerabilities for all PDEs, raising concerns about the potential misuse of this information by cybercriminals.

4.7.3 Software Bill of Materials (SBOMs)

Broadly, an SBOM is an inventory of all components, libraries, and dependencies included in a software application, somewhat resembling a list of ingredients found on food packaging [3]. It aids actors in the supply chain such as developers, manufacturers, and users in identifying, tracking, and mitigating existing and emerging vulnerabilities and risks. SBOMs play a critical role in information sharing by offering a detailed map of the software's internal structure. They help identify the origin of each component, track updates, and manage vulnerabilities effectively.[44] [3] further notes that "an SBOM lists every component of software in the finished product. This ensures that anyone who chooses the product knows its relative hygiene, and anyone who uses the software knows what is inside. When a widespread vulnerability is discovered, SBOMs enable patients or organizations such as (healthcare delivery organizations) to identify impacted technology that might be in use."

Under the CRA, manufacturers are explicitly required to incorporate a SBOM.[45] Under Article 3, an SBOM is defined as "a formal record containing details and supply chain relationships of components included in the software elements of a product with digital elements." It does not have to be made publicly available.[46] The SBOM should cover "at the very least the top-level dependencies of the products,"[47] be included in the technical documentation[48] and, upon request, provided to market surveillance authorities.[49] The Commission will likely provide further guidance on SBOMs.[50]

---

[44] CRA Recital (78) explains that: "In order to facilitate vulnerability analysis, manufacturers should identify and document components contained in the products with digital elements, including by drawing up an SBOM. An SBOM can provide those who manufacture, purchase, and operate software with information that enhances their understanding of the supply chain, which has multiple benefits, in particular it helps manufacturers and users to track known newly emerged vulnerabilities and cybersecurity risks. It is of particular importance that manufacturers ensure that their products with digital elements do not contain vulnerable components developed by third parties. Manufacturers should not be obliged to make the SBOM public.".

[45] CRA, Annex I, Part II(1).

[46] CRA Recital (78).

[47] CRA, Annex I, Part II(1).

[48] CRA, Annex VII 2(b).

[49] CRA, Annex VII 8.

[50] CRA, Recital 24 (explaining, "The Commission may, by means of implementing acts taking into account European or international standards and best practices, specify the format and elements of the software bill of materials referred to in Annex I, Part II, point (1). Those implementing acts shall be adopted in accordance with the examination procedure referred to in Article 62(2).").

The current methods for sharing SBOMs within the software supply chain are diverse and vary in sophistication [6]. There are trade-offs associated with different sharing approaches: more manual methods allow for greater control over access but lack scalability, whereas automated sharing supports discoverability and transport at scale but may require more sophisticated access controls [6]. As SBOM adoption grows, new models leveraging automation and standards are expected to emerge [6]. When the CRA comes into force, the SBOM will likely be a fundamental component of every software build moving forward and advancing SBOM sharing practices will be essential to fully realizing the benefits of software transparency throughout the entire software supply chain.

Acknowledgements This publication is based upon work from COST Action GoodBrother—Network on Privacy-Aware Audio—and Video-Based Applications for Active and Assisted Living (CA19121), supported by COST (European Cooperation in Science and Technology).

References

1. Aleksic, S., Despotovic, V., Cristina, S.: Activities of daily living (ADL) and behavior recognition. In: Salah, A.A., Colonna, L., Florez-Revuelta, F. (eds.) Privacy-Aware Monitoring for Assisted Living. Springer, Cham (2025)
2. Bygrave, L.A.: Security by design: aspirations and realities in a regulatory context. Oslo Law Rev. **3**, 126–177 (2022)
3. Carmody, S., Coravos, A., Fahs, G., Hatch, A., Medina, J., Woods, B., Corman, J.: Building resilient medical technology supply chains with a software bill of materials. NPJ Digit. Med. **4**(1), 1–6 (2021)
4. Climent-Pérez, P., Florez-Revuelta, F.: Privacy-aware video-based methods for gait and frailty recognition in active and assisted living environments. In: Salah, A.A., Colonna, L., Florez-Revuelta, F. (eds.) Privacy-Aware Monitoring for Assisted Living. Springer, Cham (2025)
5. Cristina, S., Počta, P., Zgank, A., Camilleri, K.P., Colantonio, S., Lambrinos, L.: Remote monitoring of vital signs. In: Salah, A.A., Colonna, L., Florez-Revuelta, F. (eds.) Privacy-Aware Monitoring for Assisted Living. Springer, Cham (2025)
6. Cybersecurity and Infrastructure Security Agency: SBOM sharing primer (2024). https://www.cisa.gov/resources-tools/resources/sbom-sharing-primer
7. Denecke, K.: What characterizes safety of ambient assisted living technologies? Stud. Health Technol. Inform. **281**, 704–708 (2021). https://doi.org/10.3233/SHTI210263
8. Donenfeld, J.: Zinc: minimal lightweight kernel cryptography API (2018). https://kernel-recipes.org/en/2018/talks/zinc-minimal-lightweight-kernel-cryptography-api/
9. Dong, B., Shi, Q., Yang, Y., Wen, F., Zhang, Z., Lee, C.: Technology evolution from self-powered sensors to AIoT enabled smart homes. Nano Energy **79**, 105,414 (2021). https://doi.org/10.1016/j.nanoen.2020.105414
10. Evans, D.: The Internet of Things: How the Next Evolution of the Internet Is Changing Everything. Cisco Systems (2011)
11. Gentry, C.: A Fully Homomorphic Encryption Scheme. Stanford University (2009)
12. OpenFog Consortium Architecture Working Group: Openfog reference architecture for fog computing. Technical report, OpenFog Consortium (2017)
13. Ham, J.V.D.: Toward a better understanding of "cybersecurity". Digit. Threats **2**(3) (2021). https://doi.org/10.1145/3442445

14. Iorga, M., Feldman, L., Barton, R., Martin, M., Goren, N., Mahmoudi, C.: Fog computing conceptual model (2018). https://doi.org/10.6028/NIST.SP.500-325
15. Jevremovic, A., Veinovic, M., Peraković, D.: Analyzing the efficiency of software distribution systems in AIoT environments. In: Knapčíková, L., Peraković, D. (eds.) 8th EAI International Conference on Management of Manufacturing Systems, pp. 99–108. Springer Nature Switzerland, Cham (2024)
16. Kim, Y., Daly, R., Kim, J., Fallin, C., Lee, J.H., Lee, D., Wilkerson, C., Lai, K., Mutlu, O.: Flipping bits in memory without accessing them: an experimental study of dram disturbance errors. In: 2014 ACM/IEEE 41st International Symposium on Computer Architecture (ISCA), pp. 361–372 (2014). https://doi.org/10.1109/ISCA.2014.6853210
17. Kopetz, H., Steiner, W.: Real-time systems: design principles for distributed embedded applications. Springer Nature (2022)
18. Koruyeh, E.M., Khasawneh, K.N., Song, C., Abu-Ghazaleh, N.: Spectre returns! speculation attacks using the return stack buffer. In: 12th USENIX Workshop on Offensive Technologies (WOOT 18). USENIX Association, Baltimore, MD (2018). https://www.usenix.org/conference/woot18/presentation/koruyeh
19. Lehmhus, D., Wuest, T., Wellsandt, S., Bosse, S., Kaihara, T., Thoben, K.D., Busse, M.: Cloud-based automated design and additive manufacturing: a usage data-enabled paradigm shift. Sensors **15**, 32079–32122 (2015)
20. Lipp, M., Schwarz, M., Gruss, D., Prescher, T., Haas, W., Mangard, S., Kocher, P., Genkin, D., Yarom, Y., Hamburg, M.: Meltdown (2018)
21. Lumetzberger, J., Ballester, I, Kampel, M.: Fall detection. In: Salah, A.A., Colonna, L., Florez-Revuelta, F. (eds.) Privacy-Aware Monitoring for Assisted Living. Springer, Cham (2025)
22. Mell, P.M., Grance, T.: The NIST definition of cloud computing. National Institute of Standards and Technology (2011). https://doi.org/10.6028/nist.sp.800-145
23. National Institute of Standards and Technology (U.S.): Advanced encryption standard (AES) (2001). https://doi.org/10.6028/nist.fips.197
24. Offermann-van Heek, J., Ziefle, M.: Nothing else matters! trade-offs between perceived benefits and barriers of AAL technology usage. Front. Public Health **7** (2019). https://doi.org/10.3389/fpubh.2019.00134
25. Parker, D.B.: Fighting Computer Crime: A New Framework for Protecting Information. Wiley, USA (1998)
26. Petrosyan, A.: Worldwide digital population 2024 (2024). https://www.statista.com/statistics/617136/digital-population-worldwide/
27. Regenscheid, A., Feldman, L., Witte, G.: NIST special publication 800-88, revision 1: guidelines for media sanitization (2015). https://tsapps.nist.gov/publication/get_pdf.cfm?pub_id=917935
28. Rivest, R.L., Shamir, A., Adleman, L.: A method for obtaining digital signatures and public-key cryptosystems. Commun. ACM **21**(2), 120–126 (1978)
29. Santofimia, M.J., del Toro, X., Bolaños, C., Dorado, J., Colantonio, S.: A smart mirror to your health: personalized virtual coaching for active and healthy ageing. In: Salah, A.A., Colonna, L., Florez-Revuelta, F. (eds.) Privacy-Aware Monitoring for Assisted Living. Springer, Cham (2025)
30. Schmidt, M., Obermaisser, R.: Adaptive and technology-independent architecture for fault-tolerant distributed AAL solutions. Comput. Biol. Med. **95**, 236–247 (2018). https://doi.org/10.1016/j.compbiomed.2017.11.002
31. Simmons, G.J.: Symmetric and asymmetric encryption. ACM Comput. Surv. CSUR) **11**(4), 305–330 (1979)
32. Soll, J.: The Information Master: Jean-Baptiste Colbert's Secret State Intelligence System. University of Michigan Press (2009). https://doi.org/10.3998/mpub.243021
33. Stine, K., Kissel, R., Barker, W.C., Fahlsing, J., Gulick, J.: Vol. 1 Rev. 1: Guide for mapping types of information and information systems to security categories (2008). DOI https://doi.org/10.6028/nist.sp.800-60v1r1

34. Sun, P., Shen, S., Wan, Y., Wu, Z., Fang, Z., Gao, X.Z.: A survey of IoT privacy security: architecture, technology, challenges, and trends. IEEE Internet Things J. 1–1 (2024). https://doi.org/10.1109/JIOT.2024.3372518
35. Torvalds, L.: Linus Torvalds on the importance of ECC RAM, calls out Intel's "bad policies" over ECC (2021). https://www.phoronix.com/news/Linus-Torvalds-ECC
36. Yousefnezhad, N., Malhi, A., Främling, K.: Security in product lifecycle of IoT devices: a survey. J. Netw. Comput. Appl. **171**, 102,779 (2020). https://doi.org/10.1016/j.jnca.2020.102779

Open Access This chapter is licensed under the terms of the Creative Commons Attribution 4.0 International License (http://creativecommons.org/licenses/by/4.0/), which permits use, sharing, adaptation, distribution and reproduction in any medium or format, as long as you give appropriate credit to the original author(s) and the source, provide a link to the Creative Commons license and indicate if changes were made.

The images or other third party material in this chapter are included in the chapter's Creative Commons license, unless indicated otherwise in a credit line to the material. If material is not included in the chapter's Creative Commons license and your intended use is not permitted by statutory regulation or exceeds the permitted use, you will need to obtain permission directly from the copyright holder.

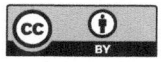

Part II
Video- and Audio-Based AAL Solutions

Chapter 5
Fall Detection

Jennifer Lumetzberger, Irene Ballester, and Martin Kampel

Abstract As the global population ages, the incidence of falls among the older adults increases, necessitating advancements in fall detection and prevention technologies. This chapter provides a comprehensive overview of the current state of these technologies in the context of Active Assisted Living (AAL). It begins by discussing the importance of fall statistics and the critical need for early detection to mitigate severe health consequences and reduce healthcare costs. Various fall detection methods are explored, distinguishing between image-based and non-image-based approaches. The chapter also examines the technological principles behind these methods, such as the use of accelerometers, pressure sensors, depth cameras, and thermal imaging. Privacy concerns are addressed, highlighting the balance between effective monitoring and maintaining user confidentiality. The usability challenges associated with false positives and false negatives are analyzed, emphasizing the importance of user-friendly systems that encourage consistent use by both older adults and caregivers. Finally, the chapter considers the ethical implications and the need for ongoing research to refine these technologies for better accuracy and user acceptance.

Keywords Active assisted living (AAL) · Fall detection · Machine learning · Sensor systems · Privacy · Usability

---

J. Lumetzberger · I. Ballester · M. Kampel (✉)
Computer Vision Lab, TU Wien, Vienna, Austria
e-mail: martin.kampel@tuwien.ac.at

J. Lumetzberger
e-mail: jlumetzberger@cvl.tuwien.ac.at

I. Ballester
e-mail: irene.ballester@tuwien.ac.at

© The Author(s) 2025
A. A. Salah et al. (eds.), *Privacy-Aware Monitoring for Assisted Living*,
Intelligent Systems Reference Library 270,
https://doi.org/10.1007/978-3-031-84158-3_5

5.1 Introduction

As the population gets older [74] and the risk of falls increases with age [34], a division of research of Active Assisted Living (AAL) focusing on the recognition and prevention of falls has evolved [22]. The European Next Generation Ambient Assisted Living Innovation Alliance (AALIANCE2) outlined the application area of fall prevention technology to range from moving safely at home and outdoors to preventive motor training and system recognition of dangerous situations [8]. Fall recognition technologies provide support by contacting care givers and informing them about a fall [8].

This chapter introduces the concepts of fall detection (Sect. 5.3) and fall prevention (Sect. 5.4). It begins with an overview of falls, including statistics (Sect. 5.2), and highlights the importance of early fall detection. The discussion covers both image-based and non-image-based methods. Following this, the chapter addresses privacy concerns related to these methods (Sect. 5.5) and examines usability aspects (Sect. 5.6).

5.2 Fall Statistics

When speaking about falls, the definition of the term is not uniform [30]. The Kellogg International Work Group on the Prevention of Falls by the Elderly [30] highlights that these varying definitions can lead to inadequate comparisons between studies on falls. Research by Zecevic et al. [86] shows that while older adults often associate falls with losing balance, healthcare providers tend to describe them in terms of their consequences. In contrast, researchers generally focus on the event itself [86]. Although a single, standardized definition may not be essential, clear communication about what constitutes a fall is vital [30]. A commonly accepted definition, provided by the Kellogg Group, describes a fall as "an event in which a person unintentionally comes to rest on the ground or other lower level and other than as a consequence of the following: sustaining a violent blow, loss of consciousness, sudden begin of paralysis, as in a stroke or an epileptic fit" [30].

5.2.1 Frequency of People Falling

Each year, approximately 28–35% of individuals aged 65 and over experience a fall [6, 57], with this percentage rising to 32–42% for those over 70 [13, 70]. Generally, the frequency of falls increases with age [34] and the level of frailty [19]. Falls lead to mild to severe injuries in 20–30% of cases and constitute 10–15% of all emergency department visits [67]. Notably, over 50% of injury-related hospitalizations involve people over 65 years old [58].

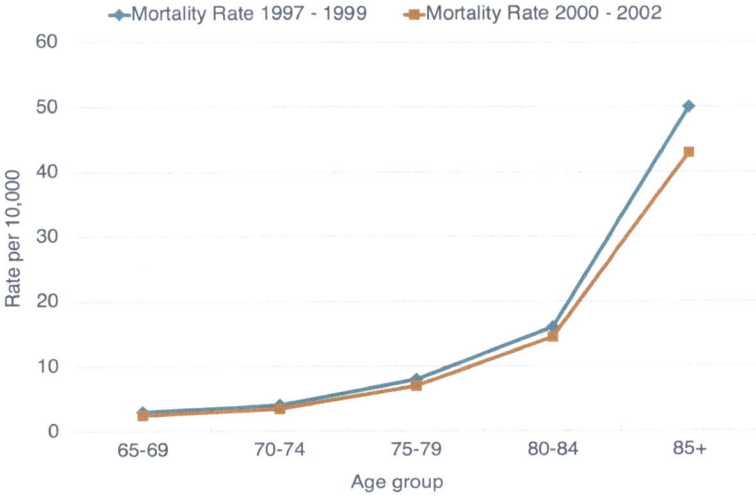

Fig. 5.1 Mortality rate due to falls by age group in Canada. (Figure adapted from [58])

Figure 5.1 highlights that fatal falls, which result in death, are particularly prevalent among older adults. This trend is further supported by studies from the Department of Health and Human Services of the United States [12] and the World Health Organization (WHO) [78].

Kannus et al. [28] explore fall-induced deaths among the older adults in Finland, uncovering a significant rise over time. Their findings show that the number of fall-related deaths for Finns aged 50 and older more than doubled between 1971 and 2002. With the aging population, similar increases are anticipated in Finland and other Western nations [28]. Moreover, Kannus et al. predict that by 2030, fall-induced cervical spine injuries among Finns aged 50 and above will be roughly twice as common as they were during 2000–2004 [27].

Beyond the health impacts, the economic burden is significant: only in 2015, the United States spent approximately 50 billion US dollars on medical costs related to both fatal and nonfatal falls, and these costs are anticipated to rise further as the population ages [18].

5.2.2 Reasons for People Falling

To develop effective solutions for preventing and detecting falls, it is essential to understand their underlying causes. The primary risk factors can be grouped into four categories: biological, behavioral, environmental, and socioeconomic factors

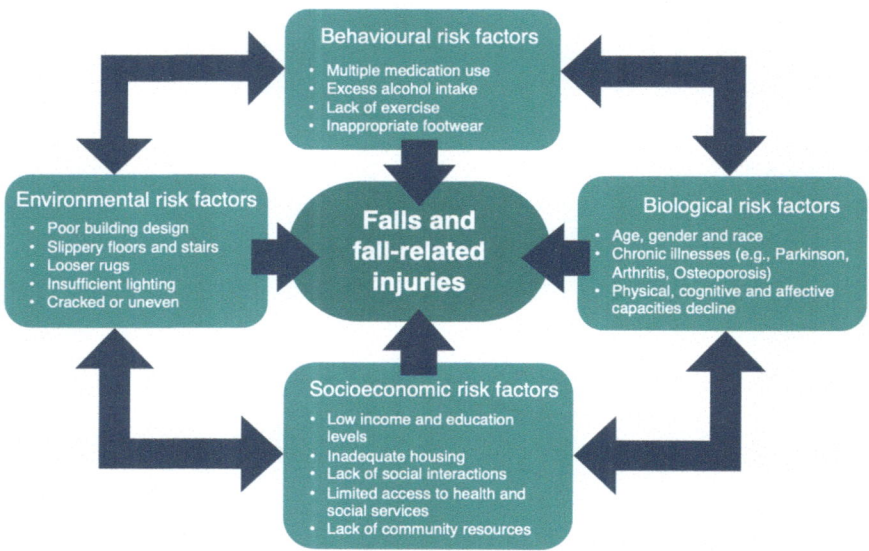

Fig. 5.2 Risk factors for falls in older age (based on [78])

[58, 78]. Examples of these risk factors are illustrated in Fig. 5.2. In addition to age and physical limitations, inappropriate footwear and poor building design can also contribute to falls [78].

As exposure to these risk factors increases, so does the likelihood of falling [78]. The 2005 Canadian Community Health Survey analyzed activities leading to falls among individuals aged 65 and over, finding that 44% of falls were due to slipping, tripping, or stumbling on various surfaces, while 26% occurred while navigating stairs. Additionally, 47% of falls in this age group that required hospital treatment happened at home [58]. This finding is corroborated by the 2005 San Diego County Elderly Falls Report, which noted that 56% of fall injuries in those over 55 occurred at home during 2000 and 2001 [71]. Moreover, older adults residing in residential care facilities experience about three times more frequent falls than those living in the community [66]. Approximately 30–50% of residents in long-term care fall each year, with 40% of these individuals falling multiple times annually [66].

5.2.3 Importance of Early Help in Falls

Studies on individuals found helpless or deceased in their homes reveal significant insights into fall-related incidents. Analysis of 367 people, averaging 73 years in age, showed that 23% were found dead, and 5% died in the hospital. The incidence of such events increased markedly with age, particularly among men over 85 living alone, who experienced the highest rates (123 per 1000 per year). The research demonstrated that the duration of helplessness was a critical factor: those who had been helpless for over 72 h faced a 67% mortality rate, compared to just 12% for those who had been waiting for less than one hour. Additionally, most individuals who were found helpless were unable to return to independent living [20].

Another study, focused on falls among older adults at home, tracked 165 individuals aged 65 and older who had fallen at home over the course of a year, comparing them with a control group. Among the fallers, 20 individuals were unable to get up by themselves for more than one hour, and four of these remained on the ground for over six hours. Follow-up visits conducted within seven days, and again at three and twelve months, revealed that 32 of these fallers had died within a year, compared to only 8 in the control group. Notably, half of those who were helpless for more than one hour had died within six months [79].

5.3 Fall Detection

Focusing on fall prevention and fall detection, different classes, based on the technology, can be distinguished [53]. In this chapter, we differentiate between image-based and non-image-based approaches.

5.3.1 Non-image-Based Fall Detection Methods

Accelerometers are a common tool used for fall detection systems [39, 77, 80]. Examples of products using accelerometers for fall detection are shown in Fig. 5.3 and Fig. 5.4. As early as 1991, Lord and Colvin [39] developed a triaxial accelerometer system to detect forces that exceeded a defined limit, alongside measuring the duration of these accelerations. The data collected were then processed and displayed on a desktop computer via a microcomputer chip [39]. In a subsequent advancement, Williams et al. [80] introduced a fall detection system incorporating a piezoelectric shock sensor combined with a mercury tilt switch. This system measured both the impact and the orientation of the patient to determine the occurrence of a fall.

Despite their low-cost technology and simple methodology, accelerometer-based wearable devices struggle with high false alarm rates due to physical activities like jumping or post-fall posture [77]. However, advancements in wearable telemedicine technology have facilitated improvements in addressing these issues [75].

Detecting the severity of a fall is crucial for deciding whether an alarm should be triggered. To enhance fall detection accuracy, Wang et al. [77] use three different inertia parameters—acceleration, angular velocity, and their combination—demonstrating a lower rate of misclassification compared to methods based on a

Fig. 5.3 Fall detection device

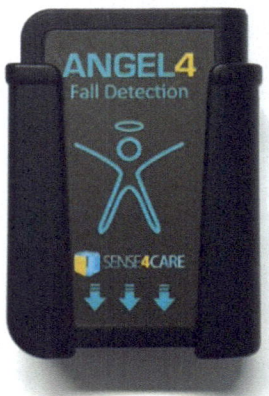

Fig. 5.4 Smart watch with fall detection function

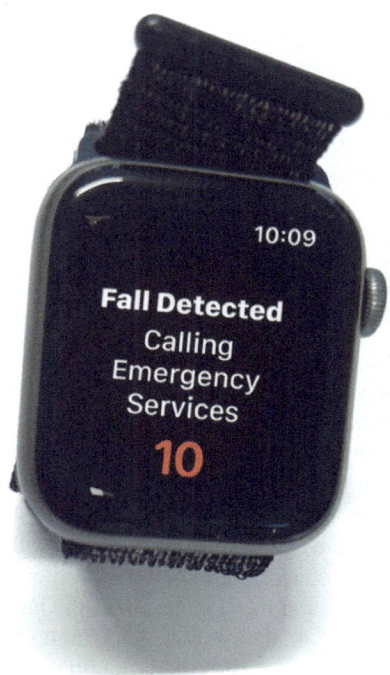

single parameter. Their chest-worn sensor effectively reduces false alarms by incorporating these multiple parameters [77]. In a different approach, Sabatini et al. [65] combine an accelerometer with a barometric altimeter to analyze both the impact of a fall and changes in posture. By measuring vertical velocity and the height of the body part to which the altimeter is attached, they apply a pre- and post-fall algorithm to improve detection accuracy [65].

Other methods are based on the use of smartphone-included sensors to detect falls and to avoid an additional device that has to be carried around [75]. For instance, smartphones' electronic compass and triaxial accelerometer can be harnessed to detect falls [29]. By analyzing tilt angles and waveform sequences, a feature sequence is generated and processed using classification techniques to identify falls. In addition, inertial measurement units combined with machine learning algorithms can classify daily activities, helping to distinguish between normal movements and falls, thereby reducing the number of false alarms [23]. However, using smartphones for fall detection comes with its own set of challenges. Issues such as limited battery life, memory constraints, and real-time processing capabilities can impact the effectiveness of the system [40]. Moreover, there is the risk that individuals might not always carry their phone, especially right after getting out of bed. This period of postural change can affect blood pressure and potentially lead to dizziness, which increases the risk of falls.

Apart from accelerometer-based methods, smartphones can also be used to detect falls by using the integrated microphone [75]. Khan et al. [32] split the audio signals coming from such a sensor into frames for extracting the frequency spectral features. With a collection of footstep sound signals and the use of a one class support vector machine method, falls are distinguished from non-falls [32]. The difficulties in this method lie in the generation of training data, since realistic fall sound signatures are difficult to design [54]. Moreover, the proper use of acoustic and vibration sensors is restricted to a certain floor type [75].

Pressure sensors are the most common type of ambient sensors [75]. Ambient sensors are not wearable devices, but attached to the surrounding area of a person, for example at home [40]. The low costs and the non-obtrusiveness of pressure sensors are in opposition to their low detection precision, which is below 90% [83].

Passive Infrared (PIR) sensors use infrared signatures to detect falls [75]. As the signal changes with the motion of a hot object in front of the sensor, a person can be recognized [84]. Falling and Activities of Daily Living (ADL) like walking can produce similar signals [84]. Hence, Yazar et al. [84] use a combination of PIR and floor vibration for fall detection. For the analysis of signals from the vibration sensors, a feature extraction method based on a single-tree complex wavelet transform is used. The PIR is integrated for reducing the number of false alarms that can occur due to falling objects or slamming doors. A major disadvantage when using PIR sensors is the restricted area where falls can be detected [75].

Doppler sensors can distinguish moving objects from background noise and have the advantage of being cheap, as well as small [38]. The drawback of this modality is that Doppler sensors are less sensitive to movements orthogonal to the irradiation direction than to movements in the irradiation direction [73]. Tomii and Ohtsuki [73] propose a method using multiple Doppler sensors to reduce the dependency on the movement direction. A support vector machine is used to classify the extracted features, which results in 95.5% of accuracy using three sensors [73]. When using Doppler sensors for fall detection, the fact that the electrometric wave signals can penetrate apartment walls has to be considered, because it limits the usage in a multi-party house [75].

Placing sensors below the floor is another approach for detecting falls. A near-field imaging system developed by Rimminen et al.[63] uses these sensors to monitor user location and movement patterns for fall detection. However, this method is constrained by the sensor's placement area, which can lead to increased costs if the area needs to be expanded. Additionally, the presence of pets or other obstructions can cause false alarms [75].

Alternatively, Velumani and Vijayakumar [76] explore fall detection through changes in channel state information from signals generated by WiFi devices in the user's environment. By analyzing variations in the phase and amplitude of these signals, it is possible to infer human activity and detect falls.

RFID tags attached to shoes are used in Toda and Shinomiya [72]. The tags transmit the pressure transition from person to ground. By analysing the movement specific sensor codes, falling of a person can be detected. Although the classification of the movements achieve 99%, this method has the drawback of the necessity of wearing shoes and the fact that falling can only be discovered when the person is standing or walking.

Finally, both Walabot Home and Vayyar Home are developed and manufactured by Vayyar Imaging Ltd.,[1] and acquire depth and motion data through radar technology. By the very nature of the data acquisition technology, both Vayyar devices are independent of lighting conditions, but according to the technology specification should be operated away from electronic devices such as TVs for instance. While Walabot Home is mainly advertised for only fall detection, the more recent Vayyar Home extends its capabilities to also include presence detection and even offers auxiliary software with which the current estimated position of the surveilled subject within the room can be viewed.

Table 5.1 summarizes the presented non-image based methods for fall detection with regard to the sensors and algorithms used.

5.3.2 Image-Based Fall Detection Methods

While stationary image-based devices can be installed almost everywhere, users might not take wearables with them while sleeping or taking a shower [10]. Getting up at night poses a risk for falling, just as well as wet bathroom floors [10]. Additionally, when using stationary devices, the user does not have to remember wearing and recharging them [10, 41, 75]. Image-based methods combining RGB with skeleton points or using depth images allow usage in day and night conditions [10].

An RGB image is a digital image composed of three color channels: red, green, and blue. Each pixel in an RGB image has a specific value for each of these three colors, which combine to produce a wide spectrum of colors. RGB images are commonly used in various applications, including fall detection systems, due to their ability to capture detailed and colorful visual information.

---

[1] https://vayyar.com/ Accessed 16 September 2024.

5 Fall Detection

Table 5.1 Non-image-based fall detection studies. Wearable approaches are marked with *

Study	Sensors	Algorithm	Privacy sensitive data
Lord and Colvin [39]	Triaxial accelerometer*	G-forces threshold	–
Williams et al. [80]	Piezoelectric shock sensor, mercury tilt switch*	Peak detection, comparing acceleration values and duration	–
Wang et al. [77]	Triaxial accelerometer, gyroscope*	Threshold for acceleration magnitude, acceleration cubic-product-root magnitude and angular velocity cubic-product-root magnitude	–
Sabatini et al. [65]	Inertial and barometric altimeter*	Two-stage decision scheme based on velocity, height and posture	–
Kau and Chen [29]	Electronic compass and triaxial accelerometer of smartphone*	Cascaded classifier with a support vector machine	–
Hakim et al. [23]	Inertial measurement unit of smartphone	Support vector machines, decision trees, nearest neighbour classifiers and discriminant analysis	–
Khan et al. [32]	2 microphones	One-class support vector machine method	Audio data
Yazar et al. [84]	Vibration and passive infrared sensors	Single-tree complex wavelet transform for feature extraction, Euclidean distance, Mahalanobis distance and support vector machine classifiers	Location and activity data
Tomii and Ohtsuki [73]	Multiple Doppler sensors	Feature combination method, support vector machine and k-nearest neighbour	Location data
Rimminen et al. [63]	Electric near field floor sensor	Feature extraction based on number of observations, longest dimension and sum of magnitudes	Location data
Velumani and Vijayakumar [76]	Carrier state information signal from Wi-Fi devices	Waveform analysis by use of a support vector machine	Activity data
Toda and Shinomiya [72]	RFID tags with sensing capabilities*	Multiclass decision forest algorithm	–

In contrast, depth images capture the distance between the camera and objects within a scene. Each pixel represents the distance from the camera to a point, allowing the creation of a three-dimensional representation. This depth information is particularly useful for fall detection as it helps discern spatial positioning and movements, even in low-light conditions. Figure 5.5 illustrates the cogvisAI system using depth images for fall detection, and Fig. 5.6 shows an example of a depth image.

Infrared images are captured using infrared cameras that detect infrared radiation, which is emitted by objects based on their temperature. Infrared imaging is beneficial for fall detection in low-light or dark environments, as it can capture thermal information and provide visibility where RGB cameras may not perform well.

By leveraging these different types of imaging technologies, stationary image-based fall detection systems can effectively monitor and detect falls in various lighting conditions and environments, ensuring continuous and reliable protection for users. Furthermore, image-based methods can monitor more than one person at a time [41]. Computer vision approaches can also more precisely distinguish between falls and ADLs [10]. On the other hand, the use of one single camera in a stationary environment can lead to a restriction in perspective [17].

A further issue arising from the use of image-based methods is the aspect of privacy [51]. Processing RGB images within the system, sending warning signals instead of pictures [10], using depth images [88] or algorithms for hiding people's identities [41] are approaches to assure privacy.

A common approach in image-based fall detection involves training algorithms with large datasets to recognize and classify specific features [17, 88]. Deep learning algorithms are increasingly popular; for example, a transformer-based approach utilizing RGB data to detect falls is presented in [50], and a CNN-based model is

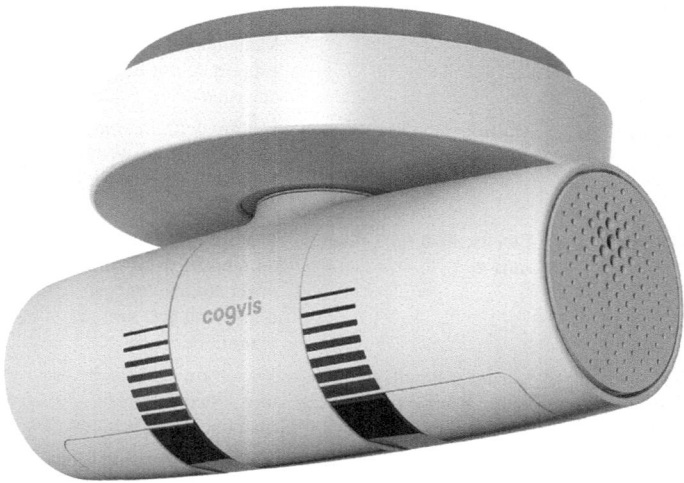

Fig. 5.5 cogvisAI fall detection system

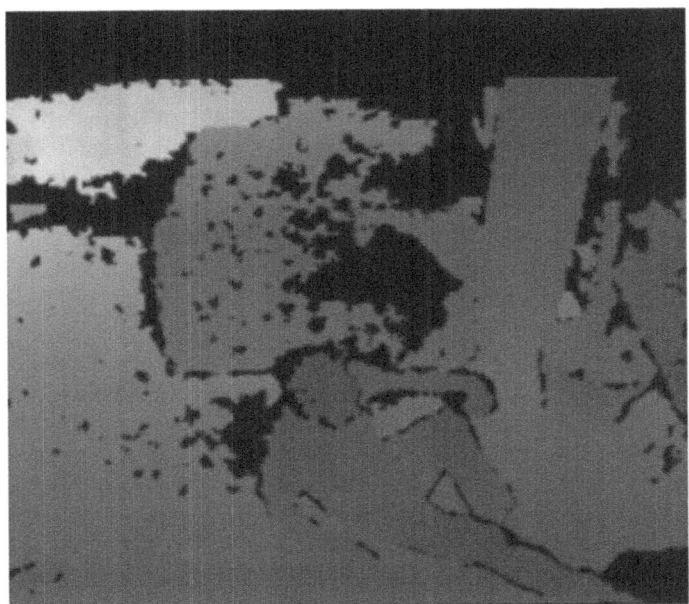

Fig. 5.6 Depth image of fall

proposed in [5]. A comprehensive review of vision-based fall detection systems using deep learning and benchmark datasets is available in [1].

Fan et al. [17] extract the human body using a background subtraction method. Six different shape features are measured to classify the human posture. A classification vector based on the squared first order temporal derivatives of the created slow features is generated. The research team uses a support vector machine to distinguish falls from other activities. Another method presented by ShanShan and Xi [68] is the Gaussian Mixed Model method to extract the human silhouette. Using semi-contour distances, the posture is quantified and classified by a support vector machine technique. Both Fan et al. [17] and ShanShan and Xi [68] extract a person's silhouette from RGB video sequences. Once extracted, only the shape of the human and not his identity is visible.

Another approach is the utilization of a depth camera with the purpose of applying privacy protection at the earliest stage. Planinc and Kampel [53] use the Kinect as a 3D depth sensor in order to calculate the orientation of different body parts. With the use of the least square algorithm, a straight line is fitted to the data points. Together with the floor orientation and the distance between the spine and the floor, a fall is separated from non-falls.

Zhao et al. [88] focus on falls from bed and use a human upper body extraction method to make the algorithm work even when human-bed interactions happen. The Large Margin Nearest Neighbour classification method is used to detect a fall from the bed. The algorithm is implemented on depth image data, using a Microsoft Kinect and a Orbbec Astra camera. The research team highlights the advantage of depth cameras to be insensitive to illumination variation [88].

A system based on the Kinect sensor and fast Fourier transformation is presented by Kong and Meng [35]. At first, the received RGB and depth image from the sensor is transformed into a skeleton image. By using fast Fourier transformation, the image is then encrypted and sent via a carrier image, which has to be decoded. In order to detect a fall, machine learning is applied. When a person is detected by the sensor, the height and width of the created skeleton image are calculated. These parameters are the basis for the classification which is done with a k-Nearest-Neighbour/Support Vector Machine approach.

Ma et al. [41] present a method using a thermal camera to determine and to extract facial regions. Visible light rays enter, controlled by a Spatial Light Modulator (Spatial Light Modulator (SLM)), an RGB camera, where only images with hidden facial regions are processed. In order to detect falls, this method combines a 3D convolutional neural network with an autoencoder. While the neural network is used for feature extraction, the autoencoder models the normal behaviour. A method presented by Kido et al. [33] uses solely a thermal camera to detect falls in bathroom environments. Normal activities in the toilet room are distinguished from falls by performing discriminant analysis. Therefore, the thermal image is split into 81 areas with known average temperature. One disadvantage of this method is that it requires visual confirmation by caregivers [33], and it needs to be trained with data from the particular location.

An alternative solution involves a wearable camera, which ensures fall detection regardless of the environment. The system proposed in [51] combines Histograms of Oriented Gradients with Gradient Local Binary Patterns to generate features, and falls are classified using a relative-entropy-based method. This approach provides flexibility and independence from specific locations [51].

Table 5.2 summarizes the presented image-based fall detection methods.

5.3.3 Collecting Fall Detection Datasets

The collection of fall detection datasets is vital for developing reliable and accurate fall detection systems. However, obtaining real-world data involves significant ethical and practical challenges [69]. It is neither practical nor ethical to ask older adults to intentionally fall for data collection purposes. Consequently, researchers use various methods to simulate falls and gather relevant data.

Typically, fall detection datasets are created using younger, healthier volunteers who can safely simulate falls. These simulations are carefully controlled to replicate various fall scenarios, such as tripping, slipping, or losing balance from different positions like standing, walking, or sitting. However, one should be aware of the potential demographic biases this may bring. The simulated falls are conducted in a variety of environments to capture diverse conditions, including different lighting,

Table 5.2 Image-based fall detection studies

Study	Camera	Algorithm	Privacy sensitive data
Kido et al. [33]	Infrared	discriminant analysis	infrared images
Planinc et al. [53]	Depth	feature extraction by use of similarity to the ground orientation and the height	depth data
Ozcan and Velipasalar [51]	Wearable RGB	relative-entropy-based classification method, HOG are combined with Gradient Local Binary Patterns to generate features	RGB images
Fan et al. [17]	RGB	background subtraction, classification vector based on slow features	RGB images
Kong and Meng [35]	RGB-D	machine learning approach based on height and width of skeleton images	RGB and depth data
ShanShan and Xi [68]	RGB	Gaussian Mixed Model, SVM classification	RGB images
Zhao et al. [88]	Depth	Human upper body extraction method, Large Margin Nearest Neighbour classification	depth data
Ma et al. [41]	RGB and infrared	combination of 3D convolutional neural network and an autoencoder	RGB and infrared images
Núñez-Marcos et al. [50]	RGB	Transformer model	RGB images

flooring, and obstacles. Researchers also use props and safety measures, such as mats and harnesses, to ensure the safety of the volunteers during these simulations.

To enhance ecological validity, researchers strive to make the simulated falls as realistic as possible. Sometimes stunt people are used to gather more realistic falls [42]. However, safety gear can alter the appearance in image-based systems, potentially affecting performance. Additionally, stuntmen are not old individuals, and their falls differ from those of older adults, who may have slower reaction times, different postural control, and varying body compositions. In [64], performing artists assisted by a physiotherapist were recruited to emulate the real fall conditions of older adults.

Despite these efforts, some limitations remain. The physical and behavioral differences between younger volunteers and old individuals can impact the accuracy of the collected data. Differences in age, height, weight, and gender can influence how falls occur and are detected. For instance, older individuals may have slower reaction times, different postural control, and varying body compositions, all of which can affect fall dynamics.

Yu et al. review the literature for fall datasets collected with wearable sensors and report 16 publicly available datasets with at least ten subjects, published between 2010–2021 [85]. A maximum of 50 subjects are included in these datasets, and the sensor setup predominantly uses accelerometers, and gyroscopes, with additional modalities coming from orientation measurements, magnetometers, and barometers. These studies typically include multiple (simulated) falls per subject, and activities of daily living, such as standing up and sitting down. [21] reviews camera-based fall detection databases, and reports RGB, infrared, and depth camera-based datasets. Often, accelerometer data are included to provide an additional modality. Some datasets are collected with multiple cameras. The UR Fall Detection dataset was obtained with two depth cameras [31]. Here, one camera provides a frontal (or side) view, and the second provides a vertical (or top) view. Similarly, the BOMNI dataset was collected via two omni-directional cameras, one at the ceiling and one side camera at person height [11]. In [64], two infrared thermal sensors were used to record very low resolution images (32×32 and 8×1, respectively). [44] lists further vision-based and multimodal datasets.

5.4 Fall Prevention

Fall prevention is about using technology to reduce risks and avoid falls. Some systems aim to recognize balance and motion abnormalities to evaluate an individual's fall risk [14]. Another approach involves detecting when a person sits up in bed or leaves the bed and sending alarms to caregivers for assistance [25]. In this context, the event of a person getting up from bed is referred to as a "getup event" or simply "getup."

5.4.1 Non-image-Based Fall Prevention

A common method to prevent patients from falling out of bed is the use of restraints such as bed rails [61]. However, the application of restraints has been associated with an increased risk of injury [16]. Alternative solutions include beds mounted close to the ground and floor mats placed in front of the bed, which aim to prevent falls and minimize the extent of injuries [25]. A significant drawback of these devices is that they do not have the capability to alert nursing staff [4].

Pressure-sensitive mats (also called smart mats) which can send alarms when the pressure exceeds a certain threshold, offer another solution [9, 36]. However, these mats can pose a tripping hazard, adding another layer of risk [15].

Hilbe et al. [25] present a pressure-based device called *Bucinator* to eliminate those drawbacks. The device mounted under the mattress alarms health workers when patients are leaving the bed. Rails filled with air are connected with a pressure sensor, which generates an electrical alarm when exceeding a predefined threshold.

In general, one can group fall prevention systems into those that detect a person in danger of falling (in the following called direct fall prevention approaches) and those that help to improve a person's balance and strength (in the following called indirect approaches) [2]. One example of an indirect approach is a robot developed by Maneeprom et al. [43]. The robot shows videos about how to prevent falls, giving advice on choosing appropriate shoes and walking assistive devices. Additionally, daily voice messages and exercise reminders are provided.

Direct approaches can be divided into two subgroups. On the one hand, there are assessments to classify a person's risk of fall based on balance and mobility tests [14]. A method developed by Yamada et al. [82] uses the Wii Fit's "Ski Slalom" and "Basic Step" games to assess the fall risk of older adults. Comparing the results with five different tests like the Timed Up & Go (TUG) under single- and dual-task conditions, the "Basic Step" game shows a significant difference between fallers and nonfallers [82]. The TUG is a commonly used method to assess the risk of a person falling by determining the time a person needs for standing up from a chair, walking three metres and returning to sit on the chair again [26, 82]. On the other hand, there are devices like the Bucinator which alarm health staff in case of an urgent risk of falling, analysing the person's posture, balance or pressure on a sensor [25].

Lee et al. [37] use ten piezoresistive pressure sensor pads positioned in a bed mattress to measure the pressure applied on the sensors. By evaluating the pressure values, a person's position and activity status is determined. When a person is about to exit the bed, an alarm is sent via a mobile application.

A method based on a body-worn accelerometer is presented by Wolf et al. [81]. An accelerometer positioned with a tape on the user's leg calculates the orientation of the sensor and the amount of movement to distinguish between lying, sitting and standing. Ribeiro et al. [62] developed a mat consisting of a pressure sensor and a 3-axial accelerometer to detect movements on the bed or armchair. A control system analyses arm as well as torso movements to detect a person getting up from bed or from a chair. A warning level loop with different states is used to offer the opportunity to manually deactivate a visual warning light before sending an acoustic alarm.

Table 5.3 summarizes the presented non-image-based methods for fall prevention.

Table 5.3 Non-image-based fall prevention studies

Study	Wearable	Principle	Privacy sensitive data
Hilbe et al. [25]	No	Pressure-sensitive device mounted under the mattress, alarm when exceeding threshold	Bed exit
Yamada et al. [82]	No	Wii Fit games for fall risk assessment	–
Wolf et al. [81]	Yes	Body-worn accelerometer	Bed exit
Lee et al. [37]	No	Pressure sensor pads in the mattress	Bed exit
Ribeiro et al. [62]	No	Pressure sensor and 3-axial accelerometer	Bed exit
Maneeprom et al. [43]	No	Robot providing videos and audio messages to prevent falls	–

5.4.2 Image-Based Fall Prevention

Image-based sensors play a role for both fall detection and fall prevention. They are used to measure balance, stability, reaction time, diversions from typical activity patterns and other physical parameters [2, 15]. Moreover, they are used for games and activities operated via a camera with the intention to improve a person's balance and strength [52].

The use of image-based sensors began with tools like the *Kinect*, which were initially employed to assess fall risk among older adults [14, 26, 59]. Today, there are numerous 3D sensor technologies and modalities, including Radar, available to enhance fall risk assessment.

In Kampel et al. [26] a 3D sensor automatically analyzes gait by calculating the start and end times of the six phases of the Timed Up and Go (TUG) test. This method uses the trajectory of the spine-shoulder joint when working with skeleton data, or the center of mass of the person when using depth data.

Also using, Dubois et al. [14] develop a method to automatically evaluate a person's fall risk by having them perform eight different balance tasks in front of the sensor. In order to assess the stability during a task, the body centroid is calculated. The horizontal dispersion of the pixel cloud is used to determine whether a person uses the arms to maintain the balance. For the final assessment of the individual fall risk, apart from the balance tasks, the age, average physical activity and gait are considered as well.

In a home environment setting, the Kinect system continuously monitors gait parameters like velocity, step length, and stride length in [59]. This allows for regular tracking of fall risk factors, with the added benefit of alerting nursing staff if the risk increases. The inclusion of Doppler radar helps prevent occlusions, ensuring continuous monitoring. Similar to bed exit alarm systems, cameras can also notify health workers when a patient at high risk of falling is about to leave their bed [4, 48].

The Kinect's depth sensor and RGB camera are integrated by Ni et al. [48] to monitor patients and alert nursing staff when necessary. They define the area around the bed as a region of interest, which is divided into eight rectangular blocks. Motion and shape features are extracted from these blocks and combined using a multiple kernel learning framework to provide a comprehensive monitoring solution.

The system *Ocuvera*, developed by Bauer et al. [4] uses the Kinect's depth sensor only. After detecting the floor and the bed, machine-learned shape models are used to find human shapes. For every person found in the scene the likelihood of bed exit is predicted in order to trigger alarms before a person exits the bed. Problems that still need to be addressed are the integration in existing alarm technology of hospitals and the improvement of the algorithm in order minimize the time between the event and the alarm [4].

Table 5.4 summarizes the presented image-based methods for fall prevention.

5.5 Dealing with Privacy

When developing new AAL devices, ethical considerations are crucial to ensure user acceptance [8]. The AALIANCE2 Consortium highlights privacy protection as one of the four key ethical issues in AAL, alongside risks of social isolation, abuse, and consent [8].

Table 5.4 Image-based fall prevention studies

Study	Cameras	Parameters	Privacy sensitive data
Ni et al. [48]	RGB-D	Motion and shape features including motion history images, histogram of optic flows and histogram of oriented gradients	RGB and depth data
Rantz et al. [59]	Depth, 2 webcams, Doppler radar	Velocity, step length, and stride length	Depth data
Bauer et al. [4]	Depth	Machine-learned shape models	Depth data
Kampel et al. [26]	Depth	Trajectory of the spine-shoulder joint, center of mass	Depth data
Dubois et al. [14]	Depth	Body centroid and dispersion depth data	Depth data
Pramerdorfer et al. [55]	Depth	Deep learning	Depth data

Privacy concerns are a major issue with image-based fall detection technologies [49]. For example, Lord and Colvin [39] developed a fall detection system that combines RGB video monitoring with an accelerometer. Although the system showed promising results, it faced low user acceptance primarily due to privacy concerns [39]. In response, several research teams are actively working on solutions that address these privacy issues while still providing effective fall detection and prevention [41, 88].

Depth cameras offer early-stage privacy protection because they capture only the distance between surfaces and the camera, which makes it impossible to directly identify individuals from the images [46, 47, 56, 88]. Similarly, thermal cameras, like the one used by Ma et al.[41], enhance privacy by masking facial regions. Thermal imaging is inherently privacy-safe as it cannot distinguish between individual faces due to similar temperature distributions among them [33, 87]. In this approach, a Spatial Light Modulator (SLM) blocks visible light from facial regions, rendering them black in the RGB image. This is achieved using a cold mirror,[2] which allows for the simultaneous capture of thermal and RGB images, ensuring that only anonymous video output is produced.

Pre-processing methods, such as altering RGB images at the capture stage, can mitigate privacy risks before hiding facial regions [41]. However, this approach relies on the accuracy of face detection algorithms [41, 49]. Kido et al. [33] address this by using only an infrared camera, bypassing the need for facial recognition. If privacy protection is applied later or involves wireless communication, encryption and data security methods must be employed [60].

The wearable RGB camera presented by Ozcan and Velipasalar [51] captures environmental images, processed locally without storage, but this method raises privacy concerns for bystanders [45]. Sabatini et al. [65] note that while wearable sensors typically do not raise privacy issues, devices using GPS or audio data can be intrusive [3]. Khan et al. [32] suggest that audio-based approaches, with active microphones, reduce privacy concerns compared to image-based methods.

Tables 5.1 and 5.4 summarize image-based and non-image-based methods for fall prevention and detection, respectively, including the types of privacy-sensitive data they process.

Additionally, fall detection from silhouettes and gait biometrics can pose privacy risks, as these methods can potentially expose individual identities. Ensuring that these biometric data are anonymized or securely handled is critical to maintaining user privacy.

In 2006, Hensel et al. [24] defined obtrusiveness as a "summary evaluation by the user based on characteristics or effects associated with the technology that are perceived as undesirable and physically and/or psychologically prominent" [24]. This work introduced categories and dimensions of obtrusiveness, laying the groundwork for its measurement. Twelve years later, Blasco et al. [7] adopted Hensel's framework,

---

[2] A cold mirror is a dichroic filter that absorbs approximately 80% of infrared rays while reflecting visible light [41].

emphasizing the subjectivity of obtrusiveness and observing that different users may perceive the same technology's impact on their privacy differently [7, 24].

5.6 Usability

Fall detection solutions based on visual sensing are typically placed on the ceiling or top view positions to see as much as possible in the room. The range of a sensor is limited (3D sensors range up to 8 m, RGB cameras see further). One sensor per room is therefore applicable, it depends on the room's size. Connectivity is important, since all sensors need a network connection to alert or to process the data acquired. The acquired data is either processed on the device, for example on a raspberry PI (see cogvisAI), or the data is streamed to a cloud service or remote server. Privacy by design aspects are better integrated in the first solution, since no (personal) data leaves the sensors.

One of the significant challenges in the usability of fall detection systems is managing false positives. Frequent false alarms can lead to alarm fatigue, where caregivers can start to ignore alerts, potentially missing real fall incidents. To address this, advanced algorithms and machine learning techniques are being developed to improve the accuracy of fall detection systems, thereby reducing the occurrence of false alarms. Systems that allow for customization of the sensitivity settings can help balance the detection accuracy according to the specific needs of the user.

Another challenge is false negatives. When the sensitivity is set too low or occlusions occur, the system might fail to detect a fall. Detecting every single fall is crucial, even if it means dealing with a few false alarms, as the consequences of a missed fall can be severe.

5.7 Conclusion

Fall detection as a research topic is considered a solved problem, and market entry and commercialization are on the way. Open issues deal with detecting falls from persons using wheelchairs, walking aids, and systems in large rooms with multiple people. Practical problems like maintenance, installation, or connectivity still need to be improved. Technology acceptance and privacy issues slow down the widespread use of fall detection solutions.

Accelerator-based fall detection systems are very unreliable since falls might occur in slow motion and take up to 2 min. Camera-based systems are hardly accepted due to privacy issues; pixeling of persons or other filtering applied to images does not change this. Camera-based systems are dependent on proper illumination, and have reduced functionality during the night. A possible future solution relies on WiFi for behavior analysis, but this technology currently still lacks domain generalization.

References

1. Alam, E., Sufian, A., Dutta, P., Leo, M.: Vision-based human fall detection systems using deep learning: a review. Comput. Biol. Med. **146**, 105,626 (2022)
2. Atoyebi, O.A., Stewart, A., Sampson, J.: Use of information technology for fall detection and prevention in the elderly. Springer Sci. Bus. Med. **40**, 277–299 (2014)
3. Avancha, S., Baxi, A., Kotz, D.: Privacy in mobile technology for personal healthcare. ACM Comput. Surv. **45**(1) (2012)
4. Bauer, P., Rush, B., Kramer, J.B., Sabalka, L.: Modeling bed exit likelihood in a camera-based automated video monitoring application. In: IEE International Conference on Electro Information Technology (EIT), pp. 56–61 (2017)
5. Bhavani, D., Ukrit, F.: Design of inception with deep convolutional neural network based fall detection and classification model. Multimed. Tools Appl. **83**, 23,799 (2024)
6. Blake, A., Morgan, K., Bendall, M.J., Dallosso, H., Ebrahim, S.B., Arie, T.H., Fentem, P.H., Bassey, E.J.: Falls by elderly people at home: prevalence and associated factors. Age Ageing **17**(6), 365–372 (1988)
7. Blasco, S.A., Llobet, D.N., Koumanakos, G.: Obtrusiveness Considerations of AAL Environments, pp. 19–32. Springer (2018)
8. van den Broek, G., Cavallo, F., Wehrmann, C.: Ambient assisted living roadmap. In: AALIANCE2—European Next Generation of Ambient Assisted Living Alliance (2014)
9. Capezuti, E., Brush, B.L., Lane, S., Rabinowitz, H.U., Secic, M.: Bed-exit alarm effectiveness. Arch. Gerontol. Geriatr. **49**(1), 27–31 (2008)
10. Dai, B., Yang, D., Ai, L., Zhang, P.: A novel video-surveillance-based algorithm of fall detection. In: 11th International Congress on Image and Signal Processing, BioMedical Engineering and Informatics (2018)
11. Demiröz, B.E., Ari, I., Eroğlu, O., Salah, A.A., Akarun, L.: Feature-based tracking on a multi-omnidirectional camera dataset. In: 2012 5th International Symposium on Communications, Control and Signal Processing, pp. 1–5. IEEE (2012)
12. Department of Health and Human Services Centers for Disease Control and Prevention: Fatalities and injuries from falls among older adults - United States, 1993–2003 and 2001–2005. Morb. Mortal. Wkly. Rep. **55**(45), 1221–1242 (2006)
13. Downton, J.H., Andrews, K.: Prevalence, characteristics and factors associated with falls among the elderly living at home. Aging Clin. Exp. Res. **3**(3), 219–228 (1991)
14. Dubois, A., Mouthon, A., Sivagnanaselvam, R.S., Bresciani, J.: Fast and automatic assessment of fall risk by coupling machine learning algorithms with a depth camera to monitor simple balance tasks. J. NeuroEng. Rehabil. **16**(1) (2019)
15. Ejupi, A.: New sensor-based methods for clinical and in-home assessment of fall risk in older people. Master's Thesis, University of Technology Vienna (2015)
16. Evans, D., Wood, J., Lamber, L., Fitzgerald, M.: Physical restraint in acute and residential care: a systematic review. The Joanna Briggs Institute (2002)
17. Fan, K., Wang, P., Zhuang, S.: Human fall detection using slow feature analysis. Multimed. Tools Appl. **78**, 9101–9128 (2019)
18. Florence, C.S., Bergen, G., Atherly, A., Burns, E., Stevens, J., Drake, S.: Medical costs of fatal and nonfatal falls in older adults. J. Am. Geriatr. Soc. **66**(4), 693–698 (2018)
19. Fried, L.P., Tangen, C.M., Walston, J., Newman, A.B., Hirsch, C., Gottdiener, J., Seeman, T., Tracy, R., Kop, W.J., Burke, G.: Frailty in older adults: evidence for a phenotype. J. Gerontol. Med. Sci. **56A**(3), M146–M156 (2001)
20. Gurley, R.J., Lum, N., Sande, M., Lo, B., Katz, M.H.: Persons found in their homes helpless or dead. New Engl. J. Med. 1710–1716 (1996)
21. Gutiérrez, J., Rodríguez, V., Martin, S.: Comprehensive review of vision-based fall detection systems. Sensors **21**(3), 947 (2021)
22. Habib, M.A., Mohktar, M.S., Kamaruzzaman, S.B., Lim, K.S., Pin, T.M., Ibrahim, F.: Smartphone-based solutions for fall detection and prevention: challenges and open issues. Sensors **14**, 7181–7208 (2014)

23. Hakim, A., Huq, M.S., Shanta, S., Ibrahim, B.: Smartphone based data mining for fall detection: analysis and design. In: 2016 IEEE International Symposium on Robotics and Intelligent Sensors, pp. 46–51 (2016)
24. Hensel, B.K., Demiris, G., Courtney, K.L.: Defining obtrusiveness in home telehealth technologies: a conceptual framework. J. Am. Med. Inform. Assoc. **13**(4), 428–431 (2006)
25. Hilbe, J., Schulc, E., Linder, B., Them, C.: Development and alarm threshold evaluation of a side rail integrated sensor technology for the prevention of falls. Int. J. Med. Inform. **79**(3), 173–180 (2010)
26. Kampel, M., Doppelbauer, S., Planinc, R.: Automated time up & go test for functional decline assessment of older adults. In: 12th EAI International Conference on Pervasive Computing Technologies for Healthcare, pp. 208–216 (2018)
27. Kannus, P., Palvanen, M., Niemi, S., Parkkari, J.: Alarming rise in the number and incidence of fall-induced cervical spine injuries among older adults. J. Gerontol. Med. Sci. **62A**(2), 180–183 (2007)
28. Kannus, P., Parkkari, J., Niemi, S., Palvanen, M.: Fall-induced deaths among elderly people. Am. J. Public Health **95**(3), 422–424 (2005)
29. Kau, L., Chen, C.: A smart phone-based pocket fall accident detection, positioning and rescue system. IEEE J. Biomed. Health Inform. **19**(1), 44–56 (2015)
30. Kennedy, T.: The prevention of falls in later life. A report of the Kellogg International Work Group on the Prevention of Falls by the Elderly. Danish Med. Bull. **34**(4), 1–24 (1987)
31. Kepski, M., Kwolek, B.: Embedded system for fall detection using body-worn accelerometer and depth sensor. In: 2015 IEEE 8th International Conference on Intelligent Data Acquisition and Advanced Computing Systems: Technology and Applications (IDAACS), vol. 2, pp. 755–759. IEEE (2015)
32. Khan, M.S., Yu, M., Feng, P., Wang, L., Chambers, J.: An unsupervised acoustic fall detection system using source separation for sound interference suppression. Signal Process. **110**, 199–210 (2015)
33. Kido, S., Miyasaka, T., Tanaka, T., Shimizu, T., Saga, T.: Fall detection in toilet rooms using thermal imaging sensors. In: Proceedings of IEEE/SICE International Symposium on System Integration (SII), pp. 83–88 (2009)
34. Kochanek, K.D., Murphy, S.L., Xu, J., Tejada-Vera, B.: National vital statistics report. Deaths: final data for 2014. Centers Dis. Control Prev. **65**(4), 44–45 (2016)
35. Kong, X., Meng, Z.: A privacy protected fall detection IoT system for elderly persons using depth camera. In: Proceedings of the International Conference on Advanced Mechatronic Systems, pp. 31–35 (2018)
36. Kumar, V., Yeo, B., Lim, W., Raja, J.E., Koh, K.: Development of electronic floor mat for fall detection and elderly care. Asian J. Sci. Res. **11**, 344–356 (2018)
37. Lee, C., Yang, S., Li, C., Liu, M., Kuo, P.: Alarm system for bed exit and prolonged bed rest. In: Proceedings of the 2018 International Conference on Machine Learning and Cybernetics, pp. 439–443 (2018)
38. Liu, L., Popescu, M., Skubic, M., Rantz, M.: An automatic fall detection framework using data fusion of doppler radar and motion sensor network. In: Conference Proceeding IEEE Engineering in Medicine and Biology Society, pp. 5940–5943 (2014)
39. Lord, C.J., Colvin, D.P.: Falls in the elderly: detection and assessment. Technol. Aging **35**(1–4), 1938–1939 (1991)
40. Luque, R., Casilari, E., Morón, M., Redondo, G.: Comparison and characterization of android-based fall detection systems. Sensors **14**, 18543–18574 (2014)
41. Ma, C., Shimada, A., Uchiyama, H., Nagahara, H., Taniguchi, R.: Fall detection using optical level anonymous image sensing system. Opt. Laser Technol. **110**, 44–61 (2019)
42. Madsen, T., Andersen, C.S., Varhelyi, A., Nilsson, M., Oskarsson, M., Jensen, M.B., Bahnsen, C.H., Christensen, M.B., Moeslund, T.: Mobile application for naturalistic walking/cycling data collection. InDeV Consortium Report (2017)
43. Maneeprom, N., Taneepanichskul, S., Panza, A., Suputtitada, A.: Effectiveness of robotics fall prevention program among elderly in senior housings, Bangkok, Thailand: a quasi-experimental study. Clin. Interv. Aging **14**, 335–346 (2019)

44. Martínez-Villaseñor, L., Ponce, H., Brieva, J., Moya-Albor, E., Núñez-Martínez, J., Peñafort-Asturiano, C.: Up-fall detection dataset: a multimodal approach. Sensors **19**(9), 1988 (2019)
45. Michael, K.: Sousveillance: implications for privacy, security, trust, and the law. IEEE Consum. Electron. Mag. 92–94 (2015)
46. Mucha, W., Kampel, M.: Addressing privacy concerns in depth sensors. In: International Conference on Computers Helping People with Special Needs, pp. 526–533. Springer (2022)
47. Mucha, W., Kampel, M.: Beyond privacy of depth sensors in active and assisted living devices. In: Proceedings of the 15th International Conference on Pervasive Technologies Related to Assistive Environments, pp. 425–429 (2022)
48. Ni, B., Dat, N.C., Moulin, P.: RGBD-camera based get-up event detection for hospital fall prevention. In: IEEE International Conference on Acoustics, Speech and Signal Processing, pp. 1405–1408 (2012)
49. Noury, N., Fleury, A., Rumeau, P., Bourke, A.K., Laighin, G.Ó., Rialle, V., Lundy, J.E.: Fall detection—principles and methods. In: Proceedings of the 29th Annual International Conference of the IEEE EMBS, pp. 1663–1666 (2007)
50. Núñez-Marcos, A., Arganda-Carreras, I.: Transformer-based fall detection in videos. Eng. Appl. Artif. Intell. **132**, 107,937 (2024)
51. Ozcan, K., Velipasalar, S.: Autonomous fall detection with wearable cameras by using relative entropy distance measure. IEEE Trans. Human Mach. Syst. **47**(1), 31–39 (2017)
52. Palestra, G., Rebiai, M., Courtial, E., Giokas, K., Koutsouris, D.: A fall prevention system for the elderly: preliminary results. In: IEEE 30th International Symposium on Computer-Based Medical Systems, pp. 550–551 (2017)
53. Planinc, R., Kampel, M.: Introducing the use of depth data for fall detection. Pers. Ubiquit. Comput. **17**(6), 1063–1072 (2013)
54. Popescu, M., Mahnot, A.: Acoustic fall detection using one-class classifiers. In: 31st Annual International Conference of the IEEE, pp. 3505–3508 (2009)
55. Pramerdorfer, C., Planinc, R., Kampel, M.: Effective deep-learning-based depth data analysis on low-power hardware for supporting elderly care. In: 2020 IEEE/CVF Conference on Computer Vision and Pattern Recognition Workshops (CVPRW), pp. 1584–1590 (2020). https://doi.org/10.1109/CVPRW50498.2020.00205
56. Pramerdorfer, C., Planinc, R., Loock, M.V., Fankhauser, D., Kampel, M., Brandstötter, M.: Fall detection based on depth-data in practice. In: European Conference on Computer Vision, pp. 195–208 (2016)
57. Prudham, D., Evans, J.G.: Factors associated with falls in the elderly: a community study. Age Ageing **10**(3), 141–146 (1981)
58. Public Health Agency of Canada: Report on seniors' falls in Canada (2005). Minister of Public Works and Government Services Canada
59. Rantz, M., Skubic, M., Abbott, C., Galambos, C., Popescu, M., Keller, J., Stone, E., Back, J., Miller, S.J., Petroski, G.F.: Automated in-home fall risk assessment and detection sensor system for elders. Gerontologist **55**(S1), 78–87 (2015)
60. Rashidi, P., Mihailidis, A.: A survey on ambient-assisted living tools for older adults. IEEE J. Biomed. Health Inform. **17**(3), 579–590 (2013)
61. von Renteln-Kruse, W., Krause, T.: Sturzereignisse stationärer geriatrischer Patienten-Ergebnisse einer 3-jährigen prospektiven Erfassung. Z. Gerontol. Geriatr. **137**, 9–14 (2004)
62. Ribeiro, A., Pereira, S., Madureira, A., Mourao, L., Coelho, L.: A low-cost automatic fall prevention system for inpatients. In: 2018 Global Medical Engineering Physics Exchanges, pp. 1–4 (2018)
63. Rimminen, H., Lindström, J., Linnavuo, M., Sepponen, R.: Detection of falls among the elderly by a floor sensor using the electric near field. IEEE Trans. Inform. Technol. Biomed. **14**(6), 1475–1476 (2010)
64. Riquelme, F., Espinoza, C., Rodenas, T., Minonzio, J.G., Taramasco, C.: eHomeSeniors dataset: an infrared thermal sensor dataset for automatic fall detection research. Sensors **19**(20), 4565 (2019)

65. Sabatini, A.M., Ligorio, G., Mannini, A., Genovese, V., Pinna, L.: Prior-to- and post-impact fall detection using inertial and barometric altimeter measurements. IEEE Trans. Neural Syst. Rehabil. Eng. **24**(7), 774–783 (2016)
66. Scott, V., Peck, S., Kendall, P.: Prevention of falls and injuries among the elderly: a special report from the office of the provincial health officer. British Columbia, Ministry of Health Planning (2004)
67. Scuffham, P., Chaplin, S., Legood, R.: Incidence and costs of unintentional falls in older people in the United Kingdom. J. Epidemiol. Community Health **57**, 740–744 (2003)
68. ShanShan, X., Xi, C.: Fall detection method based on semi-contour distances. In: Proceedings of ICSP, pp. 785–788 (2018)
69. Stack, E.: Falls are unintentional: studying simulations is a waste of faking time. J. Rehabil. Assist. Technol. Eng. **4**, 2055668317732,945 (2017)
70. Stalenhoef, P.A., Diederiks, J.P., Knottnerus, J.A., Kester, A.D., Crebolder, H.F.: A risk model for the prediction of recurrent falls in community-dwelling elderly: a prospective cohort study. J. Clin. Epidemiol. **55**(11), 1088–1094 (2002)
71. Tipirneni, R.: San Diego County elderly falls report. County of San Diego (2005)
72. Toda, K., Shinomiya, N.: Fall detection system for the elderly using RFID tags with sensing capability. In: IEEE 7th Global Conference on Consumer Electronics, pp. 475–478 (2018)
73. Tomii, S., Ohtsuki, T.: Falling detection using multiple doppler sensors. In: IEEE 14th International Conference on e-Health Networking, Applications and Services, pp. 196–201 (2012)
74. United Nations: World population ageing 2017. Department of Economic and Social Affairs Population Division, pp. 29–31 (2017)
75. Vallabh, P., Malekian, R.: Fall detection monitoring systems: a comprehensive review. J. Ambient Intell. Human Comput. **9**, 1809–1833 (2018)
76. Velumani, R., Vijayakumar, M.: Prudent automatic falls detection by analyzing the carrier state information signal using Wi-Fi devices. J. Test. Eval. **47**(4), 2947–2963 (2019)
77. Wang, F., Chan, H., Hsu, M., Lin, C., Chao, P., Chang, Y.: Threshold-based fall detection using a hybrid of tri-axial accelerometer and gyroscope. Physiol. Meas. **39**(10) (2018)
78. WHO: WHO global report on falls prevention in older age. World Health Organization (2007)
79. Wild, D., Nayak, U., Isaacs, B.: How dangerous are falls in old people at home? BMJ **282**, 266–268 (1981)
80. Williams, G., Doughty, K., Cameron, K., Bradley, D.A.: A smart fall & activity monitor for telecare applications. In: Proceedings of the 20th Annual International Conference of the IEEE Engineering in Medicine and Biology Society **20**(3), 1151–1154 (1998)
81. Wolf, K.H., Hetzer, K., zu Schwabedissen, H.M., Wiese, B., Marschollek, M.: Development and pilot study of a bed-exit alarm based on a body-worn accelerometer. Zeitschrift für Gerontologie und Geriatrie, pp. 727–733 (2013)
82. Yamada, M., Aoyama, T., Nakamura, M., Tanaka, B., Nagai, K., Tatematsu, N., Uemura, K., Nakamura, T., Tsuboyama, T., Ichihashi, N.: The reliability and preliminary validity of game-based fall risk assessment in community-dwelling older adults. Geriatr. Nurs. **32**(3), 188–194 (2011)
83. Yang, L., Ren, Y., Zhang, W.: 3D depth image analysis for indoor fall detection of elderly people. Digit. Commun. Netw. **2**, 24–34 (2016)
84. Yazar, A., Keskin, F., Töreyin, B.U., Cetin, A.E.: Fall detection using single-tree complex wavelet transform. Pattern Recogn. Lett. **34**, 1945–1952 (2013)
85. Yu, X., Jang, J., Xiong, S.: A large-scale open motion dataset (KFall) and benchmark algorithms for detecting pre-impact fall of the elderly using wearable inertial sensors. Front. Aging Neurosci. **13**, 692,865 (2021)
86. Zecevic, A.A., Salmoni, A.W., S., M., Vandervoort, A.A.: Defining a fall and reasons for falling: comparisons among the views of seniors, health care providers and the research literature. The Gerontologist **46**(3), 367–376 (2006)
87. Zhang, Y., Lu, Y., Nagahara, H., Taniguchi, R.I.: Anonymous camera for privacy protection. In: Proceedings of the 22nd International Conference on Pattern Recognition (ICPR), pp. 4170–4175 (2014)

88. Zhao, F., Cao, Z., Xiao, Y., Mao, J., Yuan, J.: Real-time detection of fall from bed using a single depth camera. IEEE Trans. Autom. Sci. Eng. (2018)

Open Access This chapter is licensed under the terms of the Creative Commons Attribution 4.0 International License (http://creativecommons.org/licenses/by/4.0/), which permits use, sharing, adaptation, distribution and reproduction in any medium or format, as long as you give appropriate credit to the original author(s) and the source, provide a link to the Creative Commons license and indicate if changes were made.

The images or other third party material in this chapter are included in the chapter's Creative Commons license, unless indicated otherwise in a credit line to the material. If material is not included in the chapter's Creative Commons license and your intended use is not permitted by statutory regulation or exceeds the permitted use, you will need to obtain permission directly from the copyright holder.

Chapter 6
Privacy-Aware Video-Based Methods for Gait and Frailty Recognition in Active and Assisted Living Environments

Pau Climent-Pérez and Francisco Florez-Revuelta

Abstract In the field of Active Assisted Living (AAL), maintaining the privacy of individuals while effectively monitoring their health and mobility status remains an unsolved question. In medicine and gerontology, several metrics have been developed to assess mobility of older adults, and the relationship between these metrics and future outcomes has been established with some success. This chapter delves into the utilization of video-based methods for gait and frailty recognition, presenting a comprehensive overview of techniques, challenges, and advancements in the field. By analysing patterns in gait, subtle changes indicative of frailty or potential health deterioration can be detected early, facilitating timely interventions and personalized care. However, the deployment of video-based gait recognition systems in AAL environments requires a delicate balance between the efficacy of monitoring and safeguarding individual privacy. This chapter analyses existing frailty metrics and their potential use in automated ecological momentary assessment from heterogeneous sensors, including video, and with a high emphasis on privacy preservation when doing so.

Keywords Active assisted living (AAL) · Gait recognition · Frailty recognition · Privacy preserving methods · Computer vision · Machine learning · Smart devices · Sensors

6.1 Introduction

The so-called 'social challenges' of the Horizon 2020 programmes, and subsequently of Horizon Europe, arise from the needs, often urgent, of European societies. These challenges determine the main lines of research to be financed due to their interest.

P. Climent-Pérez (✉) · F. Florez-Revuelta
University of Alicante, Alicante, Spain
e-mail: pau.climent@ua.es

F. Florez-Revuelta
e-mail: francisco.florez@ua.es

Among these, the first place is given to the challenge named 'Health, demographic change, and well-being'. This is easily explained by the ageing of societies, and especially its effect on European ones. The care of older people and their quality of life will be one of the main concerns in coming years due to its effects on the rest of society [79].

In response to this social challenge, the research field called Ambient Assisted Living, or subsequently Active Assisted Living (AAL) emerged, which is the topic covered in this book. The methods and techniques developed in this field aim to improve the quality of life of older adults or those with *frailty* by supporting their daily lives. Here 'frailty' can be defined as a syndrome with multiple causes characterized by a reduction in resistance, strength, and physiological functions, resulting in greater vulnerability to dependence or death. Similarly, it is an indicator of resistance to stressors, with frail individuals showing it in lower degrees. It also causes adverse effects on health and functional decline, although it is reversible through intervention, leading to the demand for methods to detect it correctly and reliably [1].

People with frailty are limited when performing activities of daily living (ADLs). In the field of AAL, multiple methods have therefore been developed for their recognition. This is done with two purposes: on one hand, to recognize activities in order to provide necessary support at each moment [23]; on the other hand, to recognize the performance of activities to identify and assess the degree of frailty.

In addition to limitations in activities, people with frailty often show mobility impairments, thus showing a higher risk of falls and hospitalization [82]. Although initially, in the AAL field, there was a strong focus on fall detection (due to limitations in technological possibilities), subsequently, prevention has been emphasized (also see Chap. 5 in this volume [66]). Therefore, different ways to evaluate frailty through gait analysis have also been developed. Gait patterns stand out as a relevant tool in assessing an individual's mobility and overall health status. By analysing these patterns, subtle changes indicative of frailty or potential health deterioration can be detected early, facilitating timely interventions and personalized care. One way to perform this analysis is through the use of wearable devices that users must wear during data collection [5, 111, 131], or through "walkways" consisting of pressure-sensing carpets [28, 82].

However, this can be inconvenient in some cases, and the use of sensors installed in the environment that are not uncomfortable or bothersome to the user is preferable. Additionally, in this way, data collection, and therefore the assessment of gait, frailty, or the presence of a medical condition, can be continuously performed in the patient's preferred environment, without requiring their attention or active interaction with the system. This achieves an ecological and momentary analysis (data capture being performed at each moment in time) [51].

Ecological momentary assessment (EMA) can be applied in the context of AAL to assess the health status, well-being, needs, and users' preferences of aforementioned technologies [118]. With EMA, parameters of physical activity (sedentary behaviour) can be measured [68], technologies that may be most useful for supporting dementia or frailty can be identified (by having data collected at times of difficulty) [83], and it can also be used to measure the behavioural and psychological symptoms of frailty states using multimodal sensors and provide personalized, tailored interventions [73]. EMA can offer a more precise and detailed insight into the needs and behaviours of AAL users than traditional self-report or observation methods. EMA can also facilitate user involvement in the design and evaluation of AAL technologies, which can improve their acceptance and satisfaction. Finally, EMA can be a useful tool for improving the quality of life and autonomy of older people or people with disabilities using AAL.

Cameras can serve this purpose since they do not require user intervention; they are simply installed in the environment and perform analysis by capturing images. In laboratory environments, precise measurements can be made using motion capture (MoCap) systems [60], although the use of reflective markers on the user is necessary for this. Therefore, since the emergence of depth cameras (RGB-D, such as Kinect and similar devices), research aimed to replicate the precision of MoCap systems in less controlled environments (laboratories, but also homes) without the need for markers [29, 74].

With the advent of complex or deep neural networks (deep learning, DL), it has become possible to even eliminate the need for capturing depth data. Initially, estimating depth with a single camera is an inherently ambiguous problem. However, it is possible to extract two-dimensional (2D) data about the coordinates in the image plane (x, y) of body joints (creating a 'skeleton' by connecting them) [19]. Additionally, more recently, and by exploiting the peculiarities of calibrated cameras or by resolving ambiguity using heuristics, it is also possible to obtain 3D data. In this case, the coordinates (x, y, z) are given either in millimetres or in units equivalent to the distance of pixels in the image [32, 42, 100].

By exploiting the data obtained in this way, it is possible to extract features of gait [106, 107]. Quantitative methods are employed to measure and analyse movements, forces, and energies involved in walking. These methods use a series of features, including spatio-temporal data (such as speed, cadence, step length and width, time and percentage of support of each leg, leg swing, and symmetry index), kinematic features (angular and linear moments of joints/segments, including flexion, extension, abduction, adduction, rotation, and translation of joints involved in walking, such as hip, knee, ankle, foot, trunk, and arms), kinetic features (forces and moments acting on the indicated joints, including flexion/rotation/torsion moment, as well as power and work of the mentioned joints), and energetic features (oxygen consumption, caloric expenditure, mechanical and metabolic efficiency, etc., during walking). Moreover, these gait features, as demonstrated in various studies, are related to metrics associated with frailty, Parkinson's Disease, dementia, among others [14, 75, 110].

Both the use of video-based methodologies, and/or advanced neural models raise questions about privacy preservation [8]. On the one hand, video-based recognition of images analyses data that might contain many other non-relevant features that might compromise the privacy of end users of these types of systems (e.g. books and newspapers around the house, exposing political views; or credit cards, debt collection letters, etc. visible in the images) [89, 117]. This is particularly relevant under the General Data Protection Regulation (GDPR), which specifies that data should be collected solely for the specific purpose of the service provided and restricts the use of collected data for other purposes. On the other hand, neural networks have been demonstrated to leak data used during training [18, 46, 136], which could potentially reveal personal and sensitive information of individuals that gave their consent for training but not for the publication of their image, or that of their relatives, or their home environment, etc.

Therefore, the deployment of video-based and/or 'deep neural network'-based gait recognition systems in AAL environments requires a delicate balance between the efficacy of monitoring and safeguarding individual privacy. Privacy-awareness is thus of utmost importance for the development of such systems. Methods for gait recognition must be designed with robust anonymization and data protection mechanisms to ensure compliance with privacy regulations and respect for individual autonomy. Techniques such as video obfuscation for gait analysis, which extracts gait features while hiding identifying information, exemplify this approach from a point of view of privacy preservation on input data (see Chap. 3 in this volume [9]). Similarly, the development of privacy-preserving training methodologies and model architectures (i.e. from the point of view of privacy preservation on model processing) is deemed necessary.

However, despite significant advancements, challenges persist in the deployment of video-based methods for gait and frailty recognition in AAL environments. While these systems often present promising results in controlled laboratory conditions, their performance may be lower when faced with the complexities of real-life settings. Real-world environments present many unforeseen challenges, including variations in camera placement, lighting conditions, and the presence of occlusions. Moreover, the concept of 'ecological' monitoring, which emphasizes the need for recognition systems that adapt to the dynamic and diverse nature of everyday living spaces, further complicates the task of accurate recognition due to the high variability among different living spaces. Variations in camera perspectives across different installations introduce additional complexities in feature extraction and model generalization, while diverse gait patterns and poses among individuals make analysis more difficult. Addressing these limitations requires ongoing research into robust feature extraction techniques (such as 3D motion encoders, either with joint coordinate information [76], or full body mesh regression [116]), adaptable algorithms capable of handling diverse viewpoints, and personalized models that account for individual variation. Therefore, in the next few years, research in these topics will be necessary in order to have video-based recognition systems that achieve higher levels of accuracy and reliability, which will open the way for effective ecological monitoring in real-world AAL scenarios.

In conclusion, effectively monitoring end users' health and mobility status while preserving their privacy remains an unsolved question. The next step is to achieve an ecological momentary analysis of these characteristics using computer vision without depth data from specialized sensors, to estimate the degree of frailty as well as the progression of certain diseases that involve specific gait deterioration. However, in the literature reviewed, existing methods have several limitations: on one hand, reviewed ecological studies are of short temporal scope and mainly use wearable sensors; on the other hand, those utilizing computer vision have restrictions such as requiring depth data or being punctual and non-ecological; finally, methods based on deep learning neural networks have been employed in many fields, for instance, for the detection and prevention of falls, even reaching commercial products in some cases (such as CogVis[1] or AltumView[2]). Yet, a detailed analysis of gait deterioration and overall frailty assessment has not been performed in realistic environments, nor applied in ecological or longitudinal studies. Furthermore, there is a need for systems that can automatically assess frailty, while upholding stringent privacy standards, since this will increase user acceptance. Additionally, these systems will prove useful for healthcare providers, caregivers, and family members better understand care needs and autonomy levels of older adults in their care.

This chapter, therefore, addresses existing metrics for frailty assessment and their potential for automation by means of heterogeneous sensory data, with an emphasis in video analytics, and a strong regard to privacy preservation. The remainder of this review chapter is structured as follows: first, a selection of existing metrics for frailty estimation will be presented, along with their potential for automation by means of sensory data collection and processing from diverse sources, including video. Then, a literature review of most recent gait analysis techniques will follow, as required by many scales. A section dedicated to privacy-awareness and preservation techniques is also included. Finally, a discussion regarding potential and future lines of work will be presented, and conclusions drawn.

6.2 Potential for Automation of Frailty Assessment Scales

To advance towards the goal of fully-automated EMA frailty assessment, it is necessary to first be able to find out the most suitable frailty scales, and be able to determine in which ways each of the items, metrics, and scores used can be automated by means of wearable or environment-deployed sensors and processing. Most of the scales, as will be seen, rely on certain physical motion patterns that have the potential to be analysed by computers in a fully automated way. Furthermore, many of the scales entail some gait analysis, to determine gait features such as speed, balance, etc. Any proposed EMA system will therefore need a reliance on the most up-to-date methods for gait analysis. Additionally, if using video, privacy preservation by means of data obfuscation against unauthorised human observers and/or remote processing deep neural models, will be required.

---

[1] See https://cogvis.ai/, Accessed 19 September 2024.
[2] See https://www.altumview.ca/, Accessed 19 September 2024.

6.2.1 Review of Frailty Scales

One of the initial works on frailty assessment is that of Tinetti [129]. The idea that many people experience a decline in mobility as they age, and that this is associated with predisposition to falls, created the urge to assess physical, social, and psychological functions as they impact on this progressive incapacity. Impairments on the locomotor, sensory and cognitive functions (all related to mobility) are potentially preventable, and their protection should be emphasized. Therefore, establishing the optimal content (i.e. items) to be assessed was a high research priority. Tinetti emphasizes how a disease-oriented or a solely gait-analytic approach is too limited in scope. In the traditional approaches, falls are a sign of underlying disease; however, falling is a clinical entity in its own right, due to the accumulated effect of multiple chronic disabilities (geriatric problems are often multifactorial), and is preventable if the causing factors are recognized. This assessment is not about diagnosing a disease, but rather about managing the symptoms and disabilities, for which something can be done. Tinetti presents their "Performance-oriented mobility assessment" (or POMA), and identifies three areas of concern: the assessment of balance, gait, as well as other factors (mental, psychologic, sensory, neurologic, musculoskeletal, etc.) contributing to mobility problems. Finally, for each of the identified limitations, Tinetti proposes rehabilitative and/or preventative measures that could potentially benefit the older adult.

Since then, two different approaches to frailty measurement have been taken: the phenotype approach by Fried et al. [33], and the frailty index (FI) or accumulation of deficits approach by Mitnitski et al. [81]. Therefore, frailty scales differ in nature and in the number of deficits (or items) accounted for, given the two contrasting conceptual models [124]: on the one hand, the phenotype approach sees frailty as a syndrome, with a small number of highly-specified deficits present being indicative of its presence; on the other, the frailty index approach sees it as an accumulation of deficits that are inter-related, therefore it accounts for a much larger number of non-specified age-associated health deficits.

Scales based on the frailty index approach usually have more than 30 items. A standard procedure for creating these indices from existing databases on ageing is described by Searle et al. [112], in which they describe a 40-item FI based on the Yale Precipitating Events Project cohort. Similarly, Theou et al. [125] create a 70-item FI based on data from the Survey of Health, Ageing and Retirement in Europe (SHARE) project database. A 44-item version based on the Comprehensive Geriatric Assessment (CGA) also exists [123].

Since the emergence of these two approaches (phenotype and FI), several other metrics have been published. Bouillon et al. [17] identify 27 scales in total, most being derived from previously existing instruments to assess functional status. Furthermore, most recent scales identified are based on either Fried's or the FI, which can be explained due to the difference in their conceptual understanding of what constitutes frailty. Furthermore, in their review of 150 papers evaluating frailty instruments they identify that 69% of studies used the Fried phenotype (FP), against 12% that used the FI and derived scales. Fried's is, therefore, the most extensively-tested tool. Nonetheless, in some cases the FP approach yields results of up to 50% less prevalence of frailty (compared to a 70-item FI) [125].

However, instead of all 27 scales in [17], Table 6.1 presents the frailty scales identified (most repeated) in the literature that is presented in this section. Along with each scale, an acronym is presented (that will be used from now onwards); as well as the year of publication; the total number of items present (e.g. questions, or metrics); the number of self-reported items in the scale (i.e. that can be answered by the older adult themselves); and a percentage of items that can be automated for the scale. This is measured according to the existence of hardware (sensors, actuators, smart devices such as smart scales, 'walkways' for gait analysis, etc.), or software (computer vision algorithms, gamified apps for vision, audition, cognitive, etc. assessment) that can be installed at-home, and with data being retrieved from the user in a fully- or semi-automated way.

Other studies have also tried to establish comparisons between several scales, either for disability, hospitalization, future health service usage or overall mortality [4, 61, 69, 123, 124]. For instance, Theou et al. [123] compare eight scales for frailty (GFI, TFI, 70-item FI, FI-CGA, CFS, FP, EFS, FRAIL) and arrive at the conclusion that the highest area under the curve (AUC) for FI and EFS is 0.77 and 0.76 for 2-year, and 0.75 for both scales, for 5-year overall mortality.

Similarly, Malmstrom et al. [69] perform a scale comparison, but in this case to measure future disability, understood as having difficulties for ADL performance at 3- and 9-year follow-ups; as well as mortality. They compared the FRAIL scale, and a 25-item FI derived from their data. They also included the Study of Osteoporotic Fractures (SOF) and the Cardiovascular Health Study (CHS, related to the FP) scales. The FI and FRAIL scales exhibited the strongest predictive validity for new disability and mortality. For instance, the AUC for new ADL difficulties after 3 years was 0.75 for FI, and 0.71 for FRAIL. Yet, the authors realised CHS and FI are not practical in busy clinics, given the length of tests that need to be performed (FI usually having more than 40 items).

A later work by Theou et al. [124] compare seven scales (EFS, FRAIL, GFI, FP, TFI, 70-item FI, 44-item FI-CGA). The 5-year mortality increased with the frailty scores. However, their conclusions show two limitations of current scales: scores are upper-bound below the theoretical limits, i.e. it is very hard to score the top theoretical values for the scales; additionally, women often have higher values than men, but their survival is better.

Aprahamian et al. [4] compare the FRAIL and CHS (FP) scales, given that their complaint is that both CHS and FI scales are impractical in clinical or large epidemiological settings: the first requires objective measures and staff training, whereas the other is based off a large database with deficits, symptoms, etc. (usually ≥ 30). They use an adapted version of FRAIL (FRAIL-BR). Their comparison shows that FRAIL generates a higher prevalence of frailty, and that the level of agreement between scales was moderate. They attribute this to the fact that FRAIL does not take an exact time of reference for answers.

Table 6.1 Frailty scales identified in this review. 'Automatable' items refers to metrics that could be gathered at home using available AAL technology

Scale name	Acronym	Year	Number of items	Self-reported items	Can be automated (%)
Performance-oriented mobility assessment [129]	POMA	1986	27	0	22/27 (81)
Short physical performance battery [44]	SPPB	1994	3	0	3/3 (100)
Frailty index [52, 81, 112, 125]	FI, FI-CGA	2001[a]	40, 70	–	–
Fried *phenotype* [33]	FP	2001	5	0	5/5 (100)
Edmonton frail scale [101, 102]	EFS	2006	11	9	3/11 (27)
Kihon checklist [6]	Kihon	2006[b]	25	25	16/25 (64)
PRISMA-7 [98]	PRISMA-7	2008	7	7	1/7 (14)
FRAIL scale [56]	FRAIL	2008	5	1	3/5 (60)
SHARE Frailty index (40-item) [103]	SHARE-FI	2012	40	7	22/40 (55)
Tilburg frailty indicator [38]	TFI	2012	15	15	8/15 (53)
Groningen frailty indicator [93]	GFI	2012	15	15	8/15 (53)
Gérontopôle screening tool [132]	GFST	2013	6	6	5/6 (83)
Frailty trait scale (FTS) [35]	FTS	2014	12	1	9/12 (75)
FTS short form (FTS-3, FTS-5) [36]	FTS-SF	2020	3 or 5	0	5/5 (100)

[a] FI based on the comprehensive geriatric assessment (CGA) is from 2005
[b] The Kihon checklist was translated into English in 2015

With regard to fall prediction in older adults, Lauretani et al. [61] compare POMA and SPPB to determine whether these are tools valid for prediction of falls. Their area under the curve (AUC) for both is under 0.70, which, although statistically significant, is of modest capacity. The SPPB was not originally designed for fall risk evaluation, but it does not underperform when compared to specific tools such as POMA, which leads the authors to conclude that both could be used for fall risk assessment.

Another approach to scale comparison, has to do with the complaints some scales receive, and that have been mentioned: the lack of time for testing in a busy setting. Therefore, Oviedo-Briones et al. [90] in their 'Frail Tools' project compare eight different scales (FP, SHARE-FI, FTS-3, FTS-5, FRAIL, a 35-item FI, GFST, CFS), and evaluate their feasibility (patients with fully-completed tests), and administration time, as well as inter-scale agreement in different settings (geriatric wards, outpatient clinics, primary care, and nursing homes). Regarding feasibility, their results show that FRAIL (Fatigue, Resistance, Ambulation, Illness, and Loss of weight scale), CFS (Clinical Frailty Scale), and GFST (Gérontopôle Frailty Screening Tool) could all be recommended for rapid screening on different settings. However, their results on scale concordance shows that agreement never reached values above 0.65 (Cohen's kappa). Their findings suggest that most tools evaluated actually assess different frailty constructs. This raises the need, according to the authors, for a combination of different scales in each setting. Also, for more cumbersome frailty metrics, automation might assist in having patient scores in a streamlined fashion.

To end this section, some conclusions are now introduced regarding the frailty metrics analysed so far. As seen in Table 6.1, several scales exist for frailty assessment. They vary in nature due to the two different approaches to frailty i.e. either as a syndrome or as an accumulation of deficits. Some frailty indices are very extensive and are not practical in busy clinical settings. Therefore, more recent scales rely on self-reported values by design, so that older adults, their families, caregivers, or other people offering support can help them complete the questionnaires. Other scales, however, depend more on physical magnitudes that can be measured, and that therefore allow more room for automation.

Some authors claim that better scales are needed, since most have AUC values that are just under or around 0.70 [61]. This of course varies from one cohort to another, in some cases leading to the adaptation of scales to ethnic or cultural differences. For instance, Japanese older adults score very high in the standard SPPB, and researchers have had to adapt it to the Japanese reality [34]. Other authors have also identified that, because of the different nature of the scales, having several non-overlapping tools for assessment might improve predictions, i.e. not one scale is enough, a combination is needed [90] but applying several, takes too much time in clinical settings. Some scales are 'short' or have a 'short form' [36] precisely because of time constraints in these settings. This supports the case for at-home, frequent measurements, and automated or semi-automated data collection with limited intervention by the end user (i.e. resident or patient).

6.2.2 Automation of Identified Frailty Scale Domains

To reach EMA frailty prediction, scale scores for each of their constituent items should be automated. Some scales, as has been seen, can be fully automated with existing well-established means. The technologies required to capture items related to each of the domains identified in Table 6.2 will now be presented. Please note that, scales which are self-reported in nature, or items that are more subjective from otherwise objective scales, need not necessarily be excluded. It is possible to retrieve the response for each item, as long as a proxy metric can automatically be extracted. An equivalence between the *actual* measurement required by the scale, and the *proxy* metric taken might need further validation by experts in the field. Discussions for data from each domain follow.

Mobility: In-house gait and balance can be retrieved by means of wristband and accelerometer data of wearable devices, computer vision, and/or smart mats and walkways that retrieve gait data. For out-of-the-house mobility, if GPS coordinates of the home dweller are retrieved, it is possible to know if they went out of the house for a walk, if they went grocery shopping (time spent at the location of a known supermarket), and if they are capable of getting there by public transport (in case it is needed). The time it took the person to reach those places can also be retrieved (walking speeds, etc.), and compared to historical data about their movements.

Nutrition: Most data regarding nutrition in the scales related to body mass index (BMI) and unexpected weight loss. A smart weighing scales with body composition calculation can be installed and data retrieved, including bone density, muscle mass, among other valuable data. For waist circumference, automated camera estimations using computer vision algorithms is possible.

Energy, Mood, and Self-reported Health: In other cases, self-reported values are about the older person's feelings. This is especially true for feelings of exhaustion (lack of energy), loneliness, sadness or depression, and generally mental state. In this case, proxy metrics might rely on the lack of activities that the person used to do, but doesn't anymore, and that are not related to physical limitations. There might be other ways to obtain this from facial expressions or other indirect cues for mental health state (sleeplessness, or getting up late from bed in the mornings). Loneliness is a tricky question, given that it is not the same to be alone as to feel lonely (one can be surrounded by people, or have daily interactions, but feel alone). This does not subtract to these scales' validity, but rather their fitness for automation in these particular set of items. Several smart devices such as voice assistants or similar could possibly collect the responses from users, and also be valuable. However, this would not allow non-interactive collection of *objective* physical assessment.

Cognition, Vision, and Hearing: The first of these domains is usually assessed in frailty scales by items such as knowing today's date, drawing certain figures (e.g. a clock), among others. These evaluations can be automated via cognitive games on a tablet, or as challenges by a voice assistant in the house. Similarly, vision and hearing impairments can be estimated from games and challenges.

Table 6.2 Frailty scale domains as identified by [124], extended to additional scales in this review

Domains	Frailty scales													
	POMA	SPPB	FI	FI-CGA	FP	EFS	Kihon	PRISMA-7	FRAIL	TFI	GFI	GFST	FTS	FTS-SF
Mobility	✓	✓	✓	✓	✓	✓	✓	✓	✓	✓	✓	✓	✓	(✓)
Nutrition			✓	✓	✓		✓		✓	✓	✓	✓	✓	✓
Energy	–		✓	✓	✓	✓	✓		✓	✓	✓	✓	–	
Cognition	–		✓	✓		✓	✓			✓	✓		✓	
Mood	–		✓	✓		✓	✓				✓			
ADL performance								✓						
Health (self-reported)			✓	✓		✓		✓		✓	✓			
Vision	–		✓	✓						✓	✓			
Hearing	–		✓	✓			✓			✓	✓			
Strength	–	–	✓	✓	✓			–		✓	✓		✓	✓
Physical activity			✓	✓		✓					✓			
Incontinence			✓	✓							✓			
Medication			✓			✓					✓			
Sleep			✓											
Hospitalization			✓						✓					
Comorbidities			✓				–	✓						
Symptoms							✓							
Social support						✓	✓					✓		
Falls			✓											

ADL Performance: This domain can be estimated directly by performing Human Activity Recognition (HAR) using computer vision or accelerometer data from wearable devices, as well as by proxy using sensors and actuators installed in the home environment (e.g. fridge usage, times when cooking appliances are used, doors open/shut, etc.).

Strength and Physical Activity: Strength is usually calculated using dynamometers, these could be 'smartified' and deployed in older adults' dwellings for their frequent use. Similarly, smart pressure balls or similar devices could be used. Physical activity can be reported from wristband data, and other accelerometers (e.g. on smartphones).

Incontinence: Several devices for automated (usually bladder) incontinence detection are available [121, 122, 133]. This item could also be self-reported or reported by formal or informal caregivers.

Medication: The first of these domains can either refer to scale items related to memory and ADL performance (i.e. remembering to take medicine), or as whether the end user has been prescribed a certain number of drugs (e.g. more than 5). The former can be detected by means of HAR (either with computer vision solutions, or with home sensor data); the latter, however, depends on either direct responses or electronic records of medicine prescription.

Sleep: Quality can currently be monitored and reported with several tools: pressure mats under the bed, smart sleep monitors, including vision-based, as well as wristband data.

Hospitalization, Co-morbidities and Symptoms: Can either all be collected from direct user responses (see "Energy, Mood, and Self-reported health" above), or be automatically extracted from patients' electronic records.

Social Support: Items in this domain can be automatically extracted by using the presence of frequent visitors in the end user's dwelling (e.g. via cameras, presence of devices from Bluetooth signals or Wi-Fi, etc.), as well as from interaction (time, frequency) with phone apps such as audio and video calls with family members of other people in the support net of the dweller. Geopositioning signals indicative of visits to others can also be used.

Falls: Last, but not least, fall prevention and detection exist in the literature and as commercial products in the market: from accelerometer-based approaches (e.g. smart watches), to camera-enabled solutions. These systems could collect this data and report it as part of the automated scoring.

6.3 Gait Analysis

The assessment of frailty, as explored through the various scales analysed, includes a component of mobility evaluation in almost every case. Among the diverse dimensions of mobility, gait and balance emerge as the most common components in these assessments, serving as vital indicators of an individual's functional status and overall frailty. This emphasis is not surprising, given that gait and balance impairments are often early manifestations of frailty, reflecting underlying vulnerabilities in musculoskeletal, neurological, and/or cardiovascular systems. As we transition into a detailed analysis of gait, this section will delve into the methodologies, technologies, and clinical implications of gait analysis, providing a comprehensive understanding of its significance in the context of frailty and its potential for enhancing automated assessments by means of ecological momentary assessment, using AAL technologies. By finding connections between gait characteristics and frailty, this section aims to further illustrate how precise gait analysis can inform and improve frailty assessment and intervention strategies.

Most research in this area was initially related to gait analysis for sports science, or for foot problems (podiatry), in laboratory conditions. Early studies mostly employed electronic walkways, accelerometers and gyroscopes installed on the leg(s) of the participants (also inertial magnetic units, or IMUs), or motion capture (MoCap) systems in ideal settings. This is far from the at-home, informal, continuous capture of gait that this review is focused on, but demonstrates early attempts at this type of system. MoCap installations require the use of reflective points on the body surface to detect the limbs and joints, and deviations in placement can lead to suboptimal results. One example of this is the work by Pogorelc et al. [94], in which they include five classes of gait, including Parkinsonian gait.

As can be observed, these are very apparent abnormal gaits, and in this, and several other studies, the gait abnormalities (or a subset of them) are feigned by healthy young adults [53, 88, 91, 94], as part of a validation step of gait detection systems. It is only in recent times that developed methodologies have been able to detect more subtle changes for early diagnosis and frailty estimation, necessitating cohorts of real, older-adult participants.

6.3.1 Use of Gait in Medical Studies

From a medical perspective, gait analysis has been used not just for frailty assessment, but for many other health conditions causing changes in gait. Table 6.3 summarises some of the ailments that have been identified in the medical literature, specifically, that use gait analysis for identification of certain patterns characteristic to said ailments. Some works in the table stand out particularly, such as that of Vavasour et al. [131] which analyses how wearable sensors have been used to determine frailty. Also, that of Varma et al. [130] since it is focused on continuous gait analysis for Alzheimer's Disease at-home evolution monitoring. In the case of Parkinson's, Mirelman et al. [80] shows there is a point to be made about in-home gait analysis during usual ADL performance since gait changes might be nuanced, and might differ from those captured in laboratory conditions. Finally, Lunardini et al. [67] make the case for the importance of differentiating usual gait (i.e. 'single-task') from 'dual-task' gait in ecological monitoring, since gait might seem artificially impaired by natural human behaviours such as smartphone usage.

Table 6.3 Ailments diagnosed via gait analysis in medical studies. MS: Multiple sclerosis. COPD: Chronic obstructive pulmonary disease. PFF: Periprosthetic femoral fracture. CHF: Congestive heart failure

Conditions or features assessed	Literature
Frailty and age-related	– Overall frailty [63, 82, 131]
	– Gait, balance, physical activity [67, 111, 120]
	– Fall risk assessment [12, 51]
Alzheimer's disease (AD)	– AD [40, 72, 130, 134]
Parkinson's disease (PD)	– PD itself [7, 20, 24, 49, 80]
	– PD w.r.t. REM sleep [25]
	– PD compared to CHF, MS, COPD, PFF [104]
Other	– Autism [39]
	– Anxiety/depression [78]
	– Hydrocephalus [135]
	– Diabetes [114]

When examining gait analysis from a computer science perspective, the literature identifies two main approaches: methods based on computer vision and video analysis; and those methods solely based on inertial magnetic units (IMUs) including accelerometers, gyroscopes, and magnetometers; with or without force sensing resistors (FSRs) as additional in-sole sensors for footfall measurement. This review will focus on the former now, since it is the main focus of this work, and then summarize key findings of non-vision IMU-based methods later, at the end of this section.

6.3.2 Gait Analysis from Video

One of the earliest works from the computer vision perspective is that of Bauckhage et al. [10, 11], in it the authors are able to distinguish normal and abnormal gait patterns (wavering, faltering, and falling) from silhouette based extracted information without specific limb detection or segmentation. This is the first work analysed that indicates the need for gait analysis not aimed at person recognition, a different field of research (gait for "biometric identification", as per the definitions set forth in the European AI Act), but to deduce physical condition. Most previous bodies of research focused on gait as a means for person identification, whereas from this point onward, the literature includes works focused on gait analysis for walking feature extraction for normal versus abnormal gait classification and/or medical condition detection. Similarly, Nieto-Hidalgo et al. [88] have the aim of early frailty assessment through gait. They use RGB-only information to detect abnormal gait in healthy adults feigning gait impairments. However, the camera setting is such that gait is observed laterally, in ideal lab conditions, for the method to perform as expected.

With the emergence of depth-enabled devices, i.e. RGB-D cameras, or cameras able to capture image as well as depth information from deviations in the bounce-back of infrared patterns emitted by the device (e.g. the Microsoft Kinect v1/v2, ASUS Xtion, etc.), several methods aimed at replicating results from MoCap systems lab conditions in more informal settings [41, 87]. These devices included software packages (MS Kinect SDK, OpenNI with NITE) that allowed the extraction of 3D joint information from subjects in the image, and thus being able to provide a 'skeleton' of the lower limbs, that could be used for, among others, gait analysis. In some occasions, RGB-D cameras can be mounted on walking machines for gait assessment, as done by André et al. [3], however, this limits exploration of gait parameters naturally at home, and requires extra equipment which might limit widespread adoption.

Earlier 'deep learning'-based techniques were unable to provide 3D joint information, due to the ambiguous nature of this problem (i.e. 3D information from monocular 2D images), but could provide 2D information in pixel coordinates of body joints [19]. With these types of methods, although limited, it has been possible to extract meaningful diagnostic information. For instance, Sabo et al. [106, 107], Ng et al. [86], and Mehdizadeh et al. [74] can find correlations of certain gait features extracted in this way with POMA gait and balance scores, with fall risk, as well as Parkinsonian severity. Although data is taken in a dementia ward, their method is marker-less and completely unobtrusive, paving the way for in-home, continued detection of gait abnormalities. Another way to extract 3D joint information from 2D joint location regressors is by using sets of calibrated cameras [57].

With the latest deep neural networks it has been possible to avoid the use of RGB-D devices providing 3D information, or even calibrated cameras, and therefore remove the 2D restriction from RGB-only methods. As said, extracting 3D information from monocular video is an ambiguous problem. However, the latest methods for full human body regression utilize heuristics and automated intrinsic camera calibration [99, 105]. By fitting a 3D human representation on top of the image, it is possible to extract 3D positions relative to the body centre, and therefore, derive metrics of gait such as step length, regardless of the camera's angle of incidence to the scene. This is exactly the approach taken by Lu et al. [65], which is the first paper in this review to actually regress Parkinson's Disease scores (MDS-UPDRS, which ranges from 0 to 3, and stands for MDS-Unified Parkinson's Disease Rating Scale) from gait data extracted in this way.

In other occasions, deep learning techniques are advantageous because recurrent models are able to take time-series information, and infer knowledge from the whole temporal sequence. Otherwise, approaches similar to motion energy or history images (MEI and MHI, respectively, [16]), that can 'compact' the time axis are required [64]. For instance, Jun et al. [53] extract body joint information from Kinect skeleton data using recurrent neural networks (RNNs), and then produce meaningful features by using autoencoders (AEs), which are finally fed to their discriminative models. With this method, they are able to classify nine gait classes (normal, and four impairments per body side, caused by adding weights or thick soles). They also perform a 5-class classification using multiple views [55]. In all cases, they use young healthy adults that have been trained to simulate the conditions [54]. Similarly, Pachon-Suescun et al. [91] use long short term memory (LSTM) recurrent networks for the classification of Parkinsonian, hemiplegic, and spastic diplegic gaits, imitated by healthy subjects who had been trained.

As mentioned above, Kaur et al. [57] use sets of calibrated cameras to extract real-world 3D joint positions from 2D joint location regressors. In their work they utilize real patients with multiple sclerosis and Parkinson's, along with a control group of older adults without impairments. They test their approach with a very comprehensive set of machine and deep learning (ML/DL) techniques, including recurrent neural networks. Finally they also perform an analysis of feature importance.

However, skeleton data is a type of graph data, and many methods do not employ graph representations for them, but rather vectors, matrices or tensors of joint coordinates. Yet, joint adjacency encodes valuable information. With this idea, Tian et al. [126] employ graph convolutional networks (GCNs) with an 'attention enhanced gait-structure' (AGS-GCN). They saturate one of the test datasets [87] (100% accuracy), thus showing that more challenging data is required, since existing datasets are too limited in number of participants and/or gait abnormality classes used (i.e. their complexity). Their work does not focus on data capture, but rather relies on skeleton data extracted by other means. As a reminder, the datasets used compare normal versus abnormal gait by introducing destabilising elements in one of the legs, e.g. thick soles or weights. To solve this issue, and be able to assess more complex scenarios, Sabo et al. [106] propose using spatio-temporal CGNs (ST-CGN) for the regression of Parkinsonian gait from 2D and 3D joint data of walking bouts in a dementia unit and independent living facilities.

6.3.3 Gait Analysis from Other Sensors

As explained above, gait can be analysed from several sensor types. In most medical studies reviewed in the literature, specifically those run in laboratory settings, IMU-based or 'electronic walkway' solutions seem to be preferred, due to their accuracy, as compared to purely video-based solutions, which, up until recently, could not compete in this regard. Furthermore, most medical studies prefer branded solutions, since these offer reliability, and have been tested and in some cases validated as medical devices. In contrast, engineer teams are more likely to use open source and bespoke sensor solutions, engineered to their specific needs.

Table 6.4 serves as a summary of the types of sensors identified in the literature. As can be seen, most reviewed works use a combination of FSRs and IMUs, with fewer using only either one. In most cases, FSRs are usually installed as in-soles in the shoes of participants [31, 48, 77]. The review by Eskofier et al. [31] covers 'smart shoes' i.e. instrumented footwear that is connected and from which several data modalities can be extracted. Further, the study by Manna et al. [70] shows the importance of correctly finding the optimal locations for IMU and FSR sensors. Sharma et al. [115] present a large non-laboratory gait dataset (using IMU sensors) with full body kinematics. Some of the activities are also recorded using egocentric vision. It contains several

Table 6.4 Identified literature regarding gait analysis from non-video-based sensors

Type of sensor	Literature
Inertial magnetic units (IMU)	[50, 58, 115]
Force sensing resistors (FSR) only	[37]
Combined FSR + IMU	[30, 31, 48, 70, 71, 77, 108]
Environmental 1-axis accelerometers	[45]
Electromyogram (EMG)	[43]

classes of gait, with and without stops, stair ambulation, obstacle avoidance, agility, etc. However, the participants were young college students, which may limit the generalizability of the findings to an older or frailer population.

Another set of works focuses on the calculation of vertical ground reaction forces (VGRF) which can be derived from worn or environmental sensors. For instance, on the one hand, in the work of Ghoreshi Beyrami et al. [37] the VGRF is derived from worn FSR sensor outputs. VGFR establishes the force of footfalls during each instant of the gait cycle, and can serve to establish differences between Amyotrophic lateral sclerosis (ALS), Parkinson's (PD), and Huntington's (HD) gaits from real patients. On the other hand, Hahm et al. [45] use single-axis accelerometers deployed in the environment for unobtrusive multi-occupant gait analysis. In their study several of these sensors are deployed in a room. The vibrations caused by footfalls are detected in this way (VGRF is estimated), and can be localised given the distance to each sensor, which detects the event with different signal strength. Therefore, multiple occupants can be walking at the same time and be detected correctly. Finally, electromyogram (EMG) sensors can also be employed for the early detection of gait abnormalities caused by age, as shown by Guo et al. [43], which compare their method to kinematic data captured from a MoCap system, and achieve similar results.

A review comparing several modalities of sensors used for gait is done by Liu et al. [62]. In their work they compare smartphones equipped with GPS, wearable sensors (IMU, EMG), and sensing fabrics (which can provide data on pressure, bio-impedance, conductivity, temperature, elongation, etc.).

6.4 Ecological Monitoring

In the original work of Stone and Shiffman [119], they present ecological momentary assessment (EMA) as a means to naturally record phenomena occurring in people's natural environments. These events can be varied, e.g. when people take medicines, when they exercise or remain seated (sedentary behaviours), etc. Historically, it has been difficult to capture these events in real-world settings. Instead of that, researchers have had to either record participants in laboratory settings, or use retrospective self-reported data. These two approaches have limitations: laboratory conditions might create biased data, or not faithfully represent real-world behaviours; asking subjects to reflect back upon past experiences is subject to a number of biases, arising from several cognitive processes that negatively affect recall. This is why EMA uses monitoring techniques, along with sampling strategies, to evaluate the events as they occur in a natural environment of the dweller. This maximises ecological validity and avoids problems associated with retrospective event recall.

According to Morris et al. [83], EMA has become widely used by researchers, particularly when studying health-related behaviours. Until recently, EMA was predominantly employed for research purposes only. However, in recent years it has been adopted for real-time data collection and observation of patients' behaviours, moods, social context, etc. Their work discusses how EMA can potentially be used for the delivery of health interventions.

In the remainder of this section, 'researchers' and 'participants' will be employed in an EMA-context, but since EMA could be deployed in non-research settings, the words 'caregiver' and 'dweller' or 'end user' could be used instead, conveying the idea of a system in which a healthcare professional, or a formal or informal caregiver can have access to the data collected from the end user of a system for overall health assessment, or specific gait, balance, fall risk, cognitive function assessments, among others. As an example, Job et al. [51] explore the idea of ecological gait assessment to boost the diagnostic accuracy of fall risk.

However, because of its nature, EMA is dependent on careful timing of assessments, given that certain behavioural patterns (e.g. alcohol drinking), happen at certain times of day. The sampling times are chosen by the researchers or practitioners, not by the subjects, as these may select times that are unrepresentative. This is why an investigator-controlled cue (an alarm, a beep, or otherwise) is used to signal when the evaluation is to be provided. Participants would then complete their assessment with pen and paper. Yet, since the appearance of EMA, Maher et al. [68], among others, have attempted to convey their 'cue' to the participant by means of other later technological advancements, such as smartphones, which also serve to complete the assessments. In this way, they have been able to collect information on physical activity and sedentary behaviour. However, for fully natural interaction, voice assistants and other environmentally-deployed sensors, actuators and IoT devices could be helpful, as the interaction with them can be perceived as more natural by older adults (e.g. not having to take out the phone for data collection).

With regards to voice assistants, Bérubé and Fleish [13] recognize these have so far been utilized for smart home control or a virtual personal assistant, but their applications in healthcare have not fully been explored. They explore a series of previous works related to mental health assessment, including feelings of isolation in older adults. Also in this field, Chen et al. [21] explore the adaptations needed to the questions in EMA assessments to be correctly deployed in these types of devices. Finally, Han et al. [47] show how EMA data can also be used to empower participants, as they can retrieve past EMA data provided to the system for their own perusal, which improves engagement in the programme.

Environmentally-deployed sensors (IoT and 'smart home' sensors) can also be utilized as sources of data for EMA assessments. For instance, Nelson and Allen [85] explore the uses of this types of sensors for psychological assessments, such as cognitive assessment, sleep, interpersonal theories, emotions, suicidality, etc. For instance, McDevitt-Murphy et al. [73] propose the use of EMA and ecological momentary intervention (EMI) as part of psychological therapy continuation outside the sessions. Smart home sensors can also be used to extract context, and therefore aim at 'cueing' participants at the right times, i.e. when they are between two activities. This increases engagement in EMA, as explored by Aminikhanghahi et al. [2]. The detection of activities, and particularly ADLs, is of use to determine the routine behaviours of older adults, so that later, deviations could potentially be detected, as done by Timon et al. [128]. Finally, Schmitter-Edgecombe et al. [109] propose the use of smart home sensors for the prediction of cognitive functioning, lifestyle behaviours, as well as contextual factors impacting health outcomes. In their study they observe that sensor usage (i.e. more ADLs detected) as well as more time out of the house correlated to better mental sharpness, social, physical, and cognitive scores.

The difference between the former (voice assistants, digitised questionnaires on tables), and the latter (environment-deployed sensors, or wearable technology) lies in that the former are still self-reported responses, whereas as discussed earlier, in the section regarding frailty assessment scales, the latter collect real objective user behaviours. This is important in behaviour analytic research, as prompted by Stinson et al. [118], who highlighted the importance of non-subjective data collection. Even further, methodologies using cameras can be completely unobtrusive as opposed to devices worn on the body [74, 86, 106, 107]. However, as reviewed, these techniques use either 3D data generated from depth images (thus requiring this type of equipment), or 2D data from earlier DL-based neural networks using RGB information only.

With regard to ecological monitoring with wearable non-video solutions, some methodologies have been already mentioned before in the previous section. It could be argued that wearable technologies are 'ecological' in nature, i.e. that they can be used always in this fashion. A focus is brought here only to those solutions that demonstrate this outside the laboratory. For instance, Duong et al. [30] present an IMU+FSR in-sole that is connected to the smartphone of the wearer and therefore captures gait continuously, which according to the authors, and as stated, can aid in the early diagnosis of neurological and musculoskeletal conditions. They can extract stride time, length, and velocity in real-life scenarios. Similarly, Salis et al. [108] propose a system combining a smart in-sole with IMU sensors for at-home non-laboratory solutions for continuous (i.e. ecological) monitoring, tested on healthy adults. In a later study, they include DL-based methodologies and real cohorts of patients with different ailments [104].

Table 6.5 summarises the outcomes for this section. It shows relevant methods for each sensor modality that perform EMA in real-world conditions, or that could potentially be used in an at-home EMA protocol without much modification, or that show how EMA could be beneficial for a specific field. Video-based works are mostly from the same research group, and present video-based EMA attempts in hospital settings that could easily be transferred to older adult living environments, since they

Table 6.5 Identified literature of works using ecological momentary assessment split by sensor modality used

Sensor modality	Performs EMA	Potentially EMA
Video-based	–	[74, 86, 106, 107]
Wearable	[30, 104, 108]	[27, 51]
Smart home sensors	[2, 109, 128]	[73, 85]

use completely unobtrusive methods, with the exception of RFID tags worn by users in order to start the recordings (and identify them) for their dataset collection.

6.5 Privacy-Awareness

If EMA-based frailty recognition systems are to be accepted by end users and the public in general, concerns about privacy need to be addressed, as stated by Morris et al. [83]. However, beyond gait analysis for health purposes, gait recognition is a whole research field that aims to identify users by their distinctive traits when walking [84, 95, 113]. This means, gait can be considered a biometric signal (i.e. "biometric data" as set forth in Article 3 (34) of the European AI Act), since it can be used to identify particular individuals, usually in combination with other biometric body and/or face features. This makes its protection a particularly challenging topic. Several reviews on the field of gait recognition exist: Nambiar et al. [84] present a general survey on personal re-identification using gait traits, whereas Rani and Kumar [95] present a comprehensive systematic review. Finally, more recently, Sepas-Moghaddam and Etemad [113] present a survey on the topic with regard to the use and evolution of 'deep learning'-based methodologies in this area. The reader is referred to these surveys for a deeper understanding of gait recognition as a biometric/identifying feature. The reader is also referred to the definitions of "biometric data", "biometric identification", and "biometric verification" as set forth in the European AI Act, Article 3 (34)–(36).[3]

Some authors, such as Bisogni et al. [15] consider that gait is somehow already less invasive than other means of identification, since it doesn't use more sensitive data such as facial cues. Similarly, for some authors, skeleton-based methodologies offer a promising approach to maintaining privacy in gait analysis, as they allow the original images or video footage to be discarded after extracting skeletal joint data. Because this approach focuses on capturing the positions and movements of key joints, it reduces the need to store identifiable visual information. Despite this, it is important to recognize that joint data itself is still a form of gait data, containing unique patterns that can potentially identify individuals. Furthermore, Kolokas et al. [59] were able

---

[3] https://eur-lex.europa.eu/legal-content/EN/TXT/PDF/?uri=OJ:L_202401689, Accessed 19 September 2024.

to match gait data from wearables to videos of the same person, thus revealing that a high correlation exists between visual and wearable data, making it possible to still associate gait data to particular individuals. Therefore, while skeleton-based methods enhance privacy by minimizing the retention of raw visual data, they still require careful handling and protection of the extracted joint information to ensure the privacy and security of individuals' biometric data.

Wearable IMU-based data is often cited as less invasive than cameras deployed in the environment for skeleton extraction. However, Rasnayaka and Sim [96] explore how gait data can be very invasive, even from wearable IMU-based devices. They also explore how sensor placement affects recognition of gait against other privacy-revealing data. IMU-based and other wearable data, commonly used for health monitoring, can also reveal a range of demographic and personal characteristics such as age, gender, and lifestyle habits. By analysing patterns in physical activity, heart rate variability, and sleep cycles, wearable devices can infer the age group of the user, as younger and older individuals often exhibit distinct physiological and activity patterns. Gender can be deduced from differences in movement patterns, body metrics, and even physiological responses captured by the wearables. Additionally, data on daily routines, exercise frequency, and activity types can provide insights into personal habits and lifestyle choices, painting a comprehensive picture of the user beyond their immediate health metrics. In fact, Climent-Pérez et al. [22] show that age and gender can be recognized from IMU-based wearable data alone, and therefore use a many-objective evolutionary algorithm to alter data in ways which affect age and gender recognition more than human activity recognition, which is the actual goal of the proposed system. This potential use of data highlights the capabilities of wearables in extracting information beyond the user's conscious choice and informed consent. This practice contradicts data protection regulations outlined in the GDPR, particularly those that limit data collection and processing to purposes explicitly agreed upon by the user. For this reason, Tieu et al. [127] developed an approach to add a 'noise gait' to a recorded gait so that it cannot be identified, while maintaining the naturalness of the gait. Similarly, Delgado-Santos et al. [26] propose a means to obfuscate sensitive information associated to gait, while maintaining user authentication capabilities. Furthermore, Parashar and Shekhawat [92] envisage a means of reversible gait anonymization that is useful against adversarial attacks. This is related to the concept, presented by Ravi et al. [97], of *dual* obfuscation required for privacy: obfuscation against human visualization, but also against model leakage during training, or adversarial attacks.

In conclusion, while EMA-based frailty recognition systems hold significant potential for health monitoring and early detection of various conditions, addressing privacy concerns is crucial for their acceptance by end users and the public. Gait recognition, as a field of research, extends beyond health applications, serving as a biometric signal capable of identifying individuals by their walking patterns. This dual-use nature of gait data makes robust privacy protections necessary. Skeleton-based methodologies, although promising in reducing identifiable visual data, still require careful handling of joint data to prevent potential privacy breaches. Similarly, wearable IMU-based data, while perceived as less invasive, can reveal a wide range of personal and demographic characteristics, further complicating privacy concerns.

Strategies such as data obfuscation and the addition of noise to gait patterns have been proposed to mitigate privacy risks. These approaches aim to balance the utility of gait data for health and authentication purposes, while safeguarding individual privacy against adversarial attacks and unauthorized access. Ultimately, ensuring the privacy and security of gait data through comprehensive and innovative solutions is essential to gaining user trust and compliance with data protection regulations like the GDPR.

6.6 Conclusion

This chapter comprehensively explores the potential for automating frailty assessment through the use of video-based methods, highlighting both the advancements and the challenges in the field. Key conclusions drawn from the analysis are discussed next.

As identified in the first section, numerous scales for frailty assessment exist, each with its own strengths and limitations. These scales vary based on whether frailty is viewed as a syndrome or an accumulation of deficits. Some scales rely on self-reported data, while others depend on measurable physical parameters that lend themselves more readily to automation. Domains of the scales which can be automated more easily have been identified, with ideas as to which types of sensors would be better suited for the task. Gait and balance analysis appear as one of the main domains that are utilized by most scales.

While controlled laboratory settings have shown promising results for video-based gait and frailty recognition systems, real-world environments introduce significant complexities. These include variations in camera placement, lighting, occlusions, and the dynamic nature of everyday living spaces. Addressing these challenges is crucial for achieving accurate and reliable monitoring in practical settings.

Furthermore, the deployment of video-based monitoring systems in AAL environments raises important privacy concerns. Ensuring data obfuscation against unauthorized human observers and secure remote processing is essential for user acceptance and compliance with privacy standards. Additionally, gait data is biometric data, and can be used for biometric identification, which raises the question as to how to anonymize the data while preserving its utility for diagnostics.

EMA has great potential in assessing the health status, well-being, and needs of older adults in AAL environments. By collecting data continuously and in real-time, EMA provides a detailed and accurate picture of the users' conditions and can help in designing tailored interventions. However, to achieve fully automated frailty assessment, it is necessary to automate the scoring of various frailty scale items. Some domains can be automated using existing technologies, while others require the development of proxy metrics and further validation. Combining multiple scales might improve predictive accuracy, but this also underscores the need for efficient data collection methods to avoid overburdening clinical settings.

Future research should focus on enhancing the robustness of feature extraction techniques and developing adaptable algorithms that can handle the diversity of real-world environments (e.g. from 3D full body models from monocular video). Integrating privacy-aware methods with obfuscation directed at human observers as well as adversarial AI models also requires further exploration. Future work should continue to advance the precision, reliability, and privacy-preserving capabilities of these technologies to ensure they meet the complex needs of real-world applications while also addressing the technical, practical, and ethical challenges associated with the deployment of automated frailty assessment systems using video-based methods in AAL environments.

Acknowledgements This publication is based upon work from COST Action GoodBrother—Network on Privacy-Aware Audio- and Video-Based Applications for Active and Assisted Living (CA19121), supported by COST (European Cooperation in Science and Technology).

References

1. Aleksic, S., Atanasov, M., Agius, J.C., Camilleri, K., Cartolovni, A., Climent-Pérez, P., Colantonio, S., Cristina, S., Despotovic, V., Ekenel, H.K., Erakin, E., Florez-Revuelta, F., Germanese, D., Grech, N., Sigurðardóttir, S.G., Emirzeoglu, M., Iliev, I., Jovanovic, M., Kampel, M., Kearns, W., Klimczuk, A., Lambrinos, L., Lumetzberger, J., Mucha, W., Noiret, S., Pajalic, Z., Peerez, R.R., Petrova, G., Petrovica, S., Pocta, P., Poli, R., Pudane, M., Spinsante, S., Salah, A.A., Santofimia, M.J., Islind, A.S., Stoicu-Tivadar, L., Tellioglu, H., Zgank, A.: State of the art of audio- and video-based solutions for AAL (2022). https://doi.org/10.48550/arXiv.2207.01487
2. Aminikhanghahi, S., Schmitter-Edgecombe, M., Cook, D.J.: Context-aware delivery of ecological momentary assessment. IEEE J. Biomed. Health Inform. **24**(4), 1206–1214 (2020). https://doi.org/10.1109/JBHI.2019.2937116
3. André, J., Lopes, J., Palermo, M., Gonçalves, D., Matias, A., Pereira, F., Afonso, J., Seabra, E., Cerqueira, J., Santos, C.: Markerless gait analysis vision system for real-time gait monitoring. In: 2020 IEEE International Conference on Autonomous Robot Systems and Competitions (ICARSC), pp. 269–274 (2020). https://doi.org/10.1109/ICARSC49921.2020.9096121
4. Aprahamian, I., Cezar, N.O.D.C., Izbicki, R., Lin, S.M., Paulo, D.L.V., Fattori, A., Biella, M.M., Jacob Filho, W., Yassuda, M.S.: Screening for frailty with the FRAIL scale: a comparison with the phenotype criteria. J. Am. Med. Dir. Assoc. **18**(7), 592–596 (2017). https://doi.org/10.1016/j.jamda.2017.01.009
5. Apsega, A., Petrauskas, L., Alekna, V., Daunoraviciene, K., Sevcenko, V., Mastaviciute, A., Vitkus, D., Tamulaitiene, M., Griskevicius, J.: Wearable sensors technology as a tool for discriminating frailty levels during instrumented gait analysis. Appl. Sci. **10**(23) (2020). https://doi.org/10.3390/app10238451
6. Arai, H., Satake, S.: English translation of the Kihon checklist. Geriatr. Gerontol. Int. **15**(4) (2015)
7. Archila, J., Manzanera, A., Martínez, F.: A multimodal Parkinson quantification by fusing eye and gait motion patterns, using covariance descriptors, from non-invasive computer vision. Comput. Methods Programs Biomed. **215**, 106,607 (2022). https://doi.org/10.1016/j.cmpb.2021.106607

8. Arning, K., Ziefle, M.: "Get that camera out of my house!" conjoint measurement of preferences for video-based healthcare monitoring systems in private and public places. In: Inclusive Smart Cities and e-Health: 13th International Conference on Smart Homes and Health Telematics, ICOST 2015, Geneva, Switzerland, June 10–12, 2015, Proceedings 13, pp. 152–164. Springer (2015)
9. Bäckström, T., Ravi, S., Florez-Revuelta, F.: Privacy preservation in audio and video. In: Salah, A.A., Colonna, L., Florez-Revuelta, F. (eds.) Privacy-Aware Monitoring for Assisted Living. Springer, Cham (2025)
10. Bauckhage, C., Tsotsos, J., Bunn, F.: Detecting Abnormal Gait. In: The 2nd Canadian Conference on Computer and Robot Vision (CRV'05), pp. 282–288. IEEE, Victoria, BC, Canada (2005). https://doi.org/10.1109/CRV.2005.32
11. Bauckhage, C., Tsotsos, J.K., Bunn, F.E.: Automatic detection of abnormal gait. Image Vis. Comput. **27**(1), 108–115 (2009). https://doi.org/10.1016/j.imavis.2006.10.004
12. Beck Jepsen, D., Robinson, K., Ogliari, G., Montero-Odasso, M., Kamkar, N., Ryg, J., Freiberger, E., Tahir, M.: Predicting falls in older adults: an umbrella review of instruments assessing gait, balance, and functional mobility. BMC Geriatr. **22**, 615 (2022). https://doi.org/10.1186/s12877-022-03271-5
13. Bérubé, C., Fleisch, E.: Voice-based conversational agents for sensing and support: examples from academia and industry. In: Digital Therapeutics for Mental Health and Addiction, pp. 113–134. Elsevier (2023). https://doi.org/10.1016/B978-0-323-90045-4.00017-4
14. Binotto, M.A., Lenardt, M.H., Rodriguez-Martinez, M.d.C.: Physical frailty and gait speed in community elderly: a systematic review. Revista da Escola de Enfermagem da USP **52**, e03,392 (2018)
15. Bisogni, C., Cimmino, L., Nappi, M., Pannese, T., Pero, C.: Walk as you feel: privacy preserving emotion recognition from gait patterns. Eng. Appl. Artif. Intell. **128**, 107,565 (2024). https://doi.org/10.1016/j.engappai.2023.107565
16. Bobick, A.F., Davis, J.W.: The recognition of human movement using temporal templates. IEEE Trans. Pattern Anal. Mach. Intell. **23**(3), 257–267 (2001)
17. Bouillon, K., Kivimaki, M., Hamer, M., Sabia, S., Fransson, E.I., Singh-Manoux, A., Gale, C.R., Batty, G.D.: Measures of frailty in population-based studies: an overview. BMC Geriatr. **13**(1), 64 (2013). https://doi.org/10.1186/1471-2318-13-64
18. Buzaglo, G., Haim, N., Yehudai, G., Vardi, G., Oz, Y., Nikankin, Y., Irani, M.: Deconstructing data reconstruction: multiclass, weight decay and general losses. In: Oh, A., Naumann, T., Globerson, A., Saenko, K., Hardt, M., Levine S. (eds.) Advances in Neural Information Processing Systems, vol. 36, pp. 51,515–51,535. Curran Associates, Inc. (2023)
19. Cao, Z., Simon, T., Wei, S.E., Sheikh, Y.: Realtime multi-person 2D pose estimation using part affinity fields. In: Proceedings of the IEEE Conference on Computer Vision and Pattern Recognition, pp. 7291–7299 (2017)
20. Carvajal-Castaño, H.A., Lemos-Duque, J.D., Orozco-Arroyave, J.R.: Effective detection of abnormal gait patterns in Parkinson's disease patients using kinematics, nonlinear, and stability gait features. Human Mov. Sci. **81**, 102,891 (2022). https://doi.org/10.1016/j.humov.2021.102891
21. Chen, C., Mrini, K., Charles, K., Lifset, E., Hogarth, M., Moore, A., Weibel, N., Farcas, E.: Toward a unified metadata schema for ecological momentary assessment with voice-first virtual assistants. In: CUI 2021 - 3rd Conference on Conversational User Interfaces, pp. 1–6. ACM, Bilbao (online) Spain (2021). https://doi.org/10.1145/3469595.3469626
22. Climent-Pérez, P., Florez-Revuelta, F.: Privacy-preserving human action recognition with a many-objective evolutionary algorithm. Sensors **22**(3), 764 (2022). https://doi.org/10.3390/s22030764
23. Climent-Pérez, P., Florez-Revuelta, F.: Improved action recognition with separable spatio-temporal attention using alternative skeletal and video pre-processing. Sensors **21**(3) (2021). https://doi.org/10.3390/s21031005
24. Del Din, S., Elshehabi, M., Galna, B., Hobert, M.A., Warmerdam, E., Suenkel, U., Brockmann, K., Metzger, F., Hansen, C., Berg, D., Rochester, L., Maetzler, W.: Gait analysis with wearables

predicts conversion to Parkinson disease. Ann. Neurol. **86**(3), 357–367 (2019). https://doi.org/10.1002/ana.25548
25. Del Din, S., Yarnall, A.J., Barber, T.R., Lo, C., Crabbe, M., Rolinski, M., Baig, F., Hu, M.T., Rochester, L.: Continuous real-world gait monitoring in idiopathic REM sleep behavior disorder. J. Parkinsons Dis. **10**(1), 283–299 (2020). https://doi.org/10.3233/JPD-191773
26. Delgado-Santos, P., Tolosana, R., Guest, R., Vera-Rodriguez, R., Deravi, F., Morales, A.: Gait-PrivacyON: privacy-preserving mobile gait biometrics using unsupervised learning. Pattern Recogn. Lett. **161**, 30–37 (2022). https://doi.org/10.1016/j.patrec.2022.07.015
27. Dion, G., Tessier-Poirier, A., Chiasson-Poirier, L., Morissette, J.F., Brassard, G., Haman, A., Turcot, K., Sylvestre, J.: In-sensor human gait analysis with machine learning in a wearable microfabricated accelerometer. Commun. Eng. **3**(1), 1–10 (2024). https://doi.org/10.1038/s44172-024-00193-5
28. Dolatabadi, E., Mansfield, A., Patterson, K.K., Taati, B., Mihailidis, A.: Mixture-model clustering of pathological gait patterns. IEEE J. Biomed. Health Inform. **21**(5), 1297–1305 (2017). https://doi.org/10.1109/JBHI.2016.2633000
29. Dolatabadi, E., Taati, B., Mihailidis, A.: An automated classification of pathological gait using unobtrusive sensing technology. IEEE Trans. Neural Syst. Rehabil. Eng. **25**(12), 2336–2346 (2017). https://doi.org/10.1109/TNSRE.2017.2736939
30. Duong, T.T.H., Uher, D., Montes, J., Zanotto, D.: Ecological validation of machine learning models for spatiotemporal gait analysis in free-living environments using instrumented insoles. IEEE Robot. Autom. Lett. **7**(4), 10834–10841 (2022). https://doi.org/10.1109/LRA.2022.3188895
31. Eskofier, B.M., Lee, S.I., Baron, M., Simon, A., Martindale, C.F., Gaßner, H., Klucken, J.: An Overview of smart shoes in the internet of health things: gait and mobility assessment in health promotion and disease monitoring. Appl. Sci. **7**(10), 986 (2017). https://doi.org/10.3390/app7100986
32. Fang, H.S., Li, J., Tang, H., Xu, C., Zhu, H., Xiu, Y., Li, Y.L., Lu, C.: AlphaPose: whole-body regional multi-person pose estimation and tracking in real-time. IEEE Trans. Pattern Anal. Mach. Intell. **45**(6), 7157–7173 (2023). https://doi.org/10.1109/TPAMI.2022.3222784
33. Fried, L.P., Tangen, C.M., Walston, J., Newman, A.B., Hirsch, C., Gottdiener, J., Seeman, T., Tracy, R., Kop, W.J., Burke, G., McBurnie, M.A.: Frailty in older adults: evidence for a phenotype. J. Gerontol. Ser. A **56**(3), M146–M157 (2001). https://doi.org/10.1093/gerona/56.3.M146
34. Fukui, K., Maeda, N., Komiya, M., Sasadai, J., Tashiro, T., Yoshimi, M., Tsutsumi, S., Arima, S., Kaneda, K., Onoue, S., Shima, T., Niitani, M., Urabe, Y.: The relationship between modified short physical performance battery and falls: a cross-sectional study of older outpatients. Geriatrics **6**(4), 106 (2021). https://doi.org/10.3390/geriatrics6040106
35. García-García, F.J., Carcaillon, L., Fernandez-Tresguerres, J., Alfaro, A., Larrion, J.L., Castillo, C., Rodriguez-Mañas, L.: A new operational definition of frailty: the frailty trait scale. J. Am. Med. Dir. Assoc. **15**(5), 371.e7–371.e13 (2014). https://doi.org/10.1016/j.jamda.2014.01.004
36. García-García, F.J., Carnicero, J.A., Losa-Reyna, J., Alfaro-Acha, A., Castillo-Gallego, C., Rosado-Artalejo, C., Gutiérrrez-Ávila, G., Rodriguez-Mañas, L.: Frailty trait scale-short form: a frailty instrument for clinical practice. J. Am. Med. Dir. Assoc. **21**(9), 1260-1266.e2 (2020). https://doi.org/10.1016/j.jamda.2019.12.008
37. Ghoreshi Beyrami, S.M., Ghaderyan, P.: A robust, cost-effective and non-invasive computer-aided method for diagnosis three types of neurodegenerative diseases with gait signal analysis. Measurement **156**, 107,579 (2020). https://doi.org/10.1016/j.measurement.2020.107579
38. Gobbens, R.J.J., van Assen, M.A.L.M.: Frailty and its prediction of disability and health care utilization: the added value of interviews and physical measures following a self-report questionnaire. Arch. Gerontol. Geriatr. **55**(2), 369–379 (2012). https://doi.org/10.1016/j.archger.2012.04.008
39. Gong, L., Liu, Y., Yi, L., Fang, J., Yang, Y., Wei, K.: Abnormal gait patterns in autism spectrum disorder and their correlations with social impairments. Autism Res. **13**(7), 1215–1226 (2020). https://doi.org/10.1002/aur.2302

40. Gras, L.Z., Kanaan, S.F., McDowd, J.M., Colgrove, Y.M., Burns, J., Pohl, P.S.: Balance and gait of adults with very mild Alzheimer disease. J. Geriatr. Phys. Therapy **38**(1), 1 (January/March 2015). https://doi.org/10.1519/JPT.0000000000000020
41. Gu, X., Guo, Y., Deligianni, F., Lo, B., Yang, G.Z.: Cross-subject and cross-modal transfer for generalized abnormal gait pattern recognition. IEEE Trans. Neural Netw. Learn. Syst. **32**(2), 546–560 (2021). https://doi.org/10.1109/TNNLS.2020.3009448
42. Güler, R.A., Neverova, N., Kokkinos, I.: DensePose: dense human pose estimation in the wild. In: Proceedings of the IEEE Conference on Computer Vision and Pattern Recognition, pp. 7297–7306 (2018)
43. Guo, Y., Gravina, R., Gu, X., Fortino, G., Yang, G.Z.: EMG-based abnormal gait detection and recognition. In: 2020 IEEE International Conference on Human-Machine Systems (ICHMS), pp. 1–6 (2020). https://doi.org/10.1109/ICHMS49158.2020.9209449
44. Guralnik, J.M., Simonsick, E.M., Ferrucci, L., Glynn, R.J., Berkman, L.F., Blazer, D.G., Scherr, P.A., Wallace, R.B.: A short physical performance battery assessing lower extremity function: association with self-reported disability and prediction of mortality and nursing home admission. J. Gerontol. **49**(2), M85–M94 (1994)
45. Hahm, K.S., Anthony, B.W.: Machine learning-based gait health monitoring for multi-occupant smart homes. Internet Things **26**, 101,154 (2024). https://doi.org/10.1016/j.iot.2024.101154
46. Haim, N., Vardi, G., Yehudai, G., Shamir, O., Irani, M.: Reconstructing training data from trained neural networks. Adv. Neural. Inf. Process. Syst. **35**, 22911–22924 (2022)
47. Han, Y., Han, C.B., Chen, C., Lee, P.W., Hogarth, M., Moore, A.A., Weibel, N., Farcas, E.: Towards visualization of time–series ecological momentary assessment (EMA) data on standalone voice–first virtual assistants. In: Proceedings of the 24th International ACM SIGACCESS Conference on Computers and Accessibility, pp. 1–4. ACM, Athens Greece (2022). https://doi.org/10.1145/3517428.3550398
48. Han, Y.C., Wong, K.I., Murray, I.: Gait phase detection for normal and abnormal gaits using IMU. IEEE Sens. J. **19**(9), 3439–3448 (2019). https://doi.org/10.1109/JSEN.2019.2894143
49. Horak, F.B., Mancini, M., Carlson-Kuhta, P., Nutt, J.G., Salarian, A.: Balance and gait represent independent domains of mobility in Parkinson disease. Phys. Ther. **96**(9), 1364–1371 (2016). https://doi.org/10.2522/ptj.20150580
50. Jeong, Y.K., Baek, K.R.: Asymmetric gait analysis using a DTW algorithm with combined gyroscope and pressure sensor. Sensors **21**(11), 3750 (2021). https://doi.org/10.3390/s21113750
51. Job, M., Dottor, A., Viceconti, A., Testa, M.: Ecological gait as a fall indicator in older adults: a systematic review. Gerontologist **60**(5), e395–e412 (2019). https://doi.org/10.1093/geront/gnz113
52. Jones, D., Song, X., Mitnitski, A., Rockwood, K.: Evaluation of a frailty index based on a comprehensive geriatric assessment in a population based study of elderly Canadians. Aging Clin. Exp. Res. **17**(6), 465–471 (2005). https://doi.org/10.1007/BF03327413
53. Jun, K., Lee, D.W., Lee, K., Lee, S., Kim, M.S.: Feature extraction using an RNN autoencoder for skeleton-based abnormal gait recognition. IEEE Access **8**, 19196–19207 (2020). https://doi.org/10.1109/ACCESS.2020.2967845
54. Jun, K., Lee, S., Lee, D.W., Kim, M.S.: Deep learning-based multimodal abnormal gait classification using a 3D skeleton and plantar foot pressure. IEEE Access **9**, 161,576–161,589 (2021). https://doi.org/10.1109/ACCESS.2021.3131613
55. Jun, K., Lee, Y., Lee, S., Lee, D.W., Kim, M.S.: Pathological gait classification using Kinect v2 and gated recurrent neural networks. IEEE Access **8**, 139,881–139,891 (2020). https://doi.org/10.1109/ACCESS.2020.3013029
56. van Kan, G.A., Rolland, Y.M., Morley, J.E., Vellas, B.: Frailty: toward a clinical definition. J. Am. Med. Dir. Assoc. **9**(2), 71–72 (2008)
57. Kaur, R., Motl, R.W., Sowers, R., Hernandez, M.E.: A vision-based framework for predicting multiple sclerosis and Parkinson's disease gait dysfunctions–a deep learning approach. IEEE J. Biomed. Health Inform. **27**(1), 190–201 (2023). https://doi.org/10.1109/JBHI.2022.3208077

58. Kiprijanovska, I., Gjoreski, H., Gams, M.: Detection of gait abnormalities for fall risk assessment using wrist-worn inertial sensors and deep learning. Sensors **20**(18), 5373 (2020). https://doi.org/10.3390/s20185373
59. Kolokas, N., Krinidis, S., Drosou, A., Ioannidis, D., Tzovaras, D.: Gait matching by mapping wearable to camera privacy-preserving recordings: experimental comparison of multiple settings. In: 2019 6th International Conference on Control, Decision and Information Technologies (CoDIT), pp. 338–343 (2019). https://doi.org/10.1109/CoDIT.2019.8820339
60. Kressig, R.W., Gregor, R.J., Oliver, A., Waddell, D., Smith, W., O'Grady, M., Curns, A.T., Kutner, M., Wolf, S.L.: Temporal and spatial features of gait in older adults transitioning to frailty. Gait Posture **20**(1), 30–35 (2004). https://doi.org/10.1016/S0966-6362(03)00089-4
61. Lauretani, F., Ticinesi, A., Gionti, L., Prati, B., Nouvenne, A., Tana, C., Meschi, T., Maggio, M.: Short-physical performance battery (SPPB) score is associated with falls in older outpatients. Aging Clin. Exp. Res. **31**(10), 1435–1442 (2019). https://doi.org/10.1007/s40520-018-1082-y
62. Liu, X., Zhao, C., Zheng, B., Guo, Q., Duan, X., Wulamu, A., Zhang, D.: Wearable devices for gait analysis in intelligent healthcare. Front. Comput. Sci. **3** (2021). https://doi.org/10.3389/fcomp.2021.661676
63. Liu, Y., He, X., Wang, R., Teng, Q., Hu, R., Qing, L., Wang, Z., He, X., Yin, B., Mou, Y., Du, Y., Li, X., Wang, H., Liu, X., Zhou, L., Deng, L., Xu, Z., Xiao, C., Ge, M., Sun, X., Jiang, J., Chen, J., Lin, X., Xia, L., Gong, H., Yu, H., Dong, B.: Application of machine vision in classifying gait frailty among older adults. Front. Aging Neurosci. **13** (2021). https://doi.org/10.3389/fnagi.2021.757823
64. Loureiro, J., Correia, P.L.: Using a Skeleton gait energy image for pathological gait classification. In: 2020 15th IEEE International Conference on Automatic Face and Gesture Recognition (FG 2020), pp. 503–507. IEEE, Buenos Aires, Argentina (2020). https://doi.org/10.1109/FG47880.2020.00064
65. Lu, M., Poston, K., Pfefferbaum, A., Sullivan, E.V., Fei-Fei, L., Pohl, K.M., Niebles, J.C., Adeli, E.: Vision-based estimation of MDS-UPDRS gait scores for assessing Parkinson's disease motor severity. In: Martel, A.L., Abolmaesumi, P., Stoyanov, D., Mateus, D., Zuluaga, M.A., Zhou, S.K., Racoceanu, D., Joskowicz, L. (eds.) Medical Image Computing and Computer Assisted Intervention—MICCAI 2020, pp. 637–647. Springer International Publishing, Cham (2020). https://doi.org/10.1007/978-3-030-59716-0_61
66. Lumetzberger, J., Ballester, I., Kampel, M.: Fall detection. In: Salah, A.A., Colonna, L., Florez-Revuelta, F. (eds.) Privacy-Aware Monitoring for Assisted Living. Springer, Cham (2025)
67. Lunardini, F., Malavolti, M., Pedrocchi, A.L.G., Borghese, N.A., Ferrante, S.: A mobile app to transparently distinguish single- from dual-task walking for the ecological monitoring of age-related changes in daily-life gait. Gait Posture **86**, 27–32 (2021). https://doi.org/10.1016/j.gaitpost.2021.02.028
68. Maher, J.P., Rebar, A.L., Dunton, G.F.: Ecological momentary assessment is a feasible and valid methodological tool to measure older adults' physical activity and sedentary behavior. Front. Psychol. **9** (2018). https://doi.org/10.3389/fpsyg.2018.01485
69. Malmstrom, T.K., Miller, D.K., Morley, J.E.: A comparison of four frailty models. J. Am. Geriatr. Soc. **62**(4), 721–726 (2014). https://doi.org/10.1111/jgs.12735
70. Manna, S.K., Hannan Bin Azhar, M., Greace, A.: Optimal locations and computational frameworks of FSR and IMU sensors for measuring gait abnormalities. Heliyon **9**(4), e15,210 (2023). https://doi.org/10.1016/j.heliyon.2023.e15210
71. Marcante, A., Di Marco, R., Gentile, G., Pellicano, C., Assogna, F., Pontieri, F.E., Spalletta, G., Macchiusi, L., Gatsios, D., Giannakis, A., Chondrogiorgi, M., Konitsiotis, S., Fotiadis, D.I., Antonini, A.: Foot pressure wearable sensors for freezing of gait detection in Parkinson's disease. Sensors **21**(1), 128 (2021). https://doi.org/10.3390/s21010128
72. Mc Ardle, R., Morris, R., Wilson, J., Galna, B., Thomas, A.J., Rochester, L.: What can quantitative gait analysis tell us about dementia and its subtypes? A structured review. J. Alzheimers Dis. **60**(4), 1295–1312 (2017). https://doi.org/10.3233/JAD-170541

73. McDevitt-Murphy, M.E., Luciano, M.T., Zakarian, R.J.: Use of ecological momentary assessment and intervention in treatment with adults. Focus **16**(4), 370–375 (2018). https://doi.org/10.1176/appi.focus.20180017. Publisher: American Psychiatric Publishing
74. Mehdizadeh, S., Dolatabadi, E., Ng, K.D., Mansfield, A., Flint, A., Taati, B., Iaboni, A.: Vision-based assessment of gait features associated with falls in people with dementia. J. Gerontol. Ser. A **75**(6), 1148–1153 (2020)
75. Mehdizadeh, S., Van Ooteghem, K., Gulka, H., Nabavi, H., Faieghi, M., Taati, B., Iaboni, A.: A systematic review of center of pressure measures to quantify gait changes in older adults. Exp. Gerontol. **143**, 111,170 (2021). https://doi.org/10.1016/j.exger.2020.111170
76. Mehraban, S., Adeli, V., Taati, B.: MotionAGFormer: enhancing 3d human pose estimation with a transformer-GCNformer network. In: Proceedings of the IEEE/CVF Winter Conference on Applications of Computer Vision (2024)
77. Meng, C., Bufu, H., Yangsheng, X.: Intelligent shoes for abnormal gait detection. In: 2008 IEEE International Conference on Robotics and Automation, pp. 2019–2024. IEEE, Pasadena, CA, USA (2008). https://doi.org/10.1109/ROBOT.2008.4543503
78. Miao, B., Liu, X., Zhu, T.: Automatic mental health identification method based on natural gait pattern. PsyCh J. **10**(3), 453–464 (2021). https://doi.org/10.1002/pchj.434
79. Mihailidis, A., Carmichael, B., Boger, J.: The use of computer vision in an intelligent environment to support aging-in-place, safety, and independence in the home. IEEE Trans. Inf Technol. Biomed. **8**(3), 238–247 (2004). https://doi.org/10.1109/TITB.2004.834386
80. Mirelman, A., Bonato, P., Camicioli, R., Ellis, T.D., Giladi, N., Hamilton, J.L., Hass, C.J., Hausdorff, J.M., Pelosin, E., Almeida, Q.J.: Gait impairments in Parkinson's disease. Lancet Neurol. **18**(7), 697–708 (2019). https://doi.org/10.1016/S1474-4422(19)30044-4
81. Mitnitski, A.B., Mogilner, A.J., Rockwood, K.: Accumulation of deficits as a proxy measure of aging. Sci. World J. **1**, 323–336 (2001). https://doi.org/10.1100/tsw.2001.58
82. Montero-Odasso, M., Muir, S.W., Hall, M., Doherty, T.J., Kloseck, M., Beauchet, O., Speechley, M.: Gait variability is associated with frailty in community-dwelling older adults. J. Gerontol. Ser. A **66A**(5), 568–576 (2011). https://doi.org/10.1093/gerona/glr007
83. Morris, I., Shiffman, S., Beckjord, E., Ferguson, S.G.: Ecological momentary assessment and technological advances in clinical care. In: The Oxford Handbook of Digital Technologies and Mental Health. Oxford University Press (2020). https://doi.org/10.1093/oxfordhb/9780190218058.013.24
84. Nambiar, A., Bernardino, A., Nascimento, J.C.: Gait-based person re-identification: a survey. ACM Comput. Surv. **52**(2), 33:1–33:34 (2019). https://doi.org/10.1145/3243043
85. Nelson, B.W., Allen, N.B.: Extending the passive-sensing toolbox: using smart-home technology in psychological science. Perspect. Psychol. Sci. **13**(6), 718–733 (2018). https://doi.org/10.1177/1745691618776008
86. Ng, K.D., Mehdizadeh, S., Iaboni, A., Mansfield, A., Flint, A., Taati, B.: Measuring gait variables using computer vision to assess mobility and fall risk in older adults with dementia. IEEE J. Transl. Eng. Health Med. **8**, 1–9 (2020). https://doi.org/10.1109/JTEHM.2020.2998326
87. Nguyen, T.N., Huynh, H.H., Meunier, J.: Skeleton-based abnormal gait detection. Sensors **16**(11), 1792 (2016). https://doi.org/10.3390/s16111792
88. Nieto-Hidalgo, M., Ferrández-Pastor, F.J., Valdivieso-Sarabia, R.J., Mora-Pascual, J., García-Chamizo, J.M.: A vision based proposal for classification of normal and abnormal gait using RGB camera. J. Biomed. Inform. **63**, 82–89 (2016). https://doi.org/10.1016/j.jbi.2016.08.003
89. Orekondy, T., Schiele, B., Fritz, M.: Towards a visual privacy advisor: understanding and predicting privacy risks in images. In: Proceedings of the IEEE International Conference on Computer Vision, pp. 3686–3695 (2017)
90. Oviedo-Briones, M., Laso, Á.R., Carnicero, J.A., Cesari, M., Grodzicki, T., Gryglewska, B., Sinclair, A., Landi, F., Vellas, B., Checa-López, M., Rodriguez-Mañas, L.: A comparison of frailty assessment instruments in different clinical and social care settings: the frailtools project. J. Am. Med. Dir. Assoc. **22**(3), 607.e7-607.e12 (2021). https://doi.org/10.1016/j.jamda.2020.09.024

91. Pachon-Suescun, C.G., Pinzon-Arenas, J.O., Jimenez-Moreno, R.: Abnormal gait detection by means of LSTM. Int. J. Electr. Comput. Eng. (IJECE) **10**(2), 1495 (2020). https://doi.org/10.11591/ijece.v10i2.pp1495-1506
92. Parashar, A., Shekhawat, R.S.: Protection of gait data set for preserving its privacy in deep learning pipeline. IET Biom. **11**(6), 557–569 (2022). https://doi.org/10.1049/bme2.12093
93. Peters, L.L., Boter, H., Buskens, E., Slaets, J.P.: Measurement properties of the Groningen frailty indicator in home-dwelling and institutionalized elderly people. J. Am. Med. Dir. Assoc. **13**(6), 546–551 (2012). https://doi.org/10.1016/j.jamda.2012.04.007
94. Pogorelc, B., Bosnić, Z., Gams, M.: Automatic recognition of gait-related health problems in the elderly using machine learning. Multimed. Tools Appl. **58**(2), 333–354 (2012). https://doi.org/10.1007/s11042-011-0786-1
95. Rani, V., Kumar, M.: Human gait recognition: a systematic review. Multimed. Tools Appl. **82**(24), 37003–37037 (2023). https://doi.org/10.1007/s11042-023-15079-5
96. Rasnayaka, S., Sim, T.: Your tattletale gait privacy invasiveness of IMU gait data. In: 2020 IEEE International Joint Conference on Biometrics (IJCB), pp. 1–10 (2020). https://doi.org/10.1109/IJCB48548.2020.9304922
97. Ravi, S., Climent-Pérez, P., Florez-Revuelta, F.: A review on visual privacy preservation techniques for active and assisted living. Multimed. Tools Appl. **83**(5), 14715–14755 (2024)
98. Raîche, M., Hébert, R., Dubois, M.F.: Prisma-7: a case-finding tool to identify older adults with moderate to severe disabilities. Arch. Gerontol. Geriatr. **47**(1), 9–18 (2008). https://doi.org/10.1016/j.archger.2007.06.004
99. Rempe, D., Birdal, T., Hertzmann, A., Yang, J., Sridhar, S., Guibas, L.J.: HUMOR: 3D human motion model for robust pose estimation. In: Proceedings of the IEEE/CVF International Conference on Computer Vision, pp. 11,488–11,499 (2021)
100. Rogez, G., Weinzaepfel, P., Schmid, C.: LCR-net++: multi-person 2d and 3d pose detection in natural images. IEEE Trans. Pattern Anal. Mach. Intell. **42**(5), 1146–1161 (2020). https://doi.org/10.1109/TPAMI.2019.2892985
101. Rolfson, D., Majumdar, S., Taher, A., Tsuyuki, R.: Development and validation of a new instrument for frailty. Clin. Invest. Med. **23** (2000)
102. Rolfson, D.B., Majumdar, S.R., Tsuyuki, R.T., Tahir, A., Rockwood, K.: Validity and reliability of the Edmonton frail scale. Age Ageing **35**(5), 526–529 (2006). https://doi.org/10.1093/ageing/afl041
103. Romero-Ortuno, R., Kenny, R.A.: The frailty index in Europeans: association with age and mortality. Age Ageing **41**(5), 684–689 (2012). https://doi.org/10.1093/ageing/afs051
104. Romijnders, R., Salis, F., Hansen, C., Küderle, A., Paraschiv-Ionescu, A., Cereatti, A., Alcock, L., Aminian, K., Becker, C., Bertuletti, S., Bonci, T., Brown, P., Buckley, E., Cantu, A., Carsin, A.E., Caruso, M., Caulfield, B., Chiari, L., D'Ascanio, I., Del Din, S., Eskofier, B., Fernstad, S.J., Fröhlich, M.S., Garcia Aymerich, J., Gazit, E., Hausdorff, J.M., Hiden, H., Hume, E., Keogh, A., Kirk, C., Kluge, F., Koch, S., Mazzà, C., Megaritis, D., Micó-Amigo, E., Müller, A., Palmerini, L., Rochester, L., Schwickert, L., Scott, K., Sharrack, B., Singleton, D., Soltani, A., Ullrich, M., Vereijken, B., Vogiatzis, I., Yarnall, A., Schmidt, G., Maetzler, W.: Ecological validity of a deep learning algorithm to detect gait events from real-life walking bouts in mobility-limiting diseases. Front. Neurol. **14** (2023). https://doi.org/10.3389/fneur.2023.1247532
105. Rong, Y., Shiratori, T., Joo, H.: Frankmocap: A monocular 3D whole-body pose estimation system via regression and integration. In: Proceedings of the IEEE/CVF International Conference on Computer Vision, pp. 1749–1759 (2021)
106. Sabo, A., Mehdizadeh, S., Iaboni, A., Taati, B.: Estimating parkinsonism severity in natural gait videos of older adults with dementia. IEEE J. Biomed. Health Inform. **26**(5), 2288–2298 (2022). https://doi.org/10.1109/JBHI.2022.3144917
107. Sabo, A., Mehdizadeh, S., Ng, K.D., Iaboni, A., Taati, B.: Assessment of Parkinsonian gait in older adults with dementia via human pose tracking in video data. J. Neuroeng. Rehabil. **17**, 1–10 (2020)

108. Salis, F., Bertuletti, S., Scott, K., Caruso, M., Bonci, T., Buckley, E., Croce, U.D., Mazzà, C., Cereatti, A.: A wearable multi-sensor system for real world gait analysis. In: 2021 43rd Annual International Conference of the IEEE Engineering in Medicine and Biology Society (EMBC), pp. 7020–7023 (2021). https://doi.org/10.1109/EMBC46164.2021.9630392
109. Schmitter-Edgecombe, M., Luna, C., Dai, S., Cook, D.J.: Predicting daily cognition and lifestyle behaviors for older adults using smart home data and ecological momentary assessment. Clin. Neuropsychol. 1–25 (2024). https://doi.org/10.1080/13854046.2024.2330143
110. Schwenk, M., Howe, C., Saleh, A., Mohler, J., Grewal, G., Armstrong, D., Najafi, B.: Frailty and technology: a systematic review of gait analysis in those with frailty. Gerontology **60**(1), 79–89 (2013)
111. Schwenk, M., Mohler, J., Wendel, C., D"Huyvetter, K., Fain, M., Taylor-Piliae, R., Najafi, B.: Wearable sensor-based in-home assessment of gait, balance, and physical activity for discrimination of frailty status: baseline results of the Arizona frailty cohort study. Gerontology **61**(3), 258–267 (2014). https://doi.org/10.1159/000369095
112. Searle, S.D., Mitnitski, A., Gahbauer, E.A., Gill, T.M., Rockwood, K.: A standard procedure for creating a frailty index. BMC Geriatr. **8**(1), 24 (2008). https://doi.org/10.1186/1471-2318-8-24
113. Sepas-Moghaddam, A., Etemad, A.: Deep gait recognition: a survey. IEEE Trans. Pattern Anal. Mach. Intell. **45**(1), 264–284 (2023). https://doi.org/10.1109/TPAMI.2022.3151865
114. Shah, V.V., Carlson-Kuhta, P., Mancini, M., Sowalsky, K., Horak, F.B.: Digital gait measures, but not the 400-meter walk time, detect abnormal gait characteristics in people with prediabetes. Gait Posture **109**, 84–88 (2024). https://doi.org/10.1016/j.gaitpost.2024.01.030
115. Sharma, A., Rai, V., Calvert, M., Dai, Z., Guo, Z., Boe, D., Rombokas, E.: A non-laboratory gait dataset of full body kinematics and egocentric vision. Sci. Data **10**(1), 26 (2023). https://doi.org/10.1038/s41597-023-01932-7
116. Shin, S., Kim, J., Halilaj, E., Black, M.J.: WHAM: reconstructing world-grounded humans with accurate 3d motion. In: Proceedings of the IEEE/CVF Conference on Computer Vision and Pattern Recognition (CVPR), pp. 2070–2080 (2024)
117. Steil, J., Koelle, M., Heuten, W., Boll, S., Bulling, A.: Privaceye: privacy-preserving head-mounted eye tracking using egocentric scene image and eye movement features. In: Proceedings of the 11th ACM Symposium on Eye Tracking Research and Applications, pp. 1–10 (2019)
118. Stinson, L., Liu, Y., Dallery, J.: Ecological momentary assessment: a systematic review of validity research. Perspect. Behavior Sci. **45**(2), 469–493 (2022). https://doi.org/10.1007/s40614-022-00339-w
119. Stone, A.A., Shiffman, S.: Ecological momentary assessment (EMA) in behavioral medicine. Ann. Behav. Med. **16**(3), 199–202 (1994). https://doi.org/10.1093/abm/16.3.199
120. Studenski, S.: Gait speed reveals clues to lifelong health. JAMA Netw. Open **2**(10), e1913,112 (2019). https://doi.org/10.1001/jamanetworkopen.2019.13112
121. Su, H., Sun, F., Lu, Z., Zhang, J., Zhang, W., Liu, J.: A wearable sensing system based on smartphone and diaper to detect urine in-situ for patients with urinary incontinence. Sens. Actuators B: Chem. **357**, 131,459 (2022). https://doi.org/10.1016/j.snb.2022.131459
122. Tamura, T., Nakajima, K., Matsushita, T., Fujimoto, T., Shimooki, S., Nakano, T.: A warning detector for urinary incontinence for home health care. Biomed. Instrum. Technol. **29**(4), 343–349 (1995)
123. Theou, O., Brothers, T.D., Mitnitski, A., Rockwood, K.: Operationalization of frailty using eight commonly used scales and comparison of their ability to predict all-cause mortality. J. Am. Geriatr. Soc. **61**(9), 1537–1551 (2013). https://doi.org/10.1111/jgs.12420
124. Theou, O., Brothers, T.D., Peña, F.G., Mitnitski, A., Rockwood, K.: Identifying common characteristics of frailty across seven scales. J. Am. Geriatr. Soc. **62**(5), 901–906 (2014). https://doi.org/10.1111/jgs.12773
125. Theou, O., Brothers, T.D., Rockwood, M.R., Haardt, D., Mitnitski, A., Rockwood, K.: Exploring the relationship between national economic indicators and relative fitness and frailty in

middle-aged and older Europeans. Age Ageing **42**(5), 614–619 (2013). https://doi.org/10.1093/ageing/aft010
126. Tian, H., Ma, X., Wu, H., Li, Y.: Skeleton-based abnormal gait recognition with spatiotemporal attention enhanced gait-structural graph convolutional networks. Neurocomputing **473**, 116–126 (2022). https://doi.org/10.1016/j.neucom.2021.12.004
127. Tieu, N.D.T., Nguyen, H.H., Nguyen-Son, H.Q., Yamagishi, J., Echizen, I.: An approach for gait anonymization using deep learning. In: 2017 IEEE Workshop on Information Forensics and Security (WIFS), pp. 1–6. IEEE, Rennes, France (2017). https://doi.org/10.1109/WIFS.2017.8267657
128. Timon, C.M., Hussey, P., Lee, H., Murphy, C., Vardan Rai, H., Smeaton, A.F.: Automatically detecting activities of daily living from in-home sensors as indicators of routine behaviour in an older population. Digital Health **9**, 20552076231184,084 (2023). https://doi.org/10.1177/20552076231184084
129. Tinetti, M.E.: Performance-oriented assessment of mobility problems in elderly patients. J. Am. Geriatr. Soc. **34**(2), 119–126 (1986)
130. Varma, V.R., Ghosal, R., Hillel, I., Volfson, D., Weiss, J., Urbanek, J., Hausdorff, J.M., Zipunnikov, V., Watts, A.: Continuous gait monitoring discriminates community-dwelling mild Alzheimer's disease from cognitively normal controls. Alzheimer's Dementia: Transl. Res. Clin. Interv. **7**(1), e12,131 (2021). https://doi.org/10.1002/trc2.12131
131. Vavasour, G., Giggins, O.M., Doyle, J., Kelly, D.: How wearable sensors have been utilised to evaluate frailty in older adults: a systematic review. J. Neuroeng. Rehabil. **18**(1), 112 (2021). https://doi.org/10.1186/s12984-021-00909-0
132. Vellas, B., Balardy, L., Gillette-Guyonnet, S., Abellan Van Kan, G., Ghisolfi-Marque, A., Subra, J., Bismuth, S., Oustric, S., Cesari, M.: Looking for frailty in community-dwelling older persons: the gérontopôle frailty screening tool (GFST). J. Nutrit. Health Aging **17**, 629–631 (2013)
133. Wang, D., Timm, G.W., Erdman, A.G., Tewfik, A.H.: Ambulatory device for urinary incontinence detection in females. In: Annual International Conference of the IEEE Engineering in Medicine and Biology Society. IEEE Engineering in Medicine and Biology Society. Annual International Conference 2009, pp. 5405–5408 (2009). https://doi.org/10.1109/IEMBS.2009.5332814
134. Webster, K.E., Merory, J.R., Wittwer, J.E.: Gait variability in community dwelling adults with Alzheimer disease. Alzheimer Dis. Assoc. Disord. **20**(1), 37 (2006-01/2006-03). https://doi.org/10.1097/01.wad.0000201849.75578.de
135. Yamada, S., Aoyagi, Y., Ishikawa, M., Yamaguchi, M., Yamamoto, K., Nozaki, K.: Gait assessment using three-dimensional acceleration of the trunk in idiopathic normal pressure hydrocephalus. Front. Aging Neurosci. **13** (2021). https://doi.org/10.3389/fnagi.2021.653964
136. Zhu, L., Liu, Z., Han, S.: Deep leakage from gradients. In: Wallach, H., Larochelle, H., Beygelzimer, A., d'Alché Buc, F., Fox, E., Garnett, R. (eds.) Advances in Neural Information Processing Systems, vol. 32. Curran Associates, Inc. (2019)

Open Access This chapter is licensed under the terms of the Creative Commons Attribution 4.0 International License (http://creativecommons.org/licenses/by/4.0/), which permits use, sharing, adaptation, distribution and reproduction in any medium or format, as long as you give appropriate credit to the original author(s) and the source, provide a link to the Creative Commons license and indicate if changes were made.

The images or other third party material in this chapter are included in the chapter's Creative Commons license, unless indicated otherwise in a credit line to the material. If material is not included in the chapter's Creative Commons license and your intended use is not permitted by statutory regulation or exceeds the permitted use, you will need to obtain permission directly from the copyright holder.

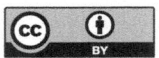

Chapter 7
Activities of Daily Living (ADL) and Behavior Recognition

Slavisa Aleksic, Vladimir Despotovic, and Stefania Cristina

Abstract This chapter addresses the state of research in human activity recognition (HAR) for active assisted living (AAL) applications. We provide a comprehensive review of the ongoing research efforts and identify future trends in this area, especially regarding the activities of daily living (ADL) and behavior recognition. The focus of this work is on privacy-preserving methods and technologies that use audio and video modalities for HAR, as well as combining them with various sensors and wearables in a multimodal setup.

Keywords Active assisted living (AAL) · Human activity recognition (HAR) · Computer vision · Audio processing · Multimodality · Privacy-preserving methods

7.1 Introduction

Human activity recognition (HAR) plays a fundamental role across a broad spectrum of applications provided by assisted living systems, including health and elderly care, human-human interaction (HHI) and human-computer interaction (HCI), smart environments, security and surveillance systems, sports and fitness tracking, or entertainment and gaming. Defined as a classification problem, HAR maps an image or a video segment into one or more activity classes. In an active assisted living (AAL)

S. Aleksic (✉)
Faculty of Digital Transformation, HTWK Leipzig, Leipzig, Germany
e-mail: slavisa.aleksic@htwk-leipzig.de

V. Despotovic
Department of Medical Informatics, Bioinformatics & AI, Luxembourg Institute of Health, Strassen, Luxembourg
e-mail: vladimir.despotovic@lih.lu

S. Cristina
Faculty of Engineering, Department of Systems and Control Engineering, University of Malta, Msida, Malta
e-mail: stefania.cristina@um.edu.mt

context, the target classes are typically activities of daily living (ADL), which are basic tasks that are necessary for independent living and personal care, such as eating, walking, sitting, bathing, etc. [53].

Technologies for recognition of ADL have experienced a fast development in the past decades [8, 23, 63, 76, 91, 99], which led to a number of new applications, components and systems that either have already found wide application, or are still in the development and/or deployment phase. Despite these advancements, several challenges still exist related to effective integration of HAR methods and systems into real-word applications and realistic scenarios.

In this chapter, we focus on HAR applications related to recognition of ADL and human behavior. ADL are often used in healthcare to assess an individual's ability to perform essential self-care tasks, particularly when evaluating older adults or people with disabilities. As shown in Fig. 7.1, one can group all ADL into general ADL and those related to healthcare applications.

HAR systems for the recognition of general ADL mostly focus on monitoring of food preparation and intake, personal hygiene activities, sport and fitness and sleeping/resting [13]. The most used sensor type for the recognition of daily activities

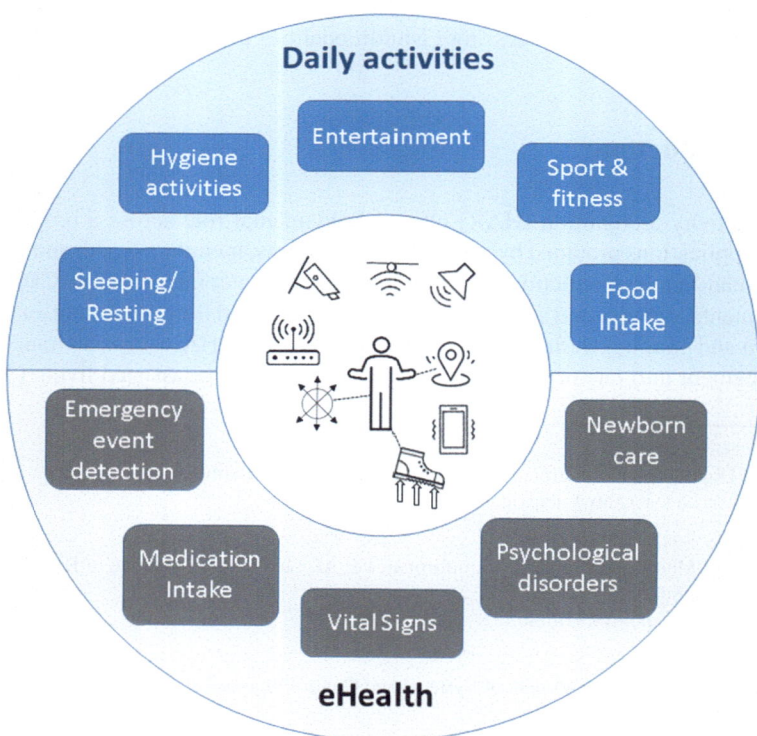

Fig. 7.1 Applications of activity/behavior recognition in assisted living environments

is the motion sensor. Other sensors used are simple contact sensors, measuring power consumption of appliances, temperature, accelerometer, light, humidity, pressure, sound as well as RGB and RGB-D cameras.

One of the most often recognized ADL is the meal preparation and food intake. According to the study results reported in [13], about 55% of the 39 reviewed systems were able to recognize either eating or meal preparation without distinguishing between these two activities. Another 18% were able to separate eating from meal preparation, while only 3% of the systems distinguished between drinking and eating, or recognized preparation of breakfast, lunch, and dinner.

Another type of activity that has attracted attention is personal hygiene. Within this activity group, mostly brushing teeth, bathing, shaving, and styling are recognized. For recognizing entertainment and gaming activities, smart switches that are able to monitor power consumption of corresponding appliances can be used. For example, power consumption of TV devices or gaming consoles can be used for recognition of the activities "watching TV" or "gaming" [112].

As presented in a recent scoping review that examined 35 articles [23], the majority of recent HAR research works in healthcare applications focus on video-based methods (71.5%), mostly using RGB cameras (see Fig. 7.3). Multimodal approaches (17%) and approaches using audio processing (11.5%) are substantially less considered. The majority of works present early experimental results (77%), whereas only 14% of the presented results are obtained in a real-world setting, suggesting a prevalent focus on algorithm development and validation in controlled environments rather than real-life deployment scenarios. Further efforts are needed to move from experimental prototypes to widespread adoption of HAR technologies in everyday environments, addressing challenges such as scalability, robustness, and user acceptance.

eHealth applications often include remote monitoring and elderly care, especially with respect to emergency event detection, dementia/Alzheimer's disease and other psychological disorders such as depression, autism, or suicidal behavior. Additionally, medication intake plays a significant role in eHealth applications. A special application is newborn care [23]. For eHealth applications mostly vision-based approaches are used (71.5%) while multimodal and audio-based systems count to only 17% and 11.5%, respectively.

Audio- and video-based HAR systems play a significant role in AAL applications. Vision-based activity recognition has gained particular attention given its potentially high performance. However, a number of factors such as the interference with the environmental light, shadowing, different angles, and privacy protection narrow its application. As shown in Fig. 7.2, vision-based activity recognition can be combined with other modalities (e.g. audio, wearables and various sensors) in order to achieve better robustness and improve performance, as well as to extend the fields of application. In this chapter, we provide an overview and classification of various video- and audio-based approaches for activity/behavior recognition, addressing the possibilities of combining these methods with other technologies and approaches, particularly in the scope of AAL systems.

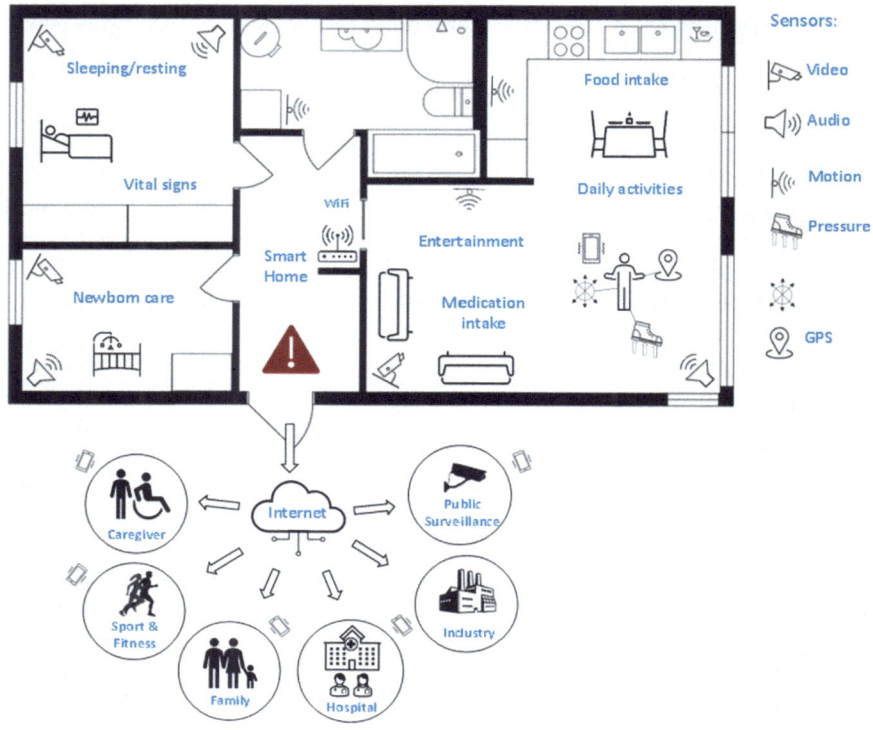

Fig. 7.2 Modalities and applications for activity/behavior recognition in assisted living environments

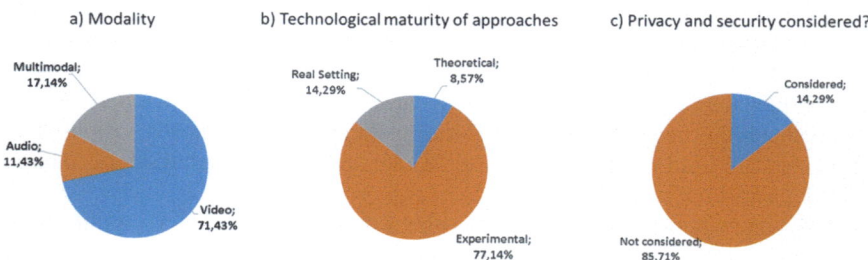

Fig. 7.3 Results of the literature analysis [23] regarding a) modality, b) technological maturity of approaches, and c) consideration of privacy and security

While privacy-aware HAR is the ultimate goal, there seems to be a lack of awareness and standardization for preserving privacy in the existing research efforts. Major challenges include the need for robust anonymisation techniques to protect sensitive data, ensuring that activity recognition algorithms operate efficiently while minimizing data collection, storage, and transmission, and addressing the trade-off between privacy preservation and model performance. The existing methods are primarily focused on protecting the user's identity while disregarding details about the living environment that could still disclose sensitive information. Additionally, designing systems that allow individuals to control the level of information they share and establishing clear guidelines and regulations for the ethical use of data are essential steps in advancing privacy-aware HAR technologies.

7.2 Activity/Behavior Recognition

7.2.1 Video-Based Approaches

Video is the most extensively used modality for activity and behavior recognition within the context of AAL. Video data is often exploited in the recognition of actions or behaviour that involve distinct body movements and postural changes, which may be clearly captured in video and recognised by means of features that can be extracted from their image frames. We have recently identified, within a scoping review [23], several application areas where video-based approaches have been exploited. The identified application areas range from the recognition of abnormal patient behaviour such as falling, the monitoring of medication intake to keep track of the patient's adherence to medication prescriptions, the identification of behaviour consistent with cognitive disorders, and in newborn care with particular interest in monitoring newborn resuscitation. Examples of healthcare-specific activities that have been targeted by video-based approaches include falling, chest clutching, head-banging, sleeping and ingestion of medication [23]. However, the video datasets that feature real-life actions stemming from specific health conditions, such as those featuring patients with dementia, collected as part of the DemCare project [6], or autistic behaviour in children [88], are often limited in number. In order to fill this gap, general purpose video datasets, such as the UCF101 [104] and the Berkeley MHAD [84], have also been used in testing and evaluating video-based approaches for HAR. Such general purpose datasets include a broader array of generic daily life activities, such as playing the guitar, biking, clapping hands and jumping in place.

In video-based HAR, the video data is captured by means of cameras that are typically placed within one's environment or, less frequently, embedded into a wearable device [65]. The two types of cameras that are most typically used in video-based HAR are visible-light and depth cameras. The advantage of using visible-light cameras lies in their ability to capture rich visual information related to shape, colour, texture and environmental context, which can provide informative cues to the problem of HAR. Nonetheless, the very characteristic of capturing rich visual information, which makes visible light cameras favourable, also leads to their downside of raising privacy concerns since there is nothing inherent to the imaging modality that can protect the user's identity. Methods that seek to protect the user's privacy often create binary silhouettes out of the raw visible-light images to hide the person's identity [4, 55], but in doing so they also lose important image information that could improve the HAR result. Depth cameras, on the other hand, offer the benefit of preserving the user's privacy from the outset, since the captured raw data consists of depth values rather than detailed visual information. They may also be less sensitive to variations in the illumination conditions when compared to visible-light cameras. Nonetheless, depth cameras usually have a limited range of operation, which may constrain the space in which HAR can be performed. Much less frequently exploited is the use of near-infrared (NIR) imagery for HAR, which however requires that the features, such as the body joint positions, on which the HAR solution is based are visible under NIR illumination [122]. Wang et al. [122] achieve this by marking the body joint positions through NIR-sensitive fabric sewn to the user's clothes, hence making them visible under NIR illumination. While such an approach can facilitate the image extraction of the body joint features, it can prove to be more complex to set up and run under real-life conditions, because it requires the use of special clothing, prepared specifically for the intended application.

In AAL setting, we typically deal with a continuous scenario, where the video acquired from the environment is not temporally segmented into isolated activities. Finding the boundaries of actions is called "action spotting" and is typically jointly solved with action recognition. However, many action recognition approaches in the literature assume that the data are pre-segmented, which means the task is made simpler. Furthermore, there is the issue of overlapping actions and activities. Finally, there are actions that are easier to spot, and those that depend heavily on the context for proper interpretation (e.g. walking vs. stalking). These issues are some of the challenges faced in HAR.

The following sections explore various classical and deep learning approaches that exploit different image information in addressing the problem of HAR.

7.2.1.1 Classical Approaches

As has been mentioned above, classical methods for HAR rely on traditional image processing and machine learning algorithms to extract the relevant image features and subsequently classify them according to activity. This section explores some of the key classical approaches that have been applied to the problem of HAR over the years.

The first step in the classical pipeline for HAR often deals with image preprocessing where the aim is to prepare the video frames for feature extraction, as the ensuing step. A common preprocessing approach for videos captured by a visible-light camera takes an image frame featuring a person performing an activity and binarises it with the aim of producing a binary silhouette, in which the pixels belonging to the human figure are assigned a foreground class label of 1, whereas all other pixels in the image are assigned a background class label of 0. This is then followed by region of interest (ROI) extraction, which crops a rectangular bounding box around the foreground pixels in the binarised video frame to be passed on to the feature extraction step. A similar preprocessing approach can be followed when working with videos captured by a depth camera, where the resulting depth silhouettes retain the depth values of pixels belonging to the human figure in the foreground and set all of the remaining depth values to 0. Typically used preprocessing methods that have been applied to visible-light images to generate a binary silhouette include Otsu thresholding [4] and background subtraction [55]. The background subtraction technique has also been applied to depth images with the aim of generating a depth silhouette [50], as well as a combination of the Chan-Vese and Bhattacharyya energy functions [97]. Alternatively, the preprocessing step may simply involve ROI detection, such as in the method of Zuo et al. [139] where the detection of a ROI in visible-light image frames is informed by the direction of the user's eye-gaze, captured while the user wore a pair of gaze-enabled smart glasses.

The next step in the classical pipeline for HAR involves manual feature engineering, where domain-specific features that are sufficiently representative of the human activities of interest are extracted from the image data. Types of features that have been exploited include features that relate to the shape [4, 55, 139] and motion [139] of the human form, and features related to the relative positioning between body joints [50, 122]. The R-transform is one technique that has been applied to extract shape features from binary silhouettes, particularly because it is also invariant to scaling, translation and rotation transformations of the input image [4, 55]. Histogram of Oriented Gradients (HOG) is another technique that has been applied for shape feature extraction directly from visible-light ROI images [139], whereas Histogram of Optical Flow (HOF) has been applied for motion feature extraction [139]. Alternatively, the relative positions and/or angles of the body joints have been exploited as features, following the reconstruction of a skeleton model from body joint markers detected under NIR illumination [122], or skeleton-fitting applied to depth silhouettes [50] or visible-light images [107].

In conjunction with feature extraction, a dimensionality reduction technique is also often applied with the aim of reducing the vector size of the feature data, hence reducing its computational complexity. Typical techniques that have been used for dimensionality reduction include Principal Component Analysis (PCA) [4, 139], Independent Component Analysis (ICA) [4] and Kernel Discriminant Analysis using a Gaussian Radial Basis kernel [55].

Once the features have been extracted from the image data and possibly reduced in dimensionality, although the latter is not always necessarily done, the last step performs activity classification. Since each activity is typically performed through a sequence of body movements, Hidden Markov Models (HMMs) have commonly been used for activity recognition due to their suitability for handling time-dependent sequential data [50, 55, 97]. Nonetheless, other machine learning methods have also been considered for activity classification of the feature data, albeit less commonly than HMMs. One of such methods is Bayesian inferencing, chosen by Wang et al. [122] due to its robustness in inferring the activity class even in the presence of missing body joint coordinates, arising from self-occlusion due to variations in body posture. In a different approach, several neural network architectures have also been investigated for activity classification, chosen based on their ease-of-use and their training and inferencing efficiency [107].

7.2.1.2 Deep Learning and Approaches

More recent video-based approaches exploit the use of deep learning models for feature extraction and activity classification, which eliminates the need for handcrafting features as in the classical approaches.

Convolutional Neural Networks (CNN) are the most widely used architectures for video-based HAR. One approach in leveraging CNNs for video-based HAR involves the application of end-to-end learning using established 2D [19, 61] or 3D [22] CNN models. In end-to-end learning, a single model takes the raw input and produces the final classification result. However, in complex tasks like HAR, this is quite challenging and either requires long training with huge datasets, or more typically, transfer learning, in which pre-trained models are used in order to adapt them to the target datasets [19, 22, 61]. End-to-end learning using 2D CNNs is typically employed when HAR is performed on each image frame individually without the aim of capturing temporal dependencies between them [22, 61], or when the temporal information across a sequence of video frames is captured into a single image to be fed into the CNN, such as by encoding skeletal joint coordinates extracted from consecutive RGB images into single spatio-temporal images [19].

The spatio-temporal information inherent in videos is more often exploited by cascading a feature extractor with a model that can capture long-range temporal dependencies [3, 38, 48, 74, 100, 124]. In such a scenario, CNN-based networks are still the most widely used for the feature extraction stage, where 2D or 3D CNNs are employed based on whether feature extraction is performed on a frame-by-frame basis [48, 100, 124, 137] or on a stack of image frames [3, 38, 74], respectively. Between the two CNN variants, the 3D CNN is often favoured for activity recognition because it is capable of capturing the spatio-temporal variations of the body movements, from which human actions are typically composed of [38, 74]. In order to capture the long-range temporal dependencies of the CNN-extracted features, most research work in the literature have applied variants of Recurrent Neural Networks (RNNs) [3, 38, 48, 71, 74, 100, 124, 137]. Of these, the traditional Long Short-Term Memory (LSTM) networks have been the most popularly used [38, 74, 100, 124, 137]. Gao et al. [38] report an improvement in the classification accuracy brought about by cascading a 3D CNN with an LSTM network, as opposed to solely using a 3D CNN for HAR. They argue that this is due to the contribution of the LSTM mechanism in capturing the temporal dependencies inherent to human actions.

Approaches based on deep learning models are often computationally costly, which can be problematic in applications, such as HAR, where timeliness is critical. Several of the reviewed methods that take this performance aspect into consideration, incorporate optimisation measures into their model design. For example, Gao et al. [38] report that the inclusion of an LSTM together with a sliding window approach, where the input video is fed into the 3D CNN for feature extraction in 10-frame batches, allowed for a reduction in the size of the 3D CNN and, consequently, its computational cost. This allowed them to reach a throughput of over 400 frames per second (fps) on a GPU-based system, without jeopardising the HAR accuracy. Similarly, Andrade-Ambriz et al. [3] experimented with different filter sizes to achieve a real-time performance of 30 fps, also on a GPU-based system.

7.2.2 Audio-Based Approaches

Audio can be used as a standalone source of information, or combined with other modalities (video, ultrasound, GPS, temperature, light and infrared sensors) to monitor behavior or ADL. The problem is challenging due to the vast amount of observations generated over time, the diverse nature of environmental sounds, and the absence of a straightforward method to correlate audio data with observed activities [1].

Audio is less extensively studied than other modalities for HAR (e.g. video, wearable sensors), although it has the potential to overcome some of their limitations. Audio signals are not affected by lighting conditions, they can propagate in indoor environments with physical obstacles, have longer range sensing, and operate with less computational cost [51]. Even from the privacy preservation point of view, audio-based HAR can be considered less intrusive than video-based methods, especially if it captures sounds not related to speech. The implementation typically requires only appropriately positioned microphones, without the need for cumbersome wearable devices and additional hardware deployment [87].

Noise exposure is common in audio-based HAR systems, as both user localization and activity detection heavily rely on acoustic conditions. This is particularly challenging for detecting activities which generate low-volume sounds that can be easily masked by background noise, or e.g. in falls where certain floor surfaces reduce the sensor's detection ability [123]. To address this, advanced noise reduction and blind source separation techniques should be applied during preprocessing [26].

Technologies for audio-based HAR incorporate various acoustic sensors integrated into Active Assisted Living (AAL) systems. These sensors can be roughly divided into active sensors that emit energy into the environment and then detect the response; and passive sensors that detect mechanical or acoustic waves that propagate through materials without emitting any energy themselves. Active acoustic sensors primarily detect sound waves traveling through the air and convert mechanical wave energy into electrical signals. This conversion can occur through either electromagnetic induction or by employing the electrostatic principle. Another type of active acoustic sensors are the ultrasonic sensors that emit and receive ultrasonic pulses, measuring the signal propagation time to the monitored object. Operating at frequencies beyond the human audible range, they are considered non-intrusive. Passive acoustic sensors, on the other hand, measure mechanical waves transmitted through solid materials, such as e.g. surface acoustic sensors [1]. Finally, the latest approaches for audio-based HAR use microphones integrated into smartphones [82], or voice assistants, such as Amazon Echo, Google Home or Apple HomePod [39], to capture the relevant acoustic cues from the environment.

Audio-based techniques for HAR can be divided into classical approaches that deploy traditional signal processing and machine learning methods for extracting relevant features and subsequent classification of activities, and deep learning approaches that use deep neural networks for end-to-end feature extraction and activity recognition directly from the raw audio signal.

7.2.2.1 Classical Approaches

Early approaches for audio-based HAR required multiple audio preprocessing steps, such as automatic audio segmentation, noise removal, silence detection, detection of abrupt feature changes or even manual annotation to recognize human activities [106]. Techniques that do not require audio segmentation usually process signals in batches (presuming a minimum duration of activities is known or can be estimated [30]), or classify short-term audio segments [45]. However, human activities can substantially vary in duration, making it difficult for the sequential models that rely on a limited signal memory, such as Hidden Markov Models (HMM) [18] that were typically used for this purpose, to perform robustly over variable-length activities. On the other hand, manual audio segmentation and annotation of activities is time consuming, therefore, approaches to automate the labeling process were recommended [39].

Selecting the relevant acoustic features that are able to generalize well across different environments is a challenging task. The most commonly used features are the time-domain features (e.g. zero-crossing rate [42, 114], energy, or entropy of energy [82, 96]), and frequency-domain features, such as spectral centroid, spectral spread, spectral entropy, spectral flux, spectral rolloff, fundamental frequency [82, 96] or total spectrum power [132]. Mel-Frequency Cepstral Coefficients (MFCC) as a compact representation of spectral features, represent the most widely used acoustic features for HAR [42, 60, 114, 136], but time-frequency representations such as Discrete Wavelet Transform features, Mel and Gammatone spectrograms are also commonly utilized [113].

Given the relatively small number of available audio datasets for HAR, early approaches to classify activities from sounds were primarily based on traditional machine learning methods, such as HMM [18, 73], Gaussian Mixture Models [5], Dynamic Time Warping [136], Support Vector Machines [42, 132], Random Forest [41, 60], or Gradient Boosting [41]. Companion robots equipped with an auditory system for speech recognition, sound localization, and sound separation in noisy environments were used for HAR of older adults living alone, applying either a dynamic Bayesian network (DBN) to model the intra- and inter-temporal constraints between the audio events and the context, or a Conditional Random Field (CRF) to predict human activities based on the recognized action, time and location [27].

7.2.2.2 Deep Learning Approaches

HAR using audio shares many similarities with the acoustic event detection task that aims to detect and classify sound events within audio recordings, or acoustic scene classification that involves categorizing entire audio scenes based on their acoustic characteristics. Sounds generated by human activities are composed of one or more different acoustic events, which can be used to distinguish the activities. On the other hand, there are also notable differences. For example, in the acoustic scene classification one scene may be composed of many activities with multiple acoustic events considered jointly, whereas in HAR the model is usually focused on a single activity in a scene or environment. However, the appearance of large scale datasets for acoustic event detection or acoustic scene classification, such as AudioSet [40], FreeSound [35], or DCASE (Detection and Classification of Acoustic Scenes and Events) challenge datasets [75], was also driving research in audio-based HAR towards the use of deep learning based approaches that require large amount of data to be trained. Although not primarily designed for HAR, these datasets contain a wide range of sounds associated with human activities relevant to AAL scenarios, such as household activities (e.g. cooking and food preparation, food intake, dishwashing, vacuum cleaning), personal care and hygiene activities (e.g. bathing and showering, tooth brushing, shaving, hair drying), or home security activities (e.g. door locking, door and window opening/closing).

The use of deep learning created also a paradigm shift towards end-to-end model training directly from raw audio recordings or their spectrograms, where CNNs are typically used to automatically learn hierarchical representations of data [51], instead of relying on handcrafted features or preprocessing steps as in classical machine learning approaches. CNN for feature extraction can be further combined with LSTM network to capture temporal dynamics [37]. Finally, the latest approaches for audio-based HAR deploy transformers that are able to model long-range dependencies and capture complex relations between the extracted features from spatial, temporal, and audio data [57].

End-to-end training also facilitates domain adaptation and transfer learning [70], where models trained in one domain where large scale data is available (e.g. the AudioSet dataset with over 2 million sound clips in the acoustic event detection domain [40]) can be fine-tuned or adapted to perform well in a related domain of HAR with limited annotated data available.

7.2.3 Multimodal Approaches

We refer here to multimodal approaches when addressing activity recognition systems relying on more than one sensing technique. The deployed sensors mostly include either audio or video information, or both. Examples of sensing modalities include pressure, video, ultrasound, passive infrared (PIR), temperature, light, accelerometers, rotation and inertial measurement units, proximity and location sensors, as well as video and audio sensors. Additionally, emerging technologies can be identified such as WiFi (IEEE 802.11) and assistive robots. These technologies have been related to various applications such as healthcare, emotion recognition, fall detection, posture recognition, localization, occupancy, mobility, and generic activity recognition applications [64, 130].

7.2.3.1 Classical Multimodal Approaches

Both classical and deep learning approaches have been extensively exploited in systems for multimodal daily activity recognition. Sometimes, these two techniques are combined to increase the performance. For example, a human activity recognition engine (HARE) for people affected by Alzheimer's disease has been developed and presented in [56]. In this work, video processing is done by applying independent component analysis (ICA) over the sequence of registered images, segmented body silhouettes, that are combined with k-means clustering and HMMs. Additionally, accelerometer data are obtained and processed using semi-Markov conditional random fields, which are used to obtain the duration of the activity. Finally, an artificial neural network (ANN) calculates the distance to the beacons for estimating location.

Dynamic Bayesian Networks, Reinforcement Q Learning and Fuzzy Partitioning are often used for classification purposes [33]. Post-processing and visualizing sensor data together with proximity charts, speech count percentage and GPS heat maps are used in [12] to identify and monitor activities and behavior of adolescent and young mothers with postpartum depression. This system combines audio recordings with passively collected proximity and activity as well as GPS data of the person's smartphone. Specially developed applications on the smartphone captures four types of information: (i) audio information, to measure social interactions through speech; (ii) movement, to obtain physical activity in contrary to sedentary behavior; (iii) GPS positioning data, to analyze movement throughout the community; and (iv) mother-infant proximity that is captured with a passive Bluetooth beacon. Another example is the system EarBit [9], which uses Random Forests for the recognition of eating episodes, while Sequential Forward Floating Selection (SFFS) was used for feature selection. EarBit is relying on a multi-modal wearable system for detecting eating events in relatively unconstrained environments with minimum restrictions on participants' behavior, i.e. in a semi-controlled lab study and outside-the-lab study. The study evaluated the usability performance of inertial, optical, and acoustic sensors with a particular focus on inertial sensing. Additionally, K-Nearest Neighbor (K-NN) and Support Vector Machine (SVM) have been applied. It has been shown that temporal features can hardly be fully extracted using the current conventional approaches. This issue has been addressed by the purely attention-based mechanism (TRASEND), which has been proposed in [11]. TRASEND is a memory access method that enables a content-dependent access to the most important parts of the input sequence.

7 Activities of Daily Living (ADL) and Behavior Recognition

Alternative approaches aim to automate the feature extraction and selection process in multi-sensor active assisted living systems [134]. By performing a generic feature engineering method, the study [134] demonstrates how automation can effectively identify robust feature sets across various sensors, leading to more accurate and efficient classification models compared to manually crafted features. The automated approach not only accelerates the discovery of optimal features but also reduces execution time and improves accuracy, making it particularly beneficial for cost-effective implementation in resource-constrained environments.

7.2.3.2 Deep Learning Approaches

Deep learning also enables automatic feature extraction in multimodal systems. It has the potential to hierarchically compose features and, thus, to obtain high-level representations. These high-level representations are superior over the handcrafted features because they are more discriminative, which leads to better results and an increase in robustness [83, 119]. Therefore, deep learning-based algorithms became popular for activity recognition using multimodal sensors [62, 66, 121].

The typical deep-learning architecture is based on convolutional neural networks (CNNs) and recurrent neural networks (RNNs) [131]. The shortcomings of RRNs are mainly with respect to learning from long input sequences [20, 47], which is in most cases addressed by applying attention models [116]. Additionally, a deep learning framework called DeepSense, which rely on commodity WiFi-enabled IoT devices, can be employed to achieve up to 97.6% activity recognition accuracy without human intervention [138]. This framework combines an autoencoder with a convolutional neural network (CNN) and a long short-term memory (LSTM) module. Similarly in [29], spatio-temporal categorization is done by applying CNN for representation learning and LSTM for determining temporal dependencies. So far, multimodal approaches for activity of daily living (ADL) applications mostly used deep learning algorithms relying on CNN and RNN, but also reverse beacon Networks (RBMs), and autoencoders have been used [77].

The application of deep learning based methods lead to a performance improvement when compared to the classical approaches. For example, applying a sensor-specific normalization technique with CNN classifiers can lead to improvements in F1 score by 4.5% points (*pp*) when using pressure-specific normalization and an additional improvement of 3.5 *pp* by using late and hybrid fusion [80]. These improvements have been achieved on the large real-world multimodal dataset obtained from the Robert Bosch Hospital (RBK). The potential of CNNs has also been shown by Zeng et al. [135]. This study investigated basic parameters such as max. weight, decay pooling, and dropout on the Skoda dataset and reported an accuracy of 88.19%. This result is 4.41% better in comparison to the best classical machine learning approach.

7.2.4 Overview of Approaches

Figure 7.4 presents an overview of approaches, sensors and devices used in systems for recognition of activities of daily living and human behaviour. HAR for ADL applications is often implemented using vision-based systems with RGB videos. However, this approach usually does not provide a comprehensive representation of actions in three-dimensional space. Using RGB-D sensors overcome a number of limitations of the monocular RGB videos by including depth maps, skeleton joints and a number of other hybrid methods, which also potentially provides an improvement regarding privacy protection [21, 32, 68]. Cameras are generally well suited to cover a certain area such as a single room and to monitor activities within this area, but the main drawback of visible-based approaches is the performance degradation due to the clutter, light and occlusion, as well as the issues related to the protection of users' privacy [86].

Audio sensors such as microphones can add an additional dimension in area-related monitoring. They are able to overcome some of the limitations of the vision-based approaches because they use less computational resources, and are able to provide a longer range, while being insensitive to changing light conditions and visual shading. However, as already mentioned in Sect. 7.2.2, they are much less studied in the literature than the vision-based approaches, mainly because of the

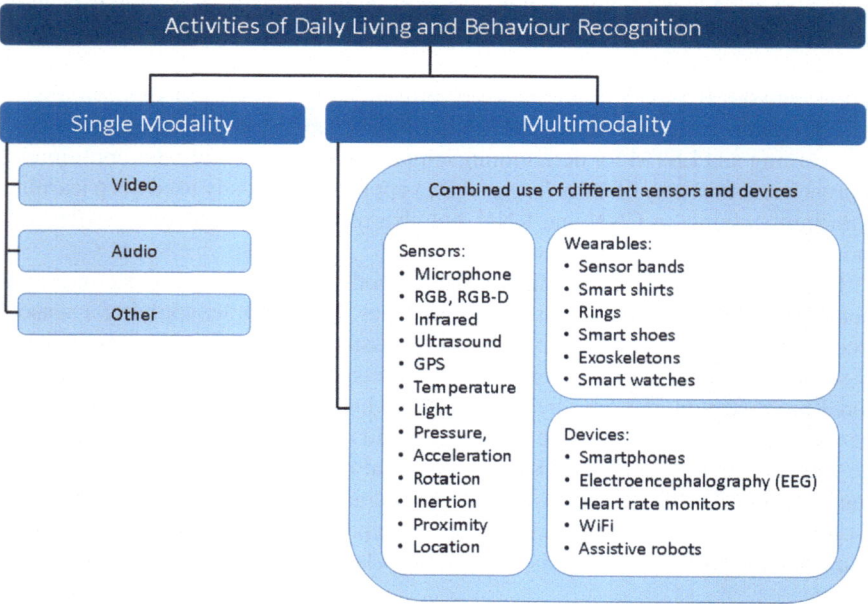

Fig. 7.4 Modalities and sensors used for activity/behavior recognition in assisted living environments

difficulty to correlate audio data with observed activities and the diverse nature of environmental sounds [1]. In many cases, microphones are combined with other sensors such as video, infrared, temperature or GPS sensors.

In a number of recent studies, inertial measurement units (IMUs) have been used as a single modality for recognizing the ADL [2, 17, 63]. Such small and effective sensor devices can easily be integrated in a number of wearables and are able to provide a relatively high level of user's privacy. These types of sensors are lightweight, low cost and can be used as a wireless sensor in bandages, rings, shirts, patches, shoes, or exoskeletons. The applications of inertial measurement units include the measurement of force, acceleration, angular rate (gyroscopes), and orientation (compasses). These sensor types are very often implemented in smartphones and smartwatches, and can be used in combination with other sensors, as well as communication and processing modules [89, 115].

Multimodal approaches can be classified into three main groups according to the sensors used: These groups are (1) approaches based on wearable sensors, (2) methods using static infrastructure-based sensors, and (3) systems relying on both wearable and external sensors [17, 25, 63]. As an external infrastructure for monitoring a certain area, cameras for recording videos and images and microphones for sound recording and processing can be used, but there are some limitations of these approaches regarding viewpoint, partial occlusion, background clutter, lighting, and appearance, as already stated above. These limitations can be partially overcome by an optimal placement of sensors and using an appropriate appearance model. For example, illumination changes and varying viewpoints can be addressed by an adaptive update of the appearance model. For object tracking, subspace-learning based methods can be applied to effectively obtain the basis vectors from target observations in order to reconstruct the target [90, 118]. An improved object tracking algorithm referred to as Partial Occlusion by Background Alignment (POBA) [129] models the candidate observation as a combination of object appearance and background region. A set of basis vectors provides a representation of object appearance, which is adaptively updated through incremental principal component analysis (PCA). Thus, POBA treats current observation as a combination of object appearance and occlusion region, while the occlusion region is constructed from the last frame based on the assumption that the appearance of background between two consecutive frames changes little. In the case of systems that rely purely on external infrastructure-based sensors, both their performance and application range can be improved by extending the system with wearable sensors.

7.2.4.1 Ongoing Challenges

Although the HAR field is constantly evolving, there are still some ongoing challenges crucial for advancing the effectiveness, reliability, and scalability of these systems.

Most HAR studies in AAL scenarios are carried out in controlled experimental environments, which can limit their ability to generalize effectively to real-world situations. Another major factor that can influence the results is the behavioral context, as participants tend to alter their behavior when they know they are being monitored. Audio, wearables or ambient sensors are less susceptible to this issue compared to video, but this remains a significant concern that needs to be addressed [26]. A solution to this problem is to use sensors and monitoring devices that are less visible or integrated into everyday objects, but transparent communication with participants is also important to clearly explain the purpose of monitoring and how the data will be used. Longitudinal monitoring over extended periods can further help participants to acclimate to the presence of monitoring devices, making them less conscious of being observed.

Certain activities in HAR are more frequent than others, and some, like sleeping, extend over a longer duration, resulting in a disproportionate number of data instances and imbalanced class distributions. This challenge can be mitigated through techniques such as over- or undersampling, employing cost-sensitive learning to assign weights to data instances based on misclassification costs [26], or synthesizing data with generative models like Generative Adversarial Networks (GAN) [28].

For multimodal approaches, there are a number of challenges and additional tasks that have to be performed in order to achieve a good functioning and accurate system. These tasks include [63]:

- Data synchronization and preprocessing: For fusing the multimodal data from a number of different sensors, an accurate time synchronization is mandatory (see for instance [101]).
- Action segmentation: Detection of the boundaries, i.e. the start and the end of an action, an efficient action segmentation has to be applied. A number of action segmentation approaches has been recently developed [58, 79, 95, 127].
- Feature extraction: Both raw sensor data and high-level feature descriptors can be obtained by a future extraction technique. In many cases, raw sensor data are not usually not sufficient for efficiently differentiating between various activities.
- Classification and Fusion: For classification, mainly classical machine learning algorithms such as SVMs and HMMs were used [31, 72]. The fusion can occur at the data, feature or decision level [125]. Combining row data from multimodal sensors and extracting features is done at the data level, while the feature level focuses on fusing the extracted features and the decisions are obtained from classifiers or decision makers as a part of the decision-level fusion. As discussed in Sect. 7.2.3, deep-learning based approaches based on CNNs, RNNs, RBMs, and autoencoders have recently become popular for multimodal activity recognition systems. However, handling data obtained from different sensors and the lack of appropriate and large data sets for multimodal systems (see Table 7.1). Most existing datasets are suited to either video or audio systems, which makes their application to multimodal approaches challenging.

7 Activities of Daily Living (ADL) and Behavior Recognition

Table 7.1 Datasets for human activity/behavior recognition

Modality	Ref.	Application	Dataset	# Subjects	Size	Instances
Audio	[52]	Emergency event detection	TUC	58	54 min	1612
Audio	[52]	Emergency event detection	Intenta	NA	4 min	704
Audio	[105]	Healthcare	BBRS	246	7 h	5166
Video (RGB)	[54]	General HAR	Kinetics-400	NA	851 h	306,245
Video (RGB)	[15]	General HAR	Kinetics-600	NA	1377 h	495,547
Video (RGB)	[102]	General HAR	Kinetics-700	NA	1806 h	650,317
Video (RGB)	[44]	General HAR	AVA	NA	108 h	430
Video (RGB)	[67]	General HAR	AVA-Kinetics	NA	NA	238,906
Video (RGB)	[43]	General HAR	Something-something	1133	121 h	108,499
Video (RGB)	[43]	General HAR	Something-something V2	1300	245 h	220,847
Video (RGB)	[78]	General HAR	Moments in time	NA	833 h	1,000,000
Video (RGB)	[46]	General HAR	ActivityNet	NA	849 h	19,994
Video (RGB)	[98]	General HAR	Charades	NA	82 h	9848
Video (RGB)	[59]	General HAR	HMDB51	NA	NA	6766
Video (RGB)	[24]	General HAR	EPIC-KITCHENS-100	45	100 h	700
Video (RGB)	[49]	General HAR	THUMOS	45	430 h	23,700
Video (RGB)	[104]	General HAR	UCF101	NA	2,7 h	13,320
Video (RGB)	[19]	General HAR	NAD	4	12 min	84
Video (RGB)	[103]	Sport	UCF Sports Action	NA	16 min	150
Video (RGB)	[126]	General HAR	IXMAS Action	10	NA	1148
Video (RGB)	[139]	Healthcare	UNN-GazeEAR	NA	5 min	50
Video (RGB)	[88]	Healthcare	SSBD	NA	112 min	75
Video (depth)	[34]	Healthcare	Nursing Home	1	72 h	NA
Video (RGB-D)	[36]	General HAR	KARD	10	1 h	2160
Video (RGB-D)	[14]	General HAR	MIVIA Action	14	NA	500
Video (RGB-D)	[34]	Healthcare	CHUN	27	NA	27
Video (RGB-D)	[34]	Healthcare	GAADRD	25	NA	25
Video (RGB-D, skeleton)	[108]	General HAR	CAD-60	4	36 min	60
Video (RGB-D, skeleton)	[120]	General HAR	MSR Daily Activity 3D	10	NA	320
Video (RGB-D, skeleton)	[133]	Human interaction	SBU Kinect Interaction	7	NA	300
Video (RGB-D, skeleton)	[85]	General HAR	MSR Action Pairs 3D	NA	21 min	360
Video (RGB-D, skeleton)	[93]	General HAR	Florence 3D	10	NA	215
Video (RGB-D, skeleton, IR)	[71]	General HAR, healthcare	NTU RGB+D 120	40	NA	56,880

7.2.4.2 Performance Evaluation

Evaluating the performance of HAR systems in AAL environments is complex and requires a comprehensive approach that balances high system performance with user-centric considerations. Traditional performance metrics such as accuracy, precision, and recall are widely used to assess the technical capabilities of the HAR systems. Given often largely imbalanced datasets, accuracy can be misleading as it may fail to account for the model's inability to detect the critical minority classes (e.g. falls, seizures, or emergency situations). Therefore, using recall (sensitivity) for performance assessment in AAL scenarios is essential to ensure that the system does not overlook important activities or events that could indicate a need for assistance. Precision in addition to recall is, on the other hand, important to correctly assess the influence of false positives in HAR systems, as they lead to false alarms and can substantially affect the user's trust in the system. If a HAR system frequently misidentifies benign activities (e.g. sitting down quickly) as critical events (e.g. fall), it can lead to unnecessary panic, and possibly desensitization to alerts over time (i.e. alarm fatigue), where users may start ignoring them, potentially missing actual critical events [81].

User acceptability and comfort need to be also taken into account, as the success of HAR systems in AAL hinges on their adoption by the end-users. Systems that are perceived as invasive or difficult to use are unlikely to be adopted, regardless of their technical performance. Therefore, performance evaluation must also include qualitative measures, such as user satisfaction and system usability.

7.3 Relevant Datasets

As audio is not commonly used independently for HAR, the available datasets created exclusively for HAR are rather scarce, and used either for emergency event detection (TUC, Intenta), by simulating critical acoustic events for older adults (e.g. calls for help, screaming, crying, whimpering, collapsing on the floor, striking the wall, trampling on carpet, or dislocating furniture [52]), or for assessment of suicidal behaviour of psychiatric patients using voice quality and speech disfluency attributes [105], as in the BBRS dataset. These datasets are limited in size ranging from 4 min (Intenta) up to 7 h of recordings (BBRS). However there are a number of large scale audio datasets not created for HAR, but which contain a variety of human activities and are utilized across multiple studies for HAR. These are datasets for audio event detection, such as AudioSet [40], with over 2 million of audio clips classified into 632 audio event classes, or DESED dataset used in DCASE task 4 Challenge with 10 event classes in domestic environment and a total duration exceeding 80 h. [94, 111]. Although they provide a comprehensive resource for audio-based human activity recognition research, they were created originally for a different purpose, so we do not list them in Table 7.1.

Video datasets for HAR contain a single video modality (RGB or depth), or a combination of multiple modalities (RGB, depth, skeleton). Most of the datasets represent general purpose HAR [10, 14, 15, 19, 24, 36, 43, 44, 46, 49, 54, 59, 67, 78, 85, 92, 93, 98, 102, 104, 120, 126], although there are also datasets specialized for applications in healthcare [34, 71, 88, 139], or sport [103] domains. SBU Kinect Interaction dataset contains synchronized video, depth and motion capture data of two person interaction activities [133], with the aim of determining causal relationships between people interacting with each other. Finally, there are datasets designed for general purpose HAR with large range of activities (120 different activities in NTU RGB+D 120), but given the substantial subset of activities related to medical conditions or mutual actions, they can be useful in healthcare, or human-to-human interactions domains, respectively [71].

The paradigm shift towards deep learning in mid 2010s required the large-scale video activity recognition data collections, which were vital for developing robust, accurate, and generalized models capable of performing well in diverse and real-world settings. These datasets were collected either via crowdsourced campaigns [43], or by web scraping videos from publicly available sources such as YouTube or other video-sharing platforms [15, 44, 54, 67, 102]. Although manual data collections allow for a high control over data collection process, they are time-consuming, expensive, and limited by the scale and scope of the manual efforts. On the other hand, the alternative methods for data collection, such as crowdsourcing or web scraping enable access to a vast amount of diverse data and are cost-effective, but can suffer from legal and ethical issues related to data usage, as well as variability in video quality and metadata accuracy.

Several large-scale video-based activity recognition datasets have become widely accepted as benchmark datasets for HAR, such as Kinetics-400 [54], Kinetics-600 [15], Kinetics-700 [102], AVA (Atomic Visual Actions) [44], or Something-Something V1 and V2 [43]. They were extensively used in the research community to evaluate and compare the performance of various activity recognition models, and to help bridge the gap from the controlled laboratory conditions to real world environments.

7.4 Privacy Preservation

Privacy and security impose significant concerns in audio- and video-based HAR systems due to the sensitive nature of data being collected and processed, especially in the AAL context where intrusion into private domains, either through cameras or audio monitoring devices is required. The major concerns are related to the misuse of data and violation of users' rights to privacy, as well as the exposure of personal data about the user, either directly (via speech in case of audio or face recognition in case of video based HAR), or indirectly (e.g. by identifying the users' daily activities and routines). However, a recent literature review [23] revealed that privacy and security concerns are largely overlooked in both audio- and video-based HAR systems, with only a few studies making efforts to properly address these issues. Even though these works propose specific measures to ensure a certain level of privacy such as using privacy-by-context methods [16], obtaining written and verbal consent [12], or utilizing silhouettes and depth cameras [4, 97], their effectiveness has not been validated in real-world scenarios.

Audio carries sensitive information that may reveal a person's identity, either related to the speaker's voice characteristics, or to the content of speech. More generally, paralinguistic audio events such as stuttering or the style of laughter, may also be considered sensitive, whereas background noise can reveal the current location [128]. Privacy-preserving audio processing is essential to remove or obfuscate sounds from the acquired signal that are not required for recognizing human activities. This can be achieved by voice masking to cover or degrade the speech, making it unintelligible, while preserving audio information relevant for HAR [69], encrypting private information while still allowing trusted processing [109, 110], or extracting only relevant sounds, while ignoring other audio sources that carry private information [117], as discussed in more detail in Chap. 3 of this volume [7].

In video-based HAR, privacy and security are mostly addressed by technical approaches, e.g. by employing depth cameras and silhouettes [4, 55, 97]. In a privacy-by-context setting, users are able to decide how, when and by whom they are watched [16], and may have their visual identity protected by image blurring and replacement with a 3D avatar. Nonetheless, such techniques focus mainly on the user, but leave the remaining image information visible and unprotected. The remaining parts of the image that are left unprotected can contain private information about a person's belongings and living environment, but may also contain cues that can be used to infer the person's location, which is one of the identifiers that can be used to identify a person or a "data subject", according to the General Data Protection Regulation (GDPR).[1] For this reason, within the context of video-based HAR, it is important that the preservation of visual privacy is broadened to also consider image cues that do not necessarily belong to the person's identity, but may still leak private information. Furthermore, the awareness of being monitored by cameras in one's personal environment may result in modifications of the natural behaviour, leading a person to perform activities in a different manner when they know they are being observed. Protecting a person's privacy may help in easing one's concerns regarding the sensitivity of the data that is being captured, while preserving their natural behaviour.

Through a number of technical innovations for AAL applications, more powerful and effective automated solutions are being developed and experimented, such as those based on conversational agents and robotic assistants. Consequently, the increasing power and pervasiveness of AAL technologies calls for a more holistic approach for privacy preservation that (1) integrates privacy-by-design principles, (2) minimizes data collection to only what is necessary, (3) anonymises data to protect user identities, (4) ensures secure data handling, and (5) prioritizes user consent and

---

[1] https://gdpr-info.eu/.

control. With these conditions, HAR systems used in AAL environments can provide the necessary support for independent living, while safeguarding the privacy and dignity of their users. An extensive survey of different methods and current initiatives in this area has recently been published by the GoodBrother consortium [1].

Acknowledgements This publication is based upon work from COST Action GoodBrother—Network on Privacy-Aware Audio- and Video-Based Applications for Active and Assisted Living (CA19121), supported by COST (European Cooperation in Science and Technology).

References

1. Aleksic, S., Colonna, L., Dantas, C., Fedosov, A., Florez-Revuelta, F., Fosch-Villaronga, E., Jevremovic Aleksandarand Msaknic, H.G., Ravi, S., Rexha, B., Tamö-Larrieux, A.: State of the art in privacy preservation in video data (2022). https://doi.org/10.5281/zenodo.6806207
2. Amor, J.D., James, C.J.: Setting the scene: mobile and wearable technology for managing healthcare and wellbeing. In: 2015 37th Annual International Conference of the IEEE Engineering in Medicine and Biology Society (EMBC), pp. 7752–7755. IEEE (2015)
3. Andrade-Ambriz, Y.A., Ledesma, S., Ibarra-Manzano, M.A., Oros-Flores, M.I., Almanza-Ojeda, D.L.: Human activity recognition using temporal convolutional neural network architecture. Expert Syst. Appl. **191**(C) (2022). https://doi.org/10.1016/j.eswa.2021.116287
4. Anitha, G., Baghavathi Priya, S.: Posture based health monitoring and unusual behavior recognition system for elderly using dynamic Bayesian network. Cluster Comput. **22**(6), 13583–13590 (2019). https://doi.org/10.1007/s10586-018-2010-9
5. Atrey, P., Maddage, N., Kankanhalli, M.: Audio based event detection for multimedia surveillance. In: 2006 IEEE International Conference on Acoustics Speech and Signal Processing Proceedings, vol. 5, pp. V–V (2006). https://doi.org/10.1109/ICASSP.2006.1661400
6. Avgerinakis, K., Kompatsiaris, Y.: DemCare action dataset for evaluating dementia patients in a home-based environment. InImpact: J. Innov. Impact **6**(1), 83 (2016)
7. Bäckström, T., Ravi, S., Florez-Revuelta, F.: Privacy preservation in audio and video. In: Salah, A.A., Colonna, L., Florez-Revuelta, F. (eds.) Privacy-Aware Monitoring for Assisted Living. Springer, Cham (2025)
8. Beddiar, D.R., Nini, B., Sabokrou, M., Hadid, A.: Vision-based human activity recognition: a survey. Multimed. Tools Appl. **79**(41), 1573–7721 (2020). https://doi.org/10.1007/s11042-020-09004-3
9. Bedri, A., Li, R., Haynes, M., Kosaraju, R.P., Grover, I., Prioleau, T., Beh, M.Y., Goel, M., Starner, T., Abowd, G.: EarBit: using wearable sensors to detect eating episodes in unconstrained environments. Proc. ACM Interact. Mob. Wearable Ubiquitous Technol. **1**(3), 1–20 (2017)
10. Blank, M., Gorelick, L., Shechtman, E., Irani, M., Basri, R.: Actions as space-time shapes. In: Tenth IEEE International Conference on Computer Vision (ICCV'05) Volume 1, vol. 2, pp. 1395–1402 (2005). https://doi.org/10.1109/ICCV.2005.28
11. Buffelli, D., Vandin, F.: Attention-based deep learning framework for human activity recognition with user adaptation. IEEE Sens. J. **21**(12), 13474–13483 (2021). https://doi.org/10.1109/JSEN.2021.3067690
12. Byanjankar, P., Poudyal, A., Kohrt, B., Maharjan, S., Hagaman, A., van Heerden, A.: Utilizing passive sensing data to provide personalized psychological care in low-resource settings. Gates Open Res. **4**(118) (2021). https://doi.org/10.12688/gatesopenres.13117.2
13. Camp, N., Lewis, M., Hunter, K., Johnston, J., Zecca, M., Di Nuovo, A., Magistro, D.: Technology used to recognize activities of daily living in community-dwelling older adults. Int. J. Environ. Res. Public Health **18**, 163 (2020). https://doi.org/10.3390/ijerph18010163

14. Carletti, V., Foggia, P., Percannella, G., Saggese, A., Vento, M.: Recognition of human actions from RGB-D videos using a reject option. In: International Workshop on Social Behaviour Analysis (SBA-2013) (2013)
15. Carreira, J., Noland, E., Banki-Horvath, A., Hillier, C., Zisserman, A.: A short note about kinetics-600. arXiv:1808.01340 (2018)
16. Chaaraoui, A.A., Padilla-López, J.R., Ferrández-Pastor, F.J., Nieto-Hidalgo, M., Flórez-Revuelta, F.: A vision-based system for intelligent monitoring: human behaviour analysis and privacy by context. Sensors **14**(5), 8895–8925 (2014). https://www.mdpi.com/1424-8220/14/5/8895
17. Chen, C., Jafari, R., Kehtarnavaz, N.: A survey of depth and inertial sensor fusion for human action recognition. Multimed. Tools Appl. **76**, 4405–4425 (2017)
18. Chen, J., Kam, A.H., Zhang, J., Liu, N., Shue, L.: Bathroom activity monitoring based on sound. In: Gellersen, H.W., Want, R., Schmidt, A. (eds.) Pervasive Computing, pp. 47–61 (2005)
19. Chen, Y., Yu, L., Ota, K., Dong, M.: Robust activity recognition for aging society. IEEE J. Biomed. Health Inform. **22**(6), 1754–1764 (2018). https://doi.org/10.1109/JBHI.2018.2819182
20. Cho, K., van Merriënboer, B., Bahdanau, D., Bengio, Y.: On the properties of neural machine translation: encoder–decoder approaches. In: Wu, D., Carpuat, M., Carreras, X., Vecchi E.M. (eds.) Proceedings of SSST-8, Eighth Workshop on Syntax, Semantics and Structure in Statistical Translation, pp. 103–111. Association for Computational Linguistics, Doha, Qatar (2014). https://doi.org/10.3115/v1/W14-4012
21. Cippitelli, E., Gambi, E., Spinsante, S., Travieso-Gonzalez, C.: Human action recognition with RGB-D sensors. Motion Track. Gesture Recognit. **97** (2017)
22. Cohen, R., Fernie, G., Fekr, A.R.: Contactless drink intake monitoring using depth data. IEEE Access **11**, 12218–12225 (2023). https://doi.org/10.1109/ACCESS.2023.3241835
23. Cristina, S., Despotovic, V., Pérez-Rodríguez, R., Aleksic, S.: Audio- and video-based human activity recognition systems in healthcare. IEEE Access **12**, 8230–8245 (2024). https://doi.org/10.1109/ACCESS.2024.3353138
24. Damen, D., Doughty, H., Farinella, G.M., Furnari, A., Ma, J., Kazakos, E., Moltisanti, D., Munro, J., Perrett, T., Price, W., Wray, M.: Rescaling egocentric vision: collection, pipeline and challenges for epic-kitchens-100. Int. J. Comput. Vis. (IJCV) **130**, 33–55 (2022)
25. De, D., Bharti, P., Das, S.K., Chellappan, S.: Multimodal wearable sensing for fine-grained activity recognition in healthcare. IEEE Internet Comput. **19**(5), 26–35 (2015)
26. Despotovic, V., Pocta, P., Zgank, A.: Audio-based active and assisted living: a review of selected applications and future trends. Comput. Biol. Med. **149**, 106,027 (2022). https://doi.org/10.1016/j.compbiomed.2022.106027
27. Do, H.M., Welch, K.C., Sheng, W.: SoHAM: a sound-based human activity monitoring framework for home service robots. IEEE Trans. Autom. Sci. Eng. **19**(3), 2369–2383 (2022). https://doi.org/10.1109/TASE.2021.3081406
28. Donahue, C., McAuley, J., Puckette, M.: Adversarial audio synthesis. In: International Conference on Learning Representations (2018)
29. Ercolano, G., Rossi, S.: Combining CNN and LSTM for activity of daily living recognition with a 3d matrix skeleton representation. Intell. Serv. Robot. **14**(2), 175–185 (2021). https://doi.org/10.1007/S11370-021-00358-7
30. Eronen, A., Peltonen, V., Tuomi, J., Klapuri, A., Fagerlund, S., Sorsa, T., Lorho, G., Huopaniemi, J.: Audio-based context recognition. IEEE Trans. Audio Speech Lang. Process. **14**(1), 321–329 (2006). https://doi.org/10.1109/TSA.2005.854103
31. Fan, H., Chang, X., Cheng, D., Yang, Y., Xu, D., Hauptmann, A.G.: Complex event detection by identifying reliable shots from untrimmed videos. In: Proceedings of the IEEE International Conference on Computer Vision, pp. 736–744 (2017)
32. Farooq, A., Won, C.S.: A survey of human action recognition approaches that use an RGB-D sensor. IEIE Trans. Smart Process. Comput. **4**(4), 281–290 (2015)

33. Feki, M.A., Biswas, J., Tolstikov, A.: Model and algorithmic framework for detection and correction of cognitive errors. Technol. Health Care **17**(3), 203–219 (2009)
34. Fernando Crispim-Junior, C., Gómez Uría, A., Strumia, C., Koperski, M., Konig, A., Negin, F., Cosar, S., Nghiem, A.T., Charpiat, G., Bremond, F., Chau, D.P.: Online recognition of daily activities by color-depth sensing and knowledge models. Sensors **17**(7), 1–15 (2017). https://doi.org/10.3390/s17071528
35. Fonseca, E., Pons, J., Favory, X., Font, F., Bogdanov, D., Ferraro, A., Oramas, S., Porter, A., Serra, X.: Freesound datasets: a platform for the creation of open audio datasets. In: Proceedings of the 18th International Society for Music Information Retrieval Conference, pp. 486–493 (2018). https://doi.org/10.5281/zenodo.1417159
36. Gaglio, S., Re, G.L., Morana, M.: Human activity recognition process using 3-d posture data. IEEE Trans. Human-Mach. Syst. **45**(5), 586–597 (2015). https://doi.org/10.1109/THMS.2014.2377111
37. Gao, R., Oh, T., Grauman, K., Torresani, L.: Listen to look: action recognition by previewing audio. In: 2020 IEEE/CVF Conference on Computer Vision and Pattern Recognition (CVPR), pp. 10,454–10,464 (2020). https://doi.org/10.1109/CVPR42600.2020.01047
38. Gao, Y., Xiang, X., Xiong, N., Huang, B., Lee, H.J., Alrifai, R., Jiang, X., Fang, Z.: Human action monitoring for healthcare based on deep learning. IEEE Access **6**, 52277–52285 (2018). https://doi.org/10.1109/ACCESS.2018.2869790
39. Garcia-Constantino, M., Beltran-Marquez, J., Cruz-Sandoval, D., Lopez-Nava, I., Favela, J., Ennis, A., Nugent, C., Rafferty, J., Cleland, I., Synnott, J., Hernandez-Cruz, N.: Semi-automated annotation of audible home activities. In: 2019 IEEE International Conference on Pervasive Computing and Communications Workshops (PerCom Workshops), pp. 40–45 (2019). https://doi.org/10.1109/PERCOMW.2019.8730729
40. Gemmeke, J.F., Ellis, D.P.W., Freedman, D., Jansen, A., Lawrence, W., Moore, R.C., Plakal, M., Ritter, M.: Audio set: an ontology and human-labeled dataset for audio events. In: 2017 IEEE International Conference on Acoustics, Speech and Signal Processing (ICASSP), pp. 776–780 (2017). https://doi.org/10.1109/ICASSP.2017.7952261
41. Giannakopoulos, T., Konstantopoulos, S.: Daily activity recognition based on meta-classification of low-level audio events. In: International Conference on Information and Communication Technologies for Ageing Well and e-Health, vol. 2, pp. 220–227 (2017)
42. Giannakopoulos, T., Siantikos, G.: A ROS framework for audio-based activity recognition. In: Proceedings of the 9th ACM International Conference on PErvasive Technologies Related to Assistive Environments, PETRA'16 (2016). https://doi.org/10.1145/2910674.2935858
43. Goyal, R., Kahou, S.E., Michalski, V., Materzynska, J., Westphal, S., Kim, H., Haenel, V., Fründ, I., Yianilos, P.N., Mueller-Freitag, M., Hoppe, F., Thurau, C., Bax, I., Memisevic, R.: The "something something" video database for learning and evaluating visual common sense. 2017 IEEE International Conference on Computer Vision (ICCV) pp. 5843–5851 (2017)
44. Gu, C., Sun, C., Vijayanarasimhan, S., Pantofaru, C., Ross, D.A., Toderici, G., Li, Y., Ricco, S., Sukthankar, R., Schmid, C., Malik, J.: AVA: a video dataset of spatio-temporally localized atomic visual actions. 2018 IEEE/CVF Conference on Computer Vision and Pattern Recognition, pp. 6047–6056 (2017)
45. Guodong, G., Hong-Jiang, Z., Li, S.: Boosting for content-based audio classification and retrieval: an evaluation. In: IEEE International Conference on Multimedia and Expo, 2001. ICME 2001, pp. 997–1000 (2001). https://doi.org/10.1109/ICME.2001.1237892
46. Heilbron, F.C., Escorcia, V., Ghanem, B., Niebles, J.C.: ActivityNet: a large-scale video benchmark for human activity understanding. In: 2015 IEEE Conference on Computer Vision and Pattern Recognition (CVPR), pp. 961–970 (2015). https://doi.org/10.1109/CVPR.2015.7298698
47. Hochreiter, S., Bengio, Y., Frasconi, P., Schmidhuber, J.: Gradient flow in recurrent nets: the difficulty of learning long-term dependencies. In: Kremer, S.C., Kolen, J.F., (eds.) A Field Guide to Dynamical Recurrent Neural Networks. IEEE Press (2001)
48. Hossain, M.S., Deb, K., Minhaz Hossain, S.M., Jo, K.H.: Daily living human activity recognition using deep neural networks. In: 2023 International Workshop on Intelligent Systems (IWIS), pp. 1–6 (2023). https://doi.org/10.1109/IWIS58789.2023.10284678

49. Idrees, H., Zamir, A.R., Jiang, Y.G., Gorban, A., Laptev, I., Sukthankar, R., Shah, M.: The THUMOS challenge on action recognition for videos "in the wild". Comput. Vis. Image Underst. **155**, 1–23 (2017). https://doi.org/10.1016/j.cviu.2016.10.018
50. Jalal, A., Kamal, S., Kim, D.: A depth video sensor-based life-logging human activity recognition system for elderly care in smart indoor environments. Sensors **14**(7), 11735–11759 (2014)
51. Jung, M., Chi, S.: Human activity classification based on sound recognition and residual convolutional neural network. Autom. Constr. **114**, 103,177 (2020). https://doi.org/10.1016/j.autcon.2020.103177
52. Kahl, S., Hussein, H., Fabian, E., Schloßhauer, J., Thangaraju, E., Kowerko, D., Eibl, M.: Acoustic event classification using convolutional neural networks. In: Eibl, M., Gaedke, M. (eds.) INFORMATIK 2017, pp. 2177–2188. Gesellschaft für Informatik, Bonn (2017). https://doi.org/10.18420/in2017_217
53. Katz, S.: Assessing self-maintenance: activities of daily living, mobility, and instrumental activities of daily living. J. Am. Geriatr. Soc. **31**(12), 721–727 (1983)
54. Kay, W., Carreira, J., Simonyan, K., Zhang, B., Hillier, C., Vijayanarasimhan, S., Viola, F., Green, T., Back, T., Natsev, P., et al.: The kinetics human action video dataset. arXiv:1705.06950 (2017)
55. Khan, Z.A., Sohn, W.: Abnormal human activity recognition system based on R-transform and kernel discriminant technique for elderly home care. IEEE Trans. Consum. Electron. **57**(4), 1843–1850 (2011)
56. Khattak, A.M., Truc, P.T.H., Hung, L.X., Vinh, L.T., Dang, V.H., Guan, D., Pervez, Z., Han, M., Lee, S., Lee, Y.K.: Towards smart homes using low level sensory data. Sensors **11**(12), 11581–11604 (2011)
57. Kim, J.H., Won, C.S.: Audio-visual action recognition using transformer fusion network. Appl. Sci. **14**(3) (2024). https://doi.org/10.3390/app14031190
58. Kong, D., Bao, Y., Chen, W.: Collaborative learning based on centroid-distance-vector for wearable devices. Knowl. Based Syst. **194**, 105,569 (2020)
59. Kuehne, H., Jhuang, H., Garrote, E., Poggio, T., Serre, T.: HMDB: a large video database for human motion recognition. In: 2011 International Conference on Computer Vision, pp. 2556–2563 (2011). https://doi.org/10.1109/ICCV.2011.6126543
60. Kumar, A., Singh, R., Raj, B.: Detecting sound objects in audio recordings. In: 2014 22nd European Signal Processing Conference (EUSIPCO), pp. 905–909 (2014)
61. Kumar, R., Kumar, S.: Light-weight deep learning model for human action recognition in videos. In: 2023 6th International Conference on Information Systems and Computer Networks (ISCON), pp. 1–6 (2023). https://doi.org/10.1109/ISCON57294.2023.10111975
62. Kumar, R., Kushwaha, N., Pandey, S., Priya, R., Mittal, J.: Superior NH_3 sensor using NI doped K-OMS-2 nanofibers. IEEE Sens. J. **18**(3), 956–961 (2018). https://doi.org/10.1109/JSEN.2017.2779327
63. Kumar Yadav, S., Tiwari, K., Pandey, H.M., Ali Akbar, S.: A review of multimodal human activity recognition with special emphasis on classification, applications, challenges and future directions. Knowl. Based Syst. **223**, 106,970 (2021). https://doi.org/10.1016/j.knosys.2021.106970
64. Kumari, P., Mathew, L., Syal, P.: Increasing trend of wearables and multimodal interface for human activity monitoring: a review. Biosens. Bioelectron. **90**, 298–307 (2017). https://doi.org/10.1016/j.bios.2016.12.001
65. Lee, H., Youm, S.: Development of a wearable camera and AI algorithm for medication behavior recognition. Sensors **21**(11) (2021). https://www.mdpi.com/1424-8220/21/11/3594
66. Lemieux, N., Noumeir, R.: A hierarchical learning approach for human action recognition. Sensors **20**(17) (2020). https://doi.org/10.3390/s20174946
67. Li, A., Thotakuri, M., Ross, D.A., Carreira, J., Vostrikov, A., Zisserman, A.: The ava-kinetics localized human actions video dataset. arXiv:2005.00214 (2020)
68. Li, W., Zhang, Z., Liu, Z.: Action recognition based on a bag of 3d points. In: 2010 IEEE Computer Society Conference on Computer Vision and Pattern Recognition-Workshops, pp. 9–14. IEEE (2010)

69. Liang, D., Song, W., Thomaz, E.: Characterizing the effect of audio degradation on privacy perception and inference performance in audio-based human activity recognition. In: 22nd International Conference on Human-Computer Interaction with Mobile Devices and Services. Association for Computing Machinery (2020). https://doi.org/10.1145/3379503.3403551
70. Liang, D., Thomaz, E.: Audio-based activities of daily living (ADL) recognition with large-scale acoustic embeddings from online videos. Proc. ACM Interact. Mob. Wearable Ubiquitous Technol. **3**(1) (2019). https://doi.org/10.1145/3314404
71. Liu, J., Shahroudy, A., Perez, M., Wang, G., Duan, L.Y., Kot, A.C.: NTU RGB+D 120: a large-scale benchmark for 3D human activity understanding. IEEE Trans. Pattern Anal. Mach. Intell. **42**(10), 2684–2701 (2020). https://doi.org/10.1109/TPAMI.2019.2916873
72. Liu, K., Chen, C., Jafari, R., Kehtarnavaz, N.: Multi-hmm classification for hand gesture recognition using two differing modality sensors. In: 2014 IEEE Dallas Circuits and Systems Conference (DCAS), pp. 1–4. IEEE (2014)
73. Ma, L., Milner, B., Smith, D.: Acoustic environment classification. ACM Trans. Speech Lang. Process. **3**(2), 1–22 (2006). https://doi.org/10.1145/1149290.1149292
74. Manocha, A., Kumar, G., Bhatia, M., Sharma, A.: Video-assisted smart health monitoring for affliction determination based on fog analytics. J. Biomed. Informat. **109**, 103,513 (2020). https://doi.org/10.1016/j.jbi.2020.103513
75. Mesaros, A., Heittola, T., Virtanen, T.: A multi-device dataset for urban acoustic scene classification. In: Proceedings of the Detection and Classification of Acoustic Scenes and Events 2018 Workshop (DCASE2018), pp. 9–13 (2018)
76. Minh Dang, L., Min, K., Wang, H., Jalil Piran, M., Hee Lee, C., Moon, H.: Sensor-based and vision-based human activity recognition: a comprehensive survey. Pattern Recognit. **108** (2020). https://doi.org/10.1016/j.patcog.2020.107561. Publisher Copyright: 2020 Elsevier Ltd
77. Miotto, R., Wang, F., Wang, S., Jiang, X., Dudley, J.T.: Deep learning for healthcare: review, opportunities and challenges. Brief. Bioinform. **19**(6), 1236–1246 (2017). https://doi.org/10.1093/bib/bbx044
78. Monfort, M., Zhou, B., Bargal, S.A., Andonian, A., Yan, T., Ramakrishnan, K., Brown, L.M., Fan, Q., Gutfreund, D., Vondrick, C., Oliva, A.: Moments in time dataset: one million videos for event understanding. IEEE Trans. Pattern Anal. Mach. Intell. **42**, 502–508 (2018)
79. Mukhopadhyay, S.C.: Wearable sensors for human activity monitoring: a review. IEEE Sens. J. **15**(3), 1321–1330 (2014)
80. Münzner, S., Schmidt, P., Reiss, A., Hanselmann, M., Stiefelhagen, R., Dürichen, R.: CNN-based sensor fusion techniques for multimodal human activity recognition. In: Proceedings of the 2017 ACM International Symposium on Wearable Computers, pp. 158–165 (2017)
81. Nguyen, D.A., Le-Khac, N.A.: SoK: behind the accuracy of complex human activity recognition using deep learning. arXiv:2405.00712 (2024)
82. Nicolini, M., Simonetta, F., Ntalampiras, S.: Lightweight audio-based human activity classification using transfer learning. In: 12th International Conference on Pattern Recognition Applications and Methods, pp. 783–789 (2023). https://doi.org/10.5220/0011647900003411
83. Nweke, H.F., Teh, Y.W., Al-garadi, M.A., Alo, U.R.: Deep learning algorithms for human activity recognition using mobile and wearable sensor networks: state of the art and research challenges. Expert Syst. Appl. **105**, 233–261 (2018). https://doi.org/10.1016/j.eswa.2018.03.056
84. Ofli, F., Chaudhry, R., Kurillo, G., Vidal, R., Bajcsy, R.: Berkeley MHAD: a comprehensive multimodal human action database. In: 2013 IEEE Workshop on Applications of Computer Vision (WACV), pp. 53–60. IEEE (2013)
85. Oreifej, O., Liu, Z.: Hon4d: Histogram of oriented 4d normals for activity recognition from depth sequences. In: 2013 IEEE Conference on Computer Vision and Pattern Recognition, pp. 716–723 (2013). https://doi.org/10.1109/CVPR.2013.98
86. Poppe, R.: A survey on vision-based human action recognition. Image Vis. Comput. **28**(6), 976–990 (2010)

87. Qu, Y., Gao, W., Liu, C.: SitPAA: sitting posture and action recognition using acoustic sensing. Electronics **13**(1) (2024). https://doi.org/10.3390/electronics13010040
88. Rajagopalan, S.S., Dhall, A., Goecke, R.: Self-stimulatory behaviours in the wild for autism diagnosis. In: 2013 IEEE International Conference on Computer Vision Workshops, pp. 755–761 (2013). https://doi.org/10.1109/ICCVW.2013.103
89. Rawassizadeh, R., Price, B.A., Petre, M.: Wearables: has the age of smartwatches finally arrived? Commun. ACM **58**(1), 45–47 (2014)
90. Ross, D.A., Lim, J., Lin, R.S., Yang, M.H.: Incremental learning for robust visual tracking. Int. J. Comput. Vision **77**, 125–141 (2008)
91. Saleem, G., Bajwa, U.I., PRaza, R.H.: Toward human activity recognition: a survey. Neural Comput. Appl. **35**(5), 4145–4182 (2023). https://doi.org/10.1007/s00521-022-07937-4
92. Schuldt, C., Laptev, I., Caputo, B.: Recognizing human actions: a local SVM approach. In: Proceedings of the 17th International Conference on Pattern Recognition, 2004. ICPR 2004., vol. 3, pp. 32–36 (2004). https://doi.org/10.1109/ICPR.2004.1334462
93. Seidenari, L., Varano, V., Berretti, S., Del Bimbo, A., Pala, P.: Recognizing actions from depth cameras as weakly aligned multi-part bag-of-poses. In: 2013 IEEE Conference on Computer Vision and Pattern Recognition Workshops, pp. 479–485 (2013). https://doi.org/10.1109/CVPRW.2013.77
94. Serizel, R., Turpault, N., Shah, A., Salamon, J.: Sound event detection in synthetic domestic environments. In: ICASSP 2020—45th International Conference on Acoustics, Speech, and Signal Processing (2020)
95. Shan, J., Akella, S.: 3d human action segmentation and recognition using pose kinetic energy. In: 2014 IEEE International Workshop on Advanced Robotics and Its Social Impacts, pp. 69–75. IEEE (2014)
96. Siantikos, G., Giannakopoulos, T., Konstantopoulos, S.: A low-cost approach for detecting activities of daily living using audio information: a use case on bathroom activity monitoring. In: ICT4AgeingWell (2016)
97. Siddiqi, M.H., Almashfi, N., Ali, A., Alruwaili, M., Alhwaiti, Y., Alanazi, S., Kamruzzaman, M.M.: A unified approach for patient activity recognition in healthcare using depth camera. IEEE Access **9**, 92300–92317 (2021). https://doi.org/10.1109/ACCESS.2021.3092403
98. Sigurdsson, G.A., Varol, G., Wang, X., Farhadi, A., Laptev, I., Gupta, A.K.: Hollywood in homes: crowdsourcing data collection for activity understanding. In: European Conference on Computer Vision (2016)
99. Singh, R., Kumar Singh Kushwaha, A., Chandni, Srivastava, R.: Recent trends in human activity recognition—a comparative study. Cogn. Syst. Res. **77**(C), 30–44 (2023). https://doi.org/10.1016/j.cogsys.2022.10.003
100. Singh, T., Vishwakarma, D.: A deeply coupled convnet for human activity recognition using dynamic and RGB images. J. Neural Comput. Appl. **33**, 469–485 (2021). https://doi.org/10.1007/s00521-020-05018-y
101. Sivrikaya, F., Yener, B.: Time synchronization in sensor networks: a survey. IEEE Netw. **18**(4), 45–50 (2004)
102. Smaira, L., Carreira, J., Noland, E., Clancy, E., Wu, A., Zisserman, A.: A short note on the kinetics-700-2020 human action dataset. arXiv:2010.10864 (2020)
103. Soomro, K., Zamir, A.R.: Action recognition in realistic sports videos. In: Moeslund, T.B., Thomas, G., Hilton, A. (eds.) Computer Vision in Sports. Springer International Publishing (2014)
104. Soomro, K., Zamir, A.R., Shah, M.: Ucf101: a dataset of 101 human actions classes from videos in the wild. arXiv:1212.0402 (2012)
105. Stasak, B., Epps, J., Schatten, H.T., Miller, I.W., Provost, E.M., Armey, M.F.: Read speech voice quality and disfluency in individuals with recent suicidal ideation or suicide attempt. Speech Commun. **132**, 10–20 (2021). https://doi.org/10.1016/j.specom.2021.05.004
106. Stork, J.A., Spinello, L., Silva, J., Arras, K.O.: Audio-based human activity recognition using non-Markovian ensemble voting. In: 2012 IEEE RO-MAN: The 21st IEEE International Symposium on Robot and Human Interactive Communication, pp. 509–514 (2012). https://doi.org/10.1109/ROMAN.2012.6343802

107. Su, M., Hayati, D.W., Tseng, S., Chen, J., Wei, H.: Smart care using a DNN-based approach for activities of daily living (ADL) recognition. Appl. Sci. **11**(1), 10 (2020)
108. Sung, J., Ponce, C., Selman, B., Saxena, A.: Unstructured human activity detection from RGBD images. In: 2012 IEEE International Conference on Robotics and Automation, pp. 842–849 (2012). https://doi.org/10.1109/ICRA.2012.6224591
109. Teixeira, F., Abad, A., Raj, B., Trancoso, I.: Towards End-to-End Private Automatic Speaker Recognition. In: Proceedings of the Interspeech, pp. 2798–2802 (2022). https://doi.org/10.21437/Interspeech.2022-10672
110. Teixeira, F., Abad, A., Raj, B., Trancoso, I.: Privacy-preserving automatic speaker diarization. In: International Conference on Acoustics, Speech and Signal Processing (ICASSP). IEEE (2023). https://doi.org/10.1109/ICASSP49357.2023.10096113
111. Turpault, N., Serizel, R., Parag Shah, A., Salamon, J.: Sound event detection in domestic environments with weakly labeled data and soundscape synthesis. In: Workshop on Detection and Classification of Acoustic Scenes and Events (2019)
112. Urwyler, P., Rampa, L., Stucki, R., Büchler, M., Müri, R., Mosimann, U., Nef, T.: Recognition of activities of daily living in healthy subjects using two ad-hoc classifiers. Biomed. Eng. Online **14** (2015). https://doi.org/10.1186/s12938-015-0050-4
113. Vafeiadis, A., Papadimitriou, I., Papanagnou, A., Giakoumis, D., Votis, K., Tzovaras, D.: Evaluating spectral magnitude representation and spectral energy for audio-based activity detection. In: 2021 IEEE 23rd International Workshop on Multimedia Signal Processing (MMSP), pp. 1–6 (2021). https://doi.org/10.1109/MMSP53017.2021.9733701
114. Vafeiadis, A., Votis, K., Giakoumis, D., Tzovaras, D., Chen, L., Hamzaoui, R.: Audio-based event recognition system for smart homes. In: 2017 IEEE SmartWorld, Ubiquitous Intelligence & Computing, Advanced & Trusted Computed, Scalable Computing & Communications, Cloud & Big Data Computing, Internet of People and Smart City Innovation (SmartWorld/SCALCOM/UIC/ATC/CBDCom/IOP/SCI), pp. 1–8 (2017). https://doi.org/10.1109/UIC-ATC.2017.8397489
115. Van Laerhoven, K., Borazio, M., Burdinski, J.H.: Wear is your mobile? Investigating phone carrying and use habits with a wearable device. Front. ICT **2**, 10 (2015)
116. Vaswani, A., Shazeer, N., Parmar, N., Uszkoreit, J., Jones, L., Gomez, A.N., Kaiser, L., Polosukhin, I.: Attention is all you need. In: Proceedings of the 31st International Conference on Neural Information Processing Systems, NIPS'17, pp. 6000–6010. Curran Associates Inc., Red Hook, NY, USA (2017)
117. Vincent, E., Virtanen, T., Gannot, S.: Audio Source Separation and Speech Enhancement. Wiley (2018). https://doi.org/10.1002/9781119279860
118. Wang, D., Lu, H., Yang, M.H.: Online object tracking with sparse prototypes. IEEE Trans. Image Process. **22**(1), 314–325 (2012)
119. Wang, J., Chen, Y., Hao, S., Peng, X., Hu, L.: Deep learning for sensor-based activity recognition: a survey. Pattern Recogn. Lett. **119**, 3–11 (2019). https://doi.org/10.1016/j.patrec.2018.02.010. Deep Learning for Pattern Recognition
120. Wang, J., Liu, Z., Wu, Y., Yuan, J.: Mining actionlet ensemble for action recognition with depth cameras. In: 2012 IEEE Conference on Computer Vision and Pattern Recognition, pp. 1290–1297 (2012). https://doi.org/10.1109/CVPR.2012.6247813
121. Wang, P., Li, W., Li, C., Hou, Y.: Action recognition based on joint trajectory maps with convolutional neural networks. Knowl. Based Syst. **158**, 43–53 (2018). https://doi.org/10.1016/j.knosys.2018.05.029
122. Wang, Y.K., Chen, H.Y., Chen, J.R.: Unobtrusive sleep monitoring using movement activity by video analysis. Electronics **8**(7) (2019). https://doi.org/10.3390/electronics8070812
123. Wang, Z., Ramamoorthy, V., Gal, U., Guez, A.: Possible life saver: a review on human fall detection technology. Robotics **9**(3) (2020)
124. Washington, P., Kline, A., Mutlu, O.C., Leblanc, E., Hou, C., Stockham, N., Paskov, K., Chrisman, B., Wall, D.: Activity recognition with moving cameras and few training examples: applications for detection of autism-related headbanging. In: Extended Abstracts of the 2021 CHI Conference on Human Factors in Computing Systems, pp. 1–7 (2021)

125. Wei, H., Jafari, R., Kehtarnavaz, N.: Fusion of video and inertial sensing for deep learning-based human action recognition. Sensors **19**(17), 3680 (2019)
126. Weinland, D., Ronfard, R., Boyer, E.: Free viewpoint action recognition using motion history volumes. Comput. Vis. Image Underst. **104**(2), 249–257 (2006). https://doi.org/10.1016/j.cviu.2006.07.013. Special Issue on Modeling People: Vision-based understanding of a person's shape, appearance, movement and behaviour
127. Weinland, D., Ronfard, R., Boyer, E.: A survey of vision-based methods for action representation, segmentation and recognition. Comput. Vis. Image Underst. **115**(2), 224–241 (2011)
128. Williams, J., Pizzi, K., Das, S., Noé, P.G.: New challenges for content privacy in speech and audio. In: Proceedings of the 2nd Symposium on Security and Privacy in Speech Communication, pp. 1–6 (2022). https://doi.org/10.21437/SPSC.2022-1
129. Wu, F., Vong, C.M., Liu, Q.: Tracking objects with partial occlusion by background alignment. Neurocomputing **402**, 1–13 (2020). https://doi.org/10.1016/j.neucom.2020.03.026
130. Yadav, S.K., Tiwari, K., Pandey, H.M., Akbar, S.A.: A review of multimodal human activity recognition with special emphasis on classification, applications, challenges and future directions. Knowl. Based Syst. **223**, 106,970 (2021). https://doi.org/10.1016/j.knosys.2021.106970
131. Yao, S., Hu, S., Zhao, Y., Zhang, A., Abdelzaher, T.: Deepsense: a unified deep learning framework for time-series mobile sensing data processing. In: Proceedings of the 26th International Conference on World Wide Web, WWW'17, pp. 351–360. International World Wide Web Conferences Steering Committee, Republic and Canton of Geneva, CHE (2017). https://doi.org/10.1145/3038912.3052577
132. Yatani, K., Truong, K.N.: Bodyscope: a wearable acoustic sensor for activity recognition. In: Proceedings of the 2012 ACM Conference on Ubiquitous Computing, UbiComp'12, pp. 341–350 (2012). https://doi.org/10.1145/2370216.2370269
133. Yun, K., Honorio, J., Chattopadhyay, D., Berg, T.L., Samaras, D.: Two-person interaction detection using body-pose features and multiple instance learning. In: 2012 IEEE Computer Society Conference on Computer Vision and Pattern Recognition Workshops, pp. 28–35 (2012). https://doi.org/10.1109/CVPRW.2012.6239234
134. Zdravevski, E., Lameski, P., Trajkovik, V., Kulakov, A., Chorbev, I., Goleva, R., Pombo, N., Garcia, N.: Improving activity recognition accuracy in ambient-assisted living systems by automated feature engineering. IEEE Access **5**, 5262–5280 (2017). https://doi.org/10.1109/ACCESS.2017.2684913
135. Zeng, M., Nguyen, L.T., Yu, B., Mengshoel, O.J., Zhu, J., Wu, P., Zhang, J.: Convolutional neural networks for human activity recognition using mobile sensors. In: 6th International Conference on Mobile Computing, Applications and Services, pp. 197–205 (2014). https://doi.org/10.4108/icst.mobicase.2014.257786
136. Zhan, Y., Miura, S., Nishimura, J., Kuroda, T.: Human activity recognition from environmental background sounds for wireless sensor networks. In: 2007 IEEE International Conference on Networking, Sensing and Control, pp. 307–312 (2007). https://doi.org/10.1109/ICNSC.2007.372796
137. Zhang, Y., Liang, W., Yuan, X., Zhang, S., Yang, G., Zeng, Z.: Deep learning-based abnormal behavior detection for elderly healthcare using consumer network cameras. IEEE Trans. Consum. Electron. **70**(1), 2414–2422 (2024). https://doi.org/10.1109/TCE.2023.3309852
138. Zou, H., Zhou, Y., Yang, J., Jiang, H., Xie, L., Spanos, C.J.: Deepsense: device-free human activity recognition via autoencoder long-term recurrent convolutional network. In: 2018 IEEE International Conference on Communications (ICC), pp. 1–6 (2018). https://doi.org/10.1109/ICC.2018.8422895
139. Zuo, Z., Yang, L., Peng, Y., Chao, F., Qu, Y.: Gaze-informed egocentric action recognition for memory aid systems. IEEE Access **6**, 12894–12904 (2018). https://doi.org/10.1109/ACCESS.2018.2808486

Open Access This chapter is licensed under the terms of the Creative Commons Attribution 4.0 International License (http://creativecommons.org/licenses/by/4.0/), which permits use, sharing, adaptation, distribution and reproduction in any medium or format, as long as you give appropriate credit to the original author(s) and the source, provide a link to the Creative Commons license and indicate if changes were made.

The images or other third party material in this chapter are included in the chapter's Creative Commons license, unless indicated otherwise in a credit line to the material. If material is not included in the chapter's Creative Commons license and your intended use is not permitted by statutory regulation or exceeds the permitted use, you will need to obtain permission directly from the copyright holder.

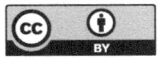

Chapter 8
Remote Monitoring of Vital Signs

Stefania Cristina, Peter Počta, Andrej Zgank, Kenneth P. Camilleri, Sara Colantonio, and Lambros Lambrinos

Abstract This chapter aims to explore state-of-the-art vision- and audio-based methods for vital sign monitoring, as applied to ambient assisted living for the older adults and people with special needs. We review different vision- and audio-based monitoring techniques, identify their advantages and limitations, explore emerging trends and open challenges, and draw recommendations for future directions. This work will serve as a starting point for beginners who are looking to gain an entry point into the area, as well as a guide to practitioners who are interested in learning more about recent developments of vision- and audio-based methods for active assisted living in general, and remote monitoring of vital signs in particular.

Keywords Active assisted living (AAL) · People with special needs · Computer vision · Audio processing · Vital sign monitoring · Multimodality

---

S. Cristina (✉) · K. P. Camilleri
Department of Systems and Control Engineering, Faculty of Engineering, University of Malta, Msida, Malta
e-mail: stefania.cristina@um.edu.mt

K. P. Camilleri
e-mail: kenneth.camilleri@um.edu.mt

P. Počta
Department of Multimedia and Information-Communication Technology, Faculty of Electrical Engineering and Information Technology, University of Žilina, Žilina, Slovakia
e-mail: peter.pocta@uniza.sk

A. Zgank
Laboratory for Digital Signal Processing, Faculty of Electrical Engineering and Computer Science, University of Maribor, Maribor, Slovenia
e-mail: andrej.zgank@um.si

S. Colantonio
Institute of Information Science and Technologies, National Research Council of Italy, Pisa, Italy
e-mail: sara.colantonio@isti.cnr.it

L. Lambrinos
Department of Communication and Internet Studies, Cyprus University of Technology, Limassol, Cyprus
e-mail: lambros.lambrinos@cut.ac.cy

© The Author(s) 2025
A. A. Salah et al. (eds.), *Privacy-Aware Monitoring for Assisted Living*, Intelligent Systems Reference Library 270,
https://doi.org/10.1007/978-3-031-84158-3_8

8.1 Introduction

The human body is characterised by several vital signs that provide measurable indicators of physiological functioning, based on which a person's overall health may be assessed. Examples of such vital signs include the heart rate and heart rate variability, the respiratory rate, and the blood oxygen saturation. These vital signs carry important information about the human body which, when monitored, can be exploited to identify abnormalities, detect medical emergencies, understand the body's responses to treatment, and generally assess the overall well-being of an individual.

Vital sign monitoring can play a significant role within the specific context of Active Assisted Living (AAL), where the aim is to enable older adults and persons with disability to lead a normal, independent and healthy life inside their own home, while alleviating their concern of not receiving timely medical assistance when required. Older adults, for instance, are at an increased risk of age-related problems that include heart complications, mobility issues, cognitive impairment and neurological conditions. Such age-related problems may be life-threatening and, hence, often require admission into a care home or hospital where an individual may be continuously monitored under the watchful eye of care or medical staff. This, however, has been placing an increasing strain on the care systems of many countries, especially in view of the skill-gap challenges presented by the global trend of lengthened life expectancy coupled with a declining birth rate. Leveraging technology-based solutions for vital sign monitoring can help reduce the in-person demand on the care workforce, and allow for early interventions that can reduce the likelihood for care home or hospital admissions.

8.2 Vital Sign Monitoring

One way of monitoring the body's vital signs is through the use of contact devices that can be attached to, or worn on the human body. The heart rate, for instance, can be measured by attaching electrodes to the chest or wearing a chest strap to record the electrical signals generated by the heart. Blood oxygen saturation, on the other hand, can be measured by placing a light-emitting probe on the finger or clipping it to the earlobe to determine the level of oxygen in the blood based on the amount of absorbed light. Such contact devices may lead to discomfort with prolonged or repeated use, or may give rise to skin health issues if they involve the use of adhesives. A further cause of concern comes from the fact that such devices for vital sign monitoring contribute to the generation of waste if they involve single-use components, such as electrode pads that are disposed of after use.

An alternative way of monitoring the body's vital signs is through the use of video or audio-based systems, which extract the necessary information from camera images or from physiological sounds coming from the body, respectively, as we will discover in the following sections. One of the main advantages of opting for video or audio-based solutions over attachable or wearable sensors is that the former typically do not require direct contact with the body, and hence can be more comfortable and flexible to use, even for prolonged periods of time. Therefore, they are perceived to be less intrusive by the end users. Furthermore, video and audio-based solutions do not typically involve single-use components, making them more cost-effective over sensor-based systems, and can possibly enable the simultaneous monitoring of multiple vital signs because they typically do not depend on specialised equipment either.

Throughout this chapter we will be exploring in greater detail the different aspects of vital sign monitoring, starting with a description of the commonly monitored parameters in Sect. 8.2.1, and followed by an investigation of different measurement modalities in Sects. 8.2.2, 8.2.3 and 8.2.4. In Sect. 8.3 we will then explore different datasets for video and audio-based monitoring, subsequently outline several privacy considerations in Sect. 8.4, as well as review the communication technologies in use by the different measurement modalities in Sect. 8.5, and finally conclude by drawing our conclusions on the challenges and future directions in Sect. 8.6.

8.2.1 Commonly Monitored Vital Sign Parameters

The most commonly monitored vital signs pertain to the respiratory, cardiovascular, blood pressure and oxygenation, and temperature regulation functions of the human body. Accurate measurement of these vital signs is required for early detection of medical conditions and timely intervention. This section provides a description of each of these vital signs together with the parameters that are typically used to monitor them.

Respiratory: The respiratory function of the human body refers to the process of breathing, which comprises an inhalation phase, during which the diaphragm contracts and moves downward to allow the intake of air through the nose or mouth as the chest cavity expands, and an exhalation phase, during which the diaphragm relaxes and moves upward to force the air back out of the lungs as the chest cavity decreases in size. This bodily function is monitored by estimating the respiratory rate in breaths per minute. The normal respiratory range for adults is reported to vary between 12 and 20 breaths per minute [22].

Cardiovascular: The heart rate is a key indicator of cardiovascular activity. Measured in beats per minute (bpm), it reflects the coordinated contraction and relaxation of the heart chambers, which enable the circulation of blood around the body to deliver oxygen and nutrients to the body's tissues and remove waste products. Another important parameter is the heart rate variability, which is a measure of the variation in the time interval between consecutive heart beats and is measured in milliseconds (ms). The normal resting heart rate in adults lies between 60 and 100 bpm.[1]

Blood Pressure: Even though the blood pressure is not a measure that is directly taken from the heart, it is still an important indicator of cardiovascular health. This is because blood pressure is a measure of the force exerted by the flowing blood against the artery walls, which therefore reflects the strength of the heart and the resistance of the blood vessels to blood flow. Blood pressure is typically represented by two values, the systolic pressure, which refers to the build up of pressure in the arteries as the heart contracts, and the diastolic pressure, which refers to the arterial pressure as the heart relaxes. These values are recorded in millimetres of mercury (mmHg). The normal range of systolic and diastolic blood pressure in adults is reported to be 120–129 and 80–84 mmHg, respectively [36].

Blood Oxygenation: The level of oxygen saturation in the blood is estimated through SpO2, which stands for peripheral capillary oxygen saturation. Within the human body, the blood oxygenation level refers to the percentage of hemoglobin, which is the protein in red blood cells that is responsible for carrying oxygen from the lungs to the tissues, which is saturated with oxygen. As such, the unit of measurement for SpO2 is a percentage (%). The normal range of oxygen saturation in the blood is stated to be 94–98% [46].

Body Temperature: The human body generates heat through metabolic processes, and regulates its temperature to ensure the stability of its internal conditions regardless of external ones. The body temperature is commonly measured in degrees Celsius (°C) or Fahrenheit (°F), and the normal axillary (armpit) body temperature is reported to range between 35.5 and 37.0 °C [64]. However, when assessing the body temperature, it is important to take note of factors such as gender, age, and the place of measurement, which may all affect the reading [64].

8.2.2 Contact and Wearable Solutions

Contact devices typically offer superior accuracy in monitoring vital sign parameters when compared to their contactless counterparts. This is due to the direct contact that these devices make with the human body, which reduces interference from external factors and allows for better signal acquisition. For this reason, contact measurement is typically preferred in clinical settings where the patients' diagnoses and treatments depend on the reliability of the measured data. One common type of such contact devices is the electrocardiogram (ECG), which is used to record the electrical activity of the heart through the use of adhesive patches that attach to the patient's chest.

---

[1] https://www.heart.org/en/health-topics/high-blood-pressure/the-facts-about-high-blood-pressure/all-about-heart-rate-pulse, Accessed: 25 September 2024.

Such contact devices are, however, primarily intended for use in a clinical setting because they often require specialised training to operate and interpret, and incur substantial costs to purchase and maintain.

Wearable devices, as a subset of contact devices, offer a more portable and affordable, easier-to-use option for continuous vital sign monitoring [25]. For this reason, the wearable devices market has grown to a billion-dollar industry [32], and continues to experience steady growth as the types of devices and their range of applications continue to expand. Some of the most ubiquitous wearables, which are also commercially available, come in the form of chest straps, armbands, smartwatches, smart rings and earbuds. With the exception of chest straps, which make use of electrodes to detect cardiac activity similar to an ECG, the other aforementioned wearables can measure several vital sign parameters that may include the heart rate, blood oxygenation and body temperature, among other bodily functions, using optical sensing techniques [69]. Among the less conventional wearables are smart textiles (also known as smart fabrics or e-textiles), which are not yet commercially available but have been drawing substantial scientific interest. These smart textiles embed sensors into the fabric itself, and can be used to create clothing that can monitor the vital signs through its contact with the human body. Even less conventional are tattoo-based wearables (also known as e-skins), which are fabricated on a flexible and stretchable substrate material and adhere to the skin to monitor physiological parameters such as the heart rate and muscular activity.

In general, all contact devices for vital sign monitoring share a common characteristic, which is the requirement for contact with the human body. While such devices may offer different levels of accuracy and portability, their direct contact with the skin can be perceived as inconvenient or uncomfortable to some who would rather not wear the sensor for prolonged periods of time. When it comes to wearables, in particular, their effectiveness also relies on user compliance and adherence to wearing the device correctly and consistently. Furthermore, as discussed later, solutions that rely on wireless transmissions of health-related data to a consumer device, such as a smartphone, may raise privacy concerns that these data may be intercepted and misused, which may prove to be yet another barrier.

8.2.3 *Video-Based Approaches*

Vision-based systems for vital sign monitoring typically follow a similar methodology, starting first with the choice of imaging modality, such as visible light [2, 9, 26, 30, 31, 49, 50, 59, 71], near-infrared [31, 62] or thermal [37, 71], based on the physical and physiological variations that are to be observed. This is followed by the acquisition of images within which regions of interest, which encompass the physical or physiological variations associated with the vital sign of interest, are then typically detected. Specific image features are subsequently extracted from the detected regions of interest using different image processing techniques. These image features are analysed to yield a measurement for the vital sign being monitored, with the aim of identifying health issues at an early stage or providing assistance if a potentially hazardous situation is detected.

The heart rate is the vital sign that is most often monitored in vision-based literature. The physiological feature that is most typically exploited is the subtle change in skin colour that occurs due to the pulsating blood flow, and which can be captured by variations in the intensity values of the pixels in visible-light [2, 9, 26, 30, 31, 50, 59, 71] or near-infrared [31] images. The face region or parts of it, such as the forehead, nose and cheek regions, typically constitute the image regions of interest from which the heart rate is estimated. One exception is the work of McGinnis et al. [41] for the treatment of panic attacks, which is based upon the use of fingertip images captured while the user presses their index finger against their smartphone lens with the flash activated. Eulerian video magnification (EMV) is sometimes applied to the image regions of interest [2], before these images are processed further. The EMV technique takes a video sequence and first decomposes it into different spatial frequency bands, followed by the application of signal amplification within a temporal frequency band of interest to magnify the subtle skin colour changes due to blood flow [70]. A sequence of such image regions of interest is then oftentimes collapsed into a one-dimensional temporal signal by, for instance, spatially averaging the pixel values within specific channels of each image frame in the sequence [30, 41, 71]. Bandpass filtering is also typically applied to the temporal signal in order to attenuate frequency components that are outside of the heart rate range, followed by peak detection on the resulting cardiac signal from which the heart rate may be estimated [30, 41, 71]. Research works that have proposed considerably different approaches include those of Qiu et al. [50] and Choi et al. [9]. Qui et al. [50] aggregate the information contained within a sequence of images into a temporal image, after decomposing the input sequence into multiple spatial frequency bands, concatenating the lowest band and temporally filtering it. This temporal image is then fed into a Convolutional Neural Network (CNN) for heart rate estimation. Choi et al. [9], on the other hand, propose to fuse visible-light (RGB) and radio-frequency information through fusion transformer modules to generate a blood volume pulse signal from which the heart rate is estimated.

Similarly, the process of estimating the respiratory rate starts with the detection of a region of interest, which may include the head and chest [2], the torso [35, 37], or the area around the nostrils [71]. If visible-light is the imaging modality of choice, then the respiratory rate is most often estimated by capturing the chest movement that occurs during breathing. Several approaches to do so have been proposed, such as the application of motion factorisation to images of the thoracic region [27], the computation of the distance between landmarks positioned on both shoulders and the nose [2], or the tracking of the thoracic area via the Kanade-Lucas-Tomasi algorithm [35]. If the resulting signal is not in one-dimensional form by default, it is usually collapsed into a one-dimensional temporal signal, such as through the use of a 3D CNN [35]. The typical subsequent steps include bandpass filtering and peak detection of the respiratory signal from which the respiratory rate is extracted [2, 30, 37], or alternatively the use of a deep neural network that takes the respiratory signal as input [9, 35]. Alternatively, the use of thermography as imaging modality can be exploited to capture the thermal variations that occur with the inhalation and exhalation of air within a region of interest below the nose [2].

Other vital signs which have been less often monitored using video-based methods include blood oxygenation (SpO2) [62], blood pressure [49] and body temperature [37, 71]. In estimating the SpO2, Stogiannopoulos et al. [62] propose a pipeline that is very similar to heart rate estimation, starting with the detection of the forehead and cheek regions of interest in near-infrared images, followed by EMV, feature extraction, and finally an investigation of different machine learning methods for SpO2 estimation. For blood pressure estimation, van Putten et al. [49] report that better performance than what has been previously achieved in the literature can be obtained if specific features and machine learning models are used for the estimation of systolic and diastolic blood pressure, independently of each other. For systolic blood pressure estimation they employ a stacked ensemble model, whereas a multiple linear regression model is used for diastolic blood pressure estimation. The estimation of body temperature is, perhaps, the most straightforward of all, since this is typically extracted from thermal images of the forehead [71] or the head [37].

In general, video-based methods for vital sign monitoring require that the user remains as stationary as possible during video acquisition, in terms of both the head pose as well as the facial expression [26, 31, 50, 62, 71]. However, given the difficulty of adhering to such a stringent condition, several of these methods still incorporate a mechanism to compensate for small head and face movements. Typical techniques applied for this purpose include facial landmark or region of interest tracking [26, 50, 71], and region of interest alignment between successive image frames via projective transformations [31]. The surrounding illumination conditions should also remain stable during video acquisition, since any variation that affects the pixel intensities in the recorded video can be erroneously interpreted as a variation of the vital sign of interest. Near-infrared illumination is often used to mitigate this problem because it is less affected by fluctuations in the surrounding lighting conditions [31, 62].

8.2.4 Audio-Based Approaches

Audio-based systems, on the other hand, exploit sounds generated by the bodily functions of interest for vital sign monitoring. Data collection is carried out via an acoustic sensor, such as a microphone, which captures sound in the form of electrical signals. The typical steps that are then involved in the analysis of such signals may include a data preparation step, whereby the audio signal is filtered, denoised and split into segments, followed by a feature extraction step, which seeks to extract a set of features that are sufficiently representative of the bodily function of interest, and finally a classification step that yields a decision regarding the vital sign being monitored.

Referring again to the diagnosis of respiratory disorders as an example, attributes of respiratory sounds that may be exploited for the diagnosis of upper respiratory conditions include the type and duration of cough, whereas crackle and wheezing may point to the presence of a lower respiratory condition [28]. Although transfer learning can be used to train audio-based models on larger datasets to then adapt them to the more specific task of respiratory condition diagnosis, to the best of the authors' knowledge, there were, at the time of writing of the chapter, no pre-trained neural networks freely available for this purpose. A typical approach for the acquisition of audio data is to place the acoustic sensor, such as a digital stethoscope, over the chest area. With advancements in technology, microphones embedded in smartphones are being increasingly employed to capture breathing sounds, replacing higher-end sensors and leading the way to more pervasive and contactless data capturing and monitoring techniques [28]. It is worth noting here that they are still supposed to be positioned as close as possible to an area of interest, i.e., a chest area in this case, to obtain audio signals of reasonable quality for further processing.

When it comes to the heart rate monitoring/estimation, Martin and Voix developed an algorithm assessing the heart rate by using physiological sounds recorded in the occluded ear-canal [40]. A rather reasonable performance (an absolute mean error of 4.3 bpm) for a further deployment in the context of AAL applications, even in the presence of ambient noise, which was, in this case, represented by broad band white noise and industrial noise, was achieved by this algorithm. A novel approach was introduced in Usman et al. [68], which estimates the individual's heart rate by applying regression algorithms to Mel-Frequency Cepstral Coefficients (MFCC) [17]. A high accuracy is claimed by the authors in the paper for the presented approach but it should be noted here that the testing presented in the paper is rather limited. To be more precise, it was done on the same dataset as deployed for the development of the presented approach, and no background noise was included in the recordings. In Tomaszewska et al. [67], the authors presented a heart rate estimation system, which identifies the heartbeat solely from tracheal audio recordings during sleep. According to the authors, the proposed system represents the precise heart rate monitoring tool that can be conveniently deployed, as a part of a home-based health monitoring system, to assess heart rate during sleep. Unfortunately, the authors did not report in the paper the performance of the system in the case when two people are sleeping side by side. Finally, Butkow et al. [4] designed the first in-ear audio-based motion-resilient heart rate monitoring approach, allowing the accurate heart rate estimation under motion artifacts caused by daily activities, i.e., walking, and running, which was proved under the controlled conditions as well as under the daily life conditions. The accuracy (a mean absolute error of 1.88 ± 2.89, 6.83 ± 5.05, and 13.19 ± 11.37 bpm for stationary, walking, and running, respectively) reported in the paper allows its further deployment in AAL applications.

Regarding the respiratory or breathing rate monitoring/estimation, the authors in Martin and Voix [40] designed an algorithm, which monitors the breathing rate by using physiological sounds recorded in the occluded ear-canal. A solid performance (an absolute mean error of 2.7 cycles per minute) for a prospective deployment in AAL applications was reported for the designed algorithm even when the ambient noise represented by industrial noise and broadband white noise was present in the recordings. In Ren et al. [51] a non-intrusive sleep monitoring system was developed, which detects the sleep events of an individual, as well as his/her respiratory rate at the same time by involving standard smartphones. When it comes to the respiratory rate detection approach, it uses the inherent correlation between breathing cycles to identify the breathing rate precisely by deploying the signal envelope detection approach. A rather high accuracy (a breathing rate error <0.5 bpm) and robustness under different scenarios were obtained for the proposed system as a result of the rather extensive testing reported in the paper. Moreover, the authors presented in Reşit Kavsaoğlu et al. [53] an innovative method to identify the breathing rate involving the adaptive filtering and speech boundary detection algorithms, obtaining a rather good accuracy. It should be noted here that the testing presented in the paper is very limited. Consequently, it is very hard to say whether this method has a reasonable performance for a further deployment in the context of AAL applications.

A contactless breathing detection system, entitled the Wi-Tracker, deploying commercial off-the-shelf smartphones was proposed in Liu et al. [34]. Breathing event is, in the proposed system, identified by capturing the Doppler effect caused by human exhaled airflow on the reflected acoustic wave. A good accuracy (a mean estimation error of 0.17 bpm) allowing its implementation in the context of AAL applications was reported for the Wi-Tracker, after the rather extensive testing, in the paper. Finally, the authors in Chara et al. [6] proposed a contactless breathing monitoring system deploying acoustic sensing with smartphones. The developed system offers a reasonable identification (a breathing median error <0.15 bpm) of breathing rates and respiration patterns, e.g., inhalation and exhalation time, in various conditions proved by the rather extensive testing reported in the paper, which allows its prospective deployment in AAL applications.

8.2.5 *Multimodal Approaches*

As far as multimodal approaches involving the audio modality are concerned, the authors in Ahmed et al. [1] developed an approach to monitor the user's respiratory rate deploying a signal processing based algorithm on motion sensors and a lightweight machine learning based algorithm on acoustic sensors from the earbuds, with the balanced data retention and accuracy. A good accuracy allowing its further deployment in the context of AAL applications was reported for the developed approach in both the lab and home environments. The lab and home testing involved 201 and 1330 sessions in different postures, i.e., sitting, standing and lying, respectively. It is worth noting here that several sessions were a bit shorter in the home environment. So, the predominance of the home sessions in the presented testing implies a high ecological validity of the corresponding study.

8.3 Video and Audio Datasets

Most recent video and audio-based vital sign monitoring solutions are based on some form of machine learning or artificial intelligence which require large amounts of data to train accurate models. The quality and diversity of datasets become critical factors to ensure that the training is unbiased and suitably generalised to ensure the system's effectiveness.

8.3.1 Video Datasets

Many video datasets for vital sign monitoring focus on the heart rate as the physiological parameter of interest, this being the vital sign that is most often monitored in the video-based literature. Nonetheless, several of these datasets may include additional ground truth physiological data, such as the respiration rate and the blood pressure, especially if such datasets would have been captured for a broader context that goes beyond the application areas of vital sign monitoring. Ground truth data refers to the real-world data that serves as a benchmark against which predictions or outputs of models, algorithms or systems can be validated to measure accuracy and reliability. A selection of the most commonly used video datasets for vital sign monitoring is as follows:

The **COHFACE** dataset [24] comprises 160 one-minute face videos collected from 40 participants. Some videos were collected in a controlled lighting environment, whereas others were recorded under natural lighting in an indoor environment. The RGB videos have been recorded using a webcam, at a resolution of 640×480 pixels and a frame rate of 20 Hz. In addition to the heart rate, this dataset also comprises ground truth data of the breathing rate as well as the blood volume pulse.

The **PURE** dataset [63] contains 60 one-minute videos from 10 participants, captured by an RGB industrial camera at a resolution of 640×480 pixels and a frame rate of 30 Hz. The participants were allowed to move their head in a controlled and well-defined manner. The videos were recorded indoors under natural lighting conditions which varied slightly due to changing cloud conditions and which streamed through a large window onto the face of the participant. The ground truth heart rate data was captured via a finger pulse oximeter.

The **MR-NIRP** (indoor) dataset [38] comprises 15 three-minute long face videos of 8 participants with varying skin tones, at a resolution of 640×640 pixels and a frame rate of 30 Hz. The videos were captured simultaneously using an RGB and a near infrared (narrow-band 940 nm) camera. Videos were captured under two conditions: during one condition the participants sat still but were allowed natural head movement; during the other condition the participants were instructed to first sit still, then carry out small out-of-plane head motions, followed by counting out loud, thus moving their mouth, and finishing with a still period. The ground truth heart rate data was captured via a finger pulse oximeter.

The **Multi-domain Mobile Video Physiology Dataset (MMPD)** [66] contains 660 one-minute face videos of 33 participants. This dataset addresses the gap of capturing video data under real-life conditions and was, therefore, collected by the camera of smartphone Samsung Galaxy S22 Ultra and comprises diverse skin tones, body motion, physical activity, and natural and artificial illumination variations. The videos have been captured at a frame rate of 30 Hz and compressed to a resolution of 320×240 pixels. In addition to the videos, the dataset contains finger photoplethysmography signals.

The **VIPL-HR** dataset [45] was also aimed at replicating daily-life conditions during data collection. For this purpose, a total of 3130 30-s face videos were recorded from 107 participants at a frame rate of 30 Hz, using a webcam, an RGB-D camera, a smartphone camera and a near infrared camera. The dataset includes various small and large head motions and diverse illumination conditions set by a filament lamp in an indoor environment. Some videos were captured with a fixed smartphone while others were captured with a hand-held smartphone. A finger pulse oximeter was used to capture the ground truth heart rate, SpO2 and blood volume pulse data.

The **BP4D+** dataset [74] is a multimodal dataset that captures spontaneous emotional states of the participants, elicited through various stimuli such as different smells and sounds. The dataset contains over 10TB of data collected from 140 participants of different ethnicity, using a data capturing system that includes 3D dynamic imaging, 2D video capture (320×240 pixels) and thermal imaging (640×480 pixels), all operating at 25 Hz, focused on the face of the participant. The collected ground truth physiological data includes the heart rate, the respiration rate, the systolic and diastolic blood pressure, and the electrodermal activity.

8.3.2 Respiratory Sound Datasets

In the context of monitoring the respiratory vital signs, audio datasets are primarily required for learning-based methods. In contrast, signal processing-based methods can estimate the respiratory rate directly from the captured audio signal without the need for an acoustic model. An approach published in Ren et al. [52], which utilises an audio signal envelope detection, can serve as a good example in this case.

Monitoring breathing sounds is challenging due to their low energy and susceptibility to interference from environmental noise and other body sounds like heart sounds, etc. Consequently, learning-based methods offer a significant advantage, as they are more robust than the signal processing ones. An audio dataset is a prerequisite for developing algorithms to estimate the respiratory rate. In addition to the audio signal, a time segmentation is essential, as it correlates the respiratory audio signal with precise time information. Many researchers, e.g., Markitantov et al. [39], Mostaani et al. [42], use in-house datasets, which often contain limited data and yield results that are not directly comparable. Examples of such in-house datasets include.

The **UCL Speech Breath Monitoring (UCL-SBM)** dataset [57], also included in the Interspeech 2020 ComParE challenge, contains audio recordings from 49 speakers, each lasting 4 min. In addition to the audio signal, the respiratory rate was recorded using a contact-based piezoelectric chest belt. This respiratory data is used for labelling and reference purposes.

Similarly, the **Philips read speech database** [43] involves 40 participants reading phonetically balanced text. Full-text transcriptions are provided along with labelled respiratory events, facilitating the development of deep-learning models for respiratory rate monitoring. Here too, piezoelectric chest belts were used in conjunction with audio recordings.

The publicly available audio datasets for respiratory rate monitoring include.

The **ICBHI Respiratory Sound Database** [55], collected as a part of the ICBHI Conference research challenge in 2017, contains 914 audio recordings labelled with inspiration and expiration intervals. This dataset facilitates respiratory rate monitoring and more complex classification tasks, such as detecting respiratory diseases.

The **SJTU Paediatric Respiratory Sound Database (SPRSound)** [73], collected in 2022, comprises 9089 respiratory sound events from 292 participants. A team of pediatric physicians manually annotated these sound recordings. The dataset is again suitable for both the respiratory rate monitoring and classifying respiratory diseases.

The **Dataset of Lung Sounds** [18] was collected using an electronic stethoscope in a clinical environment. Data from 112 participants are included, which can be utilised for the respiratory rate monitoring or disease classification.

The **Respiratory Sound Dataset** [56] is another collection that serves both respiratory rate monitoring and disease classification purposes. It contains recordings of 6898 respiratory cycles from 126 participants.

Beyond these standard audio respiratory datasets, the COVID-19 pandemic has heightened a research interest in acoustic classification as a method for pre-screening COVID-19 positive individuals based on cough sounds. The audio datasets, which were created/deployed for this type of respiratory monitoring, include among others COUGHVID [48], COVID-19 Sounds App, Coswara [58], Virufy [7], NoCoCoDa [12], and CDCVA [15].

8.3.3 Heart Sound Datasets

Cardiovascular audio datasets primarily focus on two categories. The first and most significant vital sign monitoring is heart rate monitoring, which requires high-quality time segmentation to identify specific sub-parts of heart sounds. Though more challenging, the second category has broader applicability and involves monitoring/detecting advanced cardiovascular conditions, such as murmurs and their types or outcomes of cardiovascular diseases.

The PASCAL 2011 Heart Sounds Challenge [3], the George B. Moody PhysioNet/Computing in Cardiology Challenge 2016 [11] and the George B. Moody

PhysioNet Heart Sound Challenge 2022 [54] are research challenges in the heart sound domain. They have played a significant role in popularising the field of cardiovascular audio datasets, particularly for classification tasks.

The **PASCAL** dataset [19], created in 2011, comprises 832 recordings with a total duration of 1.6 h. From today's perspective, it is considered a relatively small dataset. The heart sound recordings were taken in both medical and home environments, presenting a mix of challenging conditions. The audio files were manually segmented to detect the S1 and S2 sub-parts of the heart sounds. The recordings are categorized into normal and abnormal conditions, including murmurs, artifacts, and extra heartbeats.

The **CinC16** dataset [33], collected for the George B. Moody PhysioNet/Computing in Cardiology Challenge 2016, was sourced from nine different data sources. It consists of 3240 recordings from 1072 users, making it one of the most popular datasets currently available. The total duration of the recordings is 20.2 h. Additional segmentation information is provided to facilitate heart rate monitoring and to separate heart sounds before classification tasks. The classification objective is to categorise heart sounds as either normal or abnormal.

The **CirCor22** dataset [47], originating from the latest George B. Moody PhysioNet Heart Sound Challenge in 2022, contains 5272 recordings, totalling 33.5 h. The subjects include 1568 children and adolescents coming from Brazil. In addition to the audio data and segmentation information, the dataset also contains socio-demographic information. While this additional information can significantly enhance classification performance, it is less relevant for heart rate monitoring itself. The challenge comprised two distinct classification tasks, i.e., a murmur classification and clinical outcome classification.

Some heart sound datasets were not directly involved in the above research challenges, thus a performance reported for those datasets cannot be directly benchmark. Such audio datasets include:

The **Heart Sounds Catania 2011 (HSCT11)** dataset [60] contains audio recordings from 206 participants without any additional information about the subjects' health status. The 412 recordings were collected in a clinical environment using a digital stethoscope.

The **Ephnogram** dataset [29] is unique in that it captures heart sounds and ECG signals in parallel, allowing for the application of multi-modal approaches. Although only 24 participants were involved, the total duration of the recordings was 30.6 h.

The **Open Heart** dataset [72] comprises 1000 heart sound recordings sourced from various Internet sites. Each recording contains only three heartbeats, which limits its usability.

The **Cardiac Disease Heart Sound (CDHS)** dataset [65] focuses on heart sound quality assessment. It includes data from the PASCAL, HSCT11, and CinC16 datasets, along with additional new data coming from 76 participants, totalling 18.1 h of recordings. Each recording was manually annotated with a quality score, which can also be used to improve heart rate monitoring, particularly in acoustically complex AAL scenarios.

8.4 Privacy Considerations in Vital Sign Monitoring

Through vital sign monitoring, important information may be obtained on physiological parameters that may help determine the health status of a person. Nonetheless, whether such monitoring is done through the use of wearable or non-contact, video-based and audio-based solutions, it is imperative that privacy concerns are addressed comprehensively. This is because sensitive data collected during vital sign monitoring will likely include health information that, if not properly secured, could lead to breaches of confidentiality, potential misuse, and even physical harm thereby compromising the user's privacy, trust and well being.

As it has been previously discussed in Sect. 8.2.2, wearable devices need to establish direct contact with the human body to be able to measure the physiological parameters. While the use of wearable devices may lead to discomfort if the measurement has to happen over a prolonged period of time, their requirement for skin contact enables data collection of the source signal directly, without requiring the placement of cameras or microphones in one's environment that may pick up more data than is necessary to monitor the user's vital signs. Furthermore, while the requirement for user compliance to wearing the device consistently may be considered a disadvantage in using wearable devices for vital sign monitoring, it may alternatively be perceived as giving the user full control to use the device voluntarily, with the option of stopping data collection at any time by simply taking off the device.

In comparison, most video-based systems capture more data in their field-of-view than is necessary for vital sign monitoring, such as the full features of the face that reveal the user's identity, and potentially features in the background that may be personal to the user or revealing of the user's whereabouts. Similarly as in the video case, the user's identity and whereabouts can be again revealed by the corresponding audio features. So, the above-mentioned capture redundancy is also an issue when it comes to audio-based monitoring systems. Moreover, many video-based methods use only cropped images within regions of interest to monitor the vital sign, such as parts of the face or the torso. These cropped image regions are then typically collapsed into one-dimensional temporal signals from which the vital sign of interest is estimated. For audio-based approaches, the cropping function is replaced by spectral filtering, i.e., filtering out frequency bands, which are not relevant for vital signal monitoring. These two approaches can be considered to conceal the user's identity and to protect their privacy if the required signals are extracted on-the-fly and any unused visual and auditory information is deleted straight away, as opposed to transferring the raw image and audio data to a remote server over the Internet in order to be processed further.

The reviewed literature that works with either RGB images or with audio information rarely takes the privacy aspect of the research work into consideration, choosing alternatively to focus more on the technical aspects of processing the raw visual and audio data. One exception is the video-based work of van Putten et al. [49], which alludes to extracting the required signals locally on the smartphone to avoid transferring or storing personally identifiable images externally that could give rise to data protection concerns. Methods that rely on thermal images alone can be considered to be more robust to privacy concerns, since such images inherently obfuscate the user's identity and features in the background. However, the downside of these methods is that they require the use of specialised equipment, which can be more expensive and less straightforward to operate than consumer-grade devices such as smartphones. In general, video-based and audio-based systems can come across as more opaque to the user than a wearable, which captures only the intended signal through direct skin contact. Clear communication with the user can help mitigate suspicion and lack of technology acceptance, since the user may not necessarily be familiar with the extent of detail that is extracted from the visual and audio data to achieve the intended outcome of monitoring their vital signs.

8.5 Communication Technologies

Irrespective of the type of data captured by the different aforementioned devices and technologies, it has to be transmitted, processed, stored and displayed to end users, caregivers etc. in a meaningful way [20]. We will concentrate here on the communication technologies used by the two categories of devices we have considered in this chapter.

Wearables have specific requirements that relate to concepts such as power usage, mobility, connectivity and bandwidth among others. As such, to reduce power usage, wearable devices often have limited processing and storage capabilities. They therefore predominantly utilise low power technologies for their connectivity such as Bluetooth Low Energy (BLE) and Zigbee that have a short range and are perfectly adequate for the low data volume and relatively infrequent transmit/receive operations [61]. On the other hand, audio and video capturing devices are likely to generate continuous data streams. They will thus have a permanent power supply which allows them to utilise communication technologies more suited for large volume data such as standard WiFi and cellular or even wired connections.

As the information from both wearables and audio-video capturing devices has to reach the Internet, there are three different topologies through which this can be achieved: device-to-device, device-to-gateway, device-to-infrastructure. As one would expect, the first two are preferred by wearables whereas the last is the choice for audiovisual devices. Often, the role of the gateway is undertaken by a smartphone that utilises its own cellular Internet connection to transmit the data directly or a WiFi connection to a nearby Internet gateway. Note that the smartphone's role is two-fold, as it is also used to display data to the user in a meaningful manner. Obviously, the use of a smartphone as an intermediary has some privacy and security considerations due to various vulnerabilities. Latest advances in cellular communications may enable wearables to directly transmit their data to the Internet [14] satisfying mobility requirements seamlessly.

8.6 Trends, Challenges and Future Directions

There are several challenges that characterise audio-based and video-based vital signs monitoring. One of the primary limitations is the need for more openly available audio, video or even audiovisual datasets. State-of-the-art deep learning-based end-to-end methods typically necessitate sufficient data for effectively training deep models. The advancements achieved in other areas of audio and speech processing [16] as well as video processing [13] underscore the critical role of data, especially for more complex classification tasks. This challenge becomes particularly significant given that cardiovascular diseases pose the highest mortality risk in the developed countries [5, 8].

Another challenge in the realm of audio and visual vital sign monitoring is ensuring a robust operation in complex sound and visual environments. In a typical AAL environment, home appliances, media devices, as well as other people and animals, introduce additional audio sources that can degrade the primary vital signs' audio signal. Moreover, similarly as in the audio case, the above-mentioned appliances, devices, people and animals can decrease the performance of the developed video-based approaches. Techniques such as audio and video pre-processing and enhancement methods can mitigate these influences [21]. Moreover, it is worth noting here that data augmentation approaches (see for example Chu et al. [10], Hernández-García et al. [44], Nanni et al. [23]), involve the incorporation of noise and background audio signals or geometric transformations and colour space augmentation particularly for video-based approaches during deep learning processes to reduce over-fitting and enhance the generalisation capability of developed deep models.

As seen in Sect. 8.3.1, researchers have been developing ever more complex vital signs monitoring datasets that include various environmental factors, such as various illuminations, lighting changes and large motions [45, 66]. In addition to various environmental factors, the datasets seek to include participants with a variety of skin tones and ethnicities [66, 74]. This trend in the development of complex and varied datasets makes it more plausible to develop vision-based remote vital signs monitoring suitable for a home environment. Additional visual challenges that are presented by the home environment include the visual clutter that typically subsists in the background of home subjects and the smaller scale of face images when the subject is far from the camera.

Audio and video datasets may inadvertently contain hidden health information, often intertwined with other audible signals, such as speech due to the nature of sound propagation, and visible signals. This poses a significant privacy challenge, because the user's private information can be revealed. One approach to mitigate this issue is to ensure that users are informed about the inclusion of background speech and other potentially revealing sound and visual information when utilising audio-based and video-based vital signs monitoring services. Alternatively, employing dedicated hardware such as directed microphones and cameras can minimise the capture of ambient signals. However, preventing the inadvertent capture of hidden health information, which may be embedded within the original signal without the user's awareness, is much more challenging and sometimes impossible. If such an information is later identified, there is a serious risk that it could be exploited to harm the user. Therefore, careful consideration of privacy implications is crucial, including who has access to audio, video or even audiovisual datasets and under what circumstances. Hence, this opens up a need of new methods for privacy preservation to address these concerns.

Acknowledgements This publication is based upon work from COST Action GoodBrother—Network on Privacy-Aware Audio- and Video-Based Applications for Active and Assisted Living (CA19121), supported by COST (European Cooperation in Science and Technology).

References

1. Ahmed, T., Rahman, M.M., Nemati, E., Ahmed, M.Y., Kuang, J., Gao, A.J.: Remote breathing rate tracking in stationary position using the motion and acoustic sensors of earables. In: Proceedings of the 2023 CHI Conference on Human Factors in Computing Systems, pp. 1–22 (2023)
2. Alnaggar, M., Siam, A.I., Handosa, M., Medhat, T., Rashad, M.: Video-based real-time monitoring for heart rate and respiration rate. Expert Syst. Appl. **225**, 120,135 (2023). https://doi.org/10.1016/j.eswa.2023.120135
3. Bentley, P., Nordehn, G., Coimbra, M., Mannor, S.: The PASCAL Classifying Heart Sounds Challenge 2011 (CHSC2011) results. http://www.peterjbentley.com/heartchallenge/index.html
4. Butkow, K.J., Dang, T., Ferlini, A., Ma, D., Liu, Y., Mascolo, C.: An evaluation of heart rate monitoring with in-ear microphones under motion. Pervasive Mob. Comput. **100**, 101,913 (2024)
5. Chan, J., Rea, T., Gollakota, S., Sunshine, J.E.: Contactless cardiac arrest detection using smart devices. NPJ Digit. Med. **2**(1), 52 (2019)
6. Chara, A., Zhao, T., Wang, X., Mao, S.: Respiratory biofeedback using acoustic sensing with smartphones. Smart Health **28**, 100,387 (2023)
7. Chaudhari, G., Jiang, X., Fakhry, A., Han, A., Xiao, J., Shen, S., Khanzada, A.: Virufy: global applicability of crowdsourced and clinical datasets for AI detection of Covid-19 from cough (2020). arXiv preprint arXiv:2011.13320
8. Chen, W., Sun, Q., Chen, X., Xie, G., Wu, H., Xu, C.: Deep learning methods for heart sounds classification: a systematic review. Entropy **23**(6), 667 (2021)
9. Choi, J.H., Kang, K.B., Kim, K.T.: Fusion-vital: Video-RF fusion transformer for advanced remote physiological measurement. In: Proceedings of the AAAI Conference on Artificial Intelligence, vol. 38, issue 2, pp. 1344–1352 (2024)
10. Chu, H.C., Zhang, Y.L., Chiang, H.C.: A CNN sound classification mechanism using data augmentation. Sensors **23**(15), 6972 (2023)
11. Clifford, G.D., Liu, C., Moody, B., Springer, D., Silva, I., Li, Q., Mark, R.G.: Classification of normal/abnormal heart sound recordings: the PhysioNet/computing in cardiology challenge 2016. In: 2016 Computing in Cardiology Conference (CinC), pp. 609–612. IEEE (2016)
12. Cohen-McFarlane, M., Goubran, R., Knoefel, F.: Novel coronavirus cough database: Nococoda. IEEE Access **8**, 154,087–154,094 (2020)
13. Dang, L.M., Min, K., Wang, H., Piran, M.J., Lee, C.H., Moon, H.: Sensor-based and vision-based human activity recognition: a comprehensive survey. Pattern Recogn. **108**, 107,561 (2020)

14. Dao, N.N.: Internet of wearable things: advancements and benefits from 6G technologies. Future Gener. Comput. Syst. **138** (2022). https://doi.org/10.1016/j.future.2022.07.006
15. Despotovic, V., Ismael, M., Cornil, M., Mc Call, R., Fagherazzi, G.: Detection of Covid-19 from voice, cough and breathing patterns: dataset and preliminary results. Comput. Biol. Med. **138**, 104,944 (2021)
16. Dhanjal, A.S., Singh, W.: A comprehensive survey on automatic speech recognition using neural networks. Multimedia Tools Appl. **83**(8), 23367–23412 (2024)
17. Dwivedi, D., Ganguly, A., Haragopal, V.: Contrast between simple and complex classification algorithms. In: Statistical Modeling in Machine Learning, pp. 93–110. Elsevier (2023)
18. Fraiwan, M., Fraiwan, L., Khassawneh, B., Ibnian, A.: A dataset of lung sounds recorded from the chest wall using an electronic stethoscope. Data Brief **35**, 106,913 (2021)
19. Gomes, E.F., Bentley, P.J., Pereira, E., Coimbra, M.T., Deng, Y.: Classifying heart sounds-approaches to the PASCAL challenge. HealthInf **2013**, 337–340 (2013)
20. Haghi, M., Danyali, S., Ayasseh, S., Wang, J., Aazami, R., Deserno, T.M.: Wearable devices in health monitoring from the environmental towards multiple domains: a survey. Sensors **21**(6) (2021)
21. Halidou, A., Mohamadou, Y., Ari, A., Zacko, E.: Review of wavelet denoising algorithms. Multimedia Tools Appl. **82**(27), 41539–41569 (2023)
22. Hartley, J.: Respiratory rate 2: anatomy and physiology of breathing. Nurs. Times [Online] **114**(6), 43–44 (2018)
23. Hernández-García, A., König, P.: Further advantages of data augmentation on convolutional neural networks. In: Artificial Neural Networks and Machine Learning—ICANN 2018: 27th International Conference on Artificial Neural Networks, Rhodes, Greece, October 4–7, 2018, Proceedings, Part I 27, pp. 95–103. Springer (2018)
24. Heusch, G., Anjos, A., Marcel, S.: A reproducible study on remote heart rate measurement (2017). arXiv preprint arXiv:1709.00962
25. Iqbal, S.M., Mahgoub, I., Du, E., Leavitt, M.A., Asghar, W.: Advances in healthcare wearable devices. NPJ Flex. Electron. **5**(1), 9 (2021)
26. Jaiswal, K.B., Meenpal, T.: Continuous pulse rate monitoring from facial video using RPPG. In: 11th International Conference on Computing, Communication and Networking Technologies (ICCCNT), pp. 1–5. IEEE (2020)
27. Janssen, R., Wang, W., Moço, A., De Haan, G.: Video-based respiration monitoring with automatic region of interest detection. Physiolog. Meas. **37**(1), 100 (2015)
28. Kapetanidis, P., Kalioras, F., Tsakonas, C., Tzamalis, P., Kontogiannis, G., Karamanidou, T., Stavropoulos, T.G., Nikoletseas, S.: Respiratory diseases diagnosis using audio analysis and artificial intelligence: a systematic review. Sensors **24**(4), 1173 (2024)
29. Kazemnejad, A., Karimi, S., Gordany, P., Clifford, G.D., Sameni, R.: An open-access simultaneous electrocardiogram and phonocardiogram database. Physiol. Meas. **45**(5), 055,005 (2024)
30. Khanam, F., Al-Naji, A., Perera, A.G., Gibson, K., Chahl, J.: Non-contact automatic vital signs monitoring of neonates in NICU using video camera imaging. Comput. Methods Biomech. Biomed. Eng.: Imaging Vis. **11**(2), 278–285 (2023)
31. Kurihara, K., Sugimura, D., Hamamoto, T.: Non-contact heart rate estimation via adaptive RGB/NIR signal fusion. IEEE Trans. Image Process. **30**, 6528–6543 (2021)
32. Larios Hernández, G.J.: Wearable technology: shaping market opportunities through innovation, learning, and networking. In: Reverse Entrepreneurship in Latin America: Internationalization from Emerging Markets to Developed Economies, pp. 29–44 (2019)
33. Liu, C., Springer, D., Li, Q., Moody, B., Juan, R.A., Chorro, F.J., Castells, F., Roig, J.M., Silva, I., Johnson, A.E., et al.: An open access database for the evaluation of heart sound algorithms. Physiol. Meas. **37**(12), 2181 (2016)
34. Liu, W., Chang, S., Li, F., Xu, Y., Yan, S., Liu, Y.: Contactless breathing airflow detection on smartphone. IEEE Internet Things J. **10**(4), 3428–3439 (2022)
35. Liu, Z., Huang, B., Lin, C.L., Wu, C.L., Zhao, C., Chao, W.C., Wu, Y.C., Zheng, Y., Wang, Z.: Contactless respiratory rate monitoring for ICU patients based on unsupervised learning. In:

Proceedings of the IEEE/CVF Conference on Computer Vision and Pattern Recognition, pp. 6005–6014 (2023)
36. Luo, D., Cheng, Y., Zhang, H., Ba, M., Chen, P., Li, H., Chen, K., Sha, W., Zhang, C., Chen, H.: Association between high blood pressure and long term cardiovascular events in young adults: systematic review and meta-analysis. BMJ **370** (2020)
37. Lyra, S., Mayer, L., Ou, L., Chen, D., Timms, P., Tay, A., Chan, P.Y., Ganse, B., Leonhardt, S., Hoog Antink, C.: A deep learning-based camera approach for vital sign monitoring using thermography images for ICU patients. Sensors **21**(4), 1495 (2021)
38. Magdalena Nowara, E., Marks, T.K., Mansour, H., Veeraraghavan, A.: SparsePPG: towards driver monitoring using camera-based vital signs estimation in near-infrared. In: Proceedings of the IEEE Conference on Computer Vision and Pattern Recognition Workshops, pp. 1272–1281 (2018)
39. Markitantov, M., Dresvyanskiy, D., Mamontov, D., Kaya, H., Minker, W., Karpov, A., et al.: Ensembling end-to-end deep models for computational paralinguistics tasks: compare 2020 mask and breathing sub-challenges. In: INTERSPEECH, pp. 2072–2076 (2020)
40. Martin, A., Voix, J.: In-ear audio wearable: measurement of heart and breathing rates for health and safety monitoring. IEEE Trans. Biomed. Eng. **65**(6), 1256–1263 (2017)
41. McGinnis, R.S., McGinnis, E.W., Petrillo, C., Ferri, J., Scism, J., Price, M.: Validation of smartphone based heart rate tracking for remote treatment of panic attacks. IEEE J. Biomed. Health Inform. **25**(3), 656–662 (2020)
42. Mostaani, Z., Nallanthighal, V.S., Härmä, A., Strik, H., Magimai-Doss, M.: On the relationship between speech-based breathing signal prediction evaluation measures and breathing parameters estimation. In: IEEE International Conference on Acoustics, Speech and Signal Processing (ICASSP), pp. 1345–1349. IEEE (2021)
43. Nallanthighal, V.S., Härmä, A., Strik, H.: Speech breathing estimation using deep learning methods. In: IEEE International Conference on Acoustics, Speech and Signal Processing (ICASSP), pp. 1140–1144. IEEE (2021)
44. Nanni, L., Maguolo, G., Paci, M.: Data augmentation approaches for improving animal audio classification. Ecol. Inform. **57**, 101,084 (2020)
45. Niu, X., Han, H., Shan, S., Chen, X.: VIPL-HR: a multi-modal database for pulse estimation from less-constrained face video. In: Computer Vision—ACCV 2018: 14th Asian Conference on Computer Vision, Perth, Australia, December 2–6, 2018, Revised Selected Papers, Part V 14, pp. 562–576. Springer (2019)
46. O'Driscoll, B.R., Howard, L., Earis, J., Mak, V.: BTS guideline for oxygen use in adults in healthcare and emergency settings. Thorax **72**(Suppl. 1), ii1–ii90 (2017)
47. Oliveira, J., Renna, F., Costa, P.D., Nogueira, M., Oliveira, C., Ferreira, C., Jorge, A., Mattos, S., Hatem, T., Tavares, T., et al.: The CirCor DigiScope dataset: from murmur detection to murmur classification. IEEE J. Biomed. Health Inform. **26**(6), 2524–2535 (2021)
48. Orlandic, L., Teijeiro, T., Atienza, D.: The COUGHVID crowdsourcing dataset, a corpus for the study of large-scale cough analysis algorithms. Sci. Data **8**(1), 156 (2021)
49. van Putten, L.D., Bamford, K.E., Veleslavov, I., Wegerif, S.: From video to vital signs: using personal device cameras to measure pulse rate and predict blood pressure using explainable AI. Discov. Appl. Sci. **6**(4), 184 (2024)
50. Qiu, Y., Liu, Y., Arteaga-Falconi, J., Dong, H., El Saddik, A.: EVM-CNN: real-time contactless heart rate estimation from facial video. IEEE Trans. Multimedia **21**(7), 1778–1787 (2018)
51. Ren, Y., Wang, C., Chen, Y., Yang, J., Li, H.: Noninvasive fine-grained sleep monitoring leveraging smartphones. IEEE Internet Things J. **6**(5), 8248–8261 (2019)
52. Ren, Y., Wang, C., Yang, J., Chen, Y.: Fine-grained sleep monitoring: hearing your breathing with smartphones. In: 2015 IEEE Conference on Computer Communications (INFOCOM), pp. 1194–1202 (2015). https://doi.org/10.1109/INFOCOM.2015.7218494
53. Reşit Kavsaoğlu, A., Elhashmi, M.: An innovative respiratory rate detection system using adaptive filter with speech boundaries detection algorithm in audio signal. In: The Proceedings of the International Conference on Smart City Applications, pp. 471–480. Springer (2021)

54. Reyna, M.A., Kiarashi, Y., Elola, A., Oliveira, J., Renna, F., Gu, A., Perez Alday, E.A., Sadr, N., Sharma, A., Kpodonu, J., et al.: Heart murmur detection from phonocardiogram recordings: The George B. Moody PhysioNet challenge 2022. PLOS Digit. Health **2**(9), e0000,324 (2023)
55. Rocha, B., Filos, D., Mendes, L., Vogiatzis, I., Perantoni, E., Kaimakamis, E., Natsiavas, P., Oliveira, A., Jácome, C., Marques, A., et al.: A respiratory sound database for the development of automated classification. In: Precision Medicine Powered by pHealth and Connected Health: ICBHI 2017, Thessaloniki, Greece, 18–21 November 2017, pp. 33–37. Springer (2018)
56. Rocha, B.M., Filos, D., Mendes, L., Serbes, G., Ulukaya, S., Kahya, Y.P., Jakovljevic, N., Turukalo, T.L., Vogiatzis, I.M., Perantoni, E., et al.: An open access database for the evaluation of respiratory sound classification algorithms. Physiol. Meas. **40**(3), 035,001 (2019)
57. Schuller, B.W., Batliner, A., Bergler, C., Messner, E.M., Hamilton, A., Amiriparian, S., Baird, A., Rizos, G., Schmitt, M., Stappen, L., et al.: The interspeech 2020 computational paralinguistics challenge: elderly emotion, breathing & masks. In: Proceedings of INTERSPEECH (2020)
58. Sharma, N., Krishnan, P., Kumar, R., Ramoji, S., Chetupalli, S.R., Ghosh, P.K., Ganapathy, S., et al.: Coswara—a database of breathing, cough, and voice sounds for Covid-19 diagnosis (2020). arXiv preprint arXiv:2005.10548
59. Shoushan, M.M., Reyes, B.A., Rodriguez, A.M., Chong, J.W.: Non-contact HR monitoring via smartphone and webcam during different respiratory maneuvers and body movements. IEEE J. Biomed. Health Inform. **25**(2), 602–612 (2020)
60. Spadaccini, A., Beritelli, F.: Performance evaluation of heart sounds biometric systems on an open dataset. In: 2013 18th International Conference on Digital Signal Processing (DSP), pp. 1–5. IEEE (2013)
61. Stiller, B., Schiller, E., Schmitt, C.: An overview of network communication technologies for IoT. In: Ziegler, S., Radócz, R., Quesada Rodriguez, A., Matheu Garcia, S.N. (eds.) Handbook of Internet-of-Things, pp. 1–31 (2020)
62. Stogiannopoulos, T., Cheimariotis, G.A., Mitianoudis, N.: A non-contact SpO2 estimation using video magnification and infrared data. In: IEEE International Conference on Acoustics, Speech and Signal Processing (ICASSP), pp. 1–5. IEEE (2023)
63. Stricker, R., Müller, S., Gross, H.M.: Non-contact video-based pulse rate measurement on a mobile service robot. In: The 23rd IEEE International Symposium on Robot and Human Interactive Communication, pp. 1056–1062. IEEE (2014)
64. Sund-Levander, M., Forsberg, C., Wahren, L.K.: Normal oral, rectal, tympanic and axillary body temperature in adult men and women: a systematic literature review. Scand. J. Caring Sci. **16**(2), 122–128 (2002)
65. Tang, H., Wang, M., Hu, Y., Guo, B., Li, T.: Automated signal quality assessment for heart sound signal by novel features and evaluation in open public datasets. BioMed Res. Int. **2021**(1), 7565,398 (2021)
66. Tang, J., Chen, K., Wang, Y., Shi, Y., Patel, S., McDuff, D., Liu, X.: MMPD: multi-domain mobile video physiology dataset. In: 45th Annual International Conference of the IEEE Engineering in Medicine & Biology Society (EMBC), pp. 1–5. IEEE (2023)
67. Tomaszewska, J.Z., Młyńczak, M., Georgakis, A., Chousidis, C., Ładogórska, M., Kukwa, W.: Automatic heart rate detection during sleep using tracheal audio recordings from wireless acoustic sensor. Diagnostics **13**(18), 2914 (2023)
68. Usman, M., Zubair, M., Ahmad, Z., Zaidi, M., Ijyas, T., Parayangat, M., Wajid, M., Shiblee, M., Ali, S.J.: Heart rate detection and classification from speech spectral features using machine learning. Arch. Acoust. **46**(1), 41–53 (2021)
69. Vavrinsky, E., Esfahani, N.E., Hausner, M., Kuzma, A., Rezo, V., Donoval, M., Kosnacova, H.: The current state of optical sensors in medical wearables. Biosensors **12**(4), 217 (2022)
70. Wu, H.Y., Rubinstein, M., Shih, E., Guttag, J., Durand, F., Freeman, W.: Eulerian video magnification for revealing subtle changes in the world. ACM Trans. Graph. (TOG) **31**(4), 1–8 (2012)
71. Yang, F., He, S., Sadanand, S., Yusuf, A., Bolic, M.: Contactless measurement of vital signs using thermal and RGB cameras: a study of Covid 19-related health monitoring. Sensors **22**(2), 627 (2022)

72. Yaseen, Son, G.Y., Kwon, S.: Classification of heart sound signal using multiple features. Appl. Sci. **8**(12), 2344 (2018)
73. Zhang, Q., Zhang, J., Yuan, J., Huang, H., Zhang, Y., Zhang, B., Lv, G., Lin, S., Wang, N., Liu, X., et al.: SPRSound: open-source STJU paediatric respiratory sound database. IEEE Trans. Biomed. Circ. Syst. **16**(5), 867–881 (2022)
74. Zhang, Z., Girard, J.M., Wu, Y., Zhang, X., Liu, P., Ciftci, U., Canavan, S., Reale, M., Horowitz, A., Yang, H., et al.: Multimodal spontaneous emotion corpus for human behavior analysis. In: Proceedings of the IEEE Conference on Computer Vision and Pattern Recognition, pp. 3438–3446 (2016)

Open Access This chapter is licensed under the terms of the Creative Commons Attribution 4.0 International License (http://creativecommons.org/licenses/by/4.0/), which permits use, sharing, adaptation, distribution and reproduction in any medium or format, as long as you give appropriate credit to the original author(s) and the source, provide a link to the Creative Commons license and indicate if changes were made.

The images or other third party material in this chapter are included in the chapter's Creative Commons license, unless indicated otherwise in a credit line to the material. If material is not included in the chapter's Creative Commons license and your intended use is not permitted by statutory regulation or exceeds the permitted use, you will need to obtain permission directly from the copyright holder.

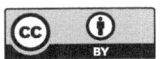

Chapter 9
Affective Computing in Active Assisted Living

Albert Ali Salah, Deniz Iren, and Heysem Kaya

Abstract Emotions play an important role in human behavior, and their analysis is often a necessary step in correct interpretation of said behaviors, providing context and depth. In active assisted living (AAL) applications, affective computing methods are used to understand a user's affective state, as well as provide systems interacting with the user with improved communication capabilities. In this chapter, we provide an overview of affective computing and its uses in AAL, discuss issues of trust and responsible AI, as well as provide a short overview of the AI Act as an example legal framework that regulates the use of affective computing in AAL.

Keywords Affective computing · Active assisted living (AAL) · Responsible AI · AI act

9.1 Introduction

In recent years, artificial intelligence (AI) technologies have seen a noticeable improvement, leading to their widespread adoption in many aspects of life. The prevalence of AI applications has led most societal stakeholders to perceive the significance of the ethical concerns of AI and take necessary actions to ensure that AI is developed and deployed in alignment with human values. Companies adopt human-centered design principles to create and deploy AI systems that deliver value to their customers by trying to understand precisely how the users respond to different design

---

A. A. Salah (✉) · H. Kaya
Department of Information and Computing Sciences, Utrecht University,
Utrecht, The Netherlands
e-mail: a.a.salah@uu.nl

H. Kaya
e-mail: h.kaya@uu.nl

D. Iren
Department of Information Science, Open Universiteit, Heerlen, The Netherlands
e-mail: deniz.iren@ou.nl

elements [5]. Researchers explore the ethical dimensions of AI, conducting studies to understand the implications of AI on society, and developing models that are more accurate, explainable, and transparent [16]. Policymakers play a key role in setting the ethical and legal frameworks to ensure that AI systems are safe, transparent, accountable, and fair. This comprises a complex dynamic ecosystem that gives rise to overlaps and conflicts in the goals and practices of these stakeholders.

AI systems operating under conditions where human rights, safety, and privacy are at stake require special attention. By design, Active Assisted Living (AAL) systems are deployed in settings such as homes and offices, and may access affective and behavioral signals that potentially carry sensitive and private information. Therefore, the ethical and responsible design and deployment of AAL technologies must be carefully studied, especially in light of AI regulations [23] such as the General Data Protection Regulation (GDPR)[1] and the European Union (EU) AI Act.[2]

This chapter aims to provide information on affective computing use cases in AAL and to explore the challenges and concerns regarding the trustworthy and responsible design of such systems. Affective computing (AC) is an interdisciplinary field dealing with computational systems that can recognize, interpret, process, and simulate human emotions [77]. Since human behavior analysis is incomplete without understanding the emotional state of the studied human, AC has a lot of potential in AAL. Yet, AC may involve sensitive information, which for example reveals responses of a person that are not purposefully communicated, or if aggregated over long periods of time, may be conducive to inferences about the person that go beyond the purposes of the monitoring systems.

In this chapter, we briefly summarize the main technologies of affective computing (Sect. 9.2), emphasizing its interdisciplinary and multimodal aspects. Section 9.3 discusses the use cases of AC in AAL, laying out the characteristic differences of these use cases. Section 9.4 explores the trustworthy and responsible design of AC in AAL. Section 9.5 covers an overview of a recent legal framework related to AC in AAL, highlighting the potentially impactful AC regulations in AAL. Finally, Sect. 9.6 concludes the chapter.

---

[1] Regulation (EU) 2016/679 of the European Parliament and of the Council of 27 April 2016 on the protection of natural persons with regard to the processing of personal data and on the free movement of such data, and repealing Directive 95/46/EC (General Data Protection Regulation), http://data.europa.eu/eli/reg/2016/679/oj, Accessed: 2024-09-24.

[2] Regulation (EU) 2024/1689 of the European Parliament and of the Council of 13 June 2024 laying down harmonised rules on artificial intelligence and amending Regulations (EC) No 300/2008, (EU) No 167/2013, (EU) No 168/2013, (EU) 2018/858, (EU) 2018/1139 and (EU) 2019/2144 and Directives 2014/90/EU, (EU) 2016/797 and (EU) 2020/1828 (Artificial Intelligence Act), https://eur-lex.europa.eu/eli/reg/2024/1689/oj, Accessed 2024-09-24.

9.2 What Is Affective Computing?

In the Introduction, we gave a definition of AC that included multiple capabilities, which were disjoint, but related. Having a computer system that can recognize the affective state of a monitored person is different from a system that can also appear to the user as having some emotions, for example interacting with a happy or sad voice. But what is affect in general?

Affect can encompass emotions, moods, feelings. Wundt provided a distinction between emotions and feelings; "An emotion is a unitary whole which is distinguished from a composite feeling only through the two characteristics that it has a definite temporal course and that it exercises a more intense present and subsequent effect on the interconnection of psychical processes" [105]. Furthermore, the literature on emotions distinguishes "basic emotions" from more complex or composite emotions. These are defined as discrete and primitive categories, corresponding to a fixed set of neural and bodily expressed components, and a stable feeling or motivational component that is evolved via natural selection because of its direct relevance (such as fear or disgust) [95]. The most widely used basic emotion model in AC is popularized with the research of Paul Ekman, and includes six basic emotions (i.e. happiness, sadness, fear, anger, surprise, disgust, respectively) [34]. Ekman observes that these emotions have certain characteristics, such as "rapid onset, short duration, unbidden occurrence, automatic appraisal, and coherence among responses" [34]. This list is occasionally extended with a seventh emotion, "contempt," and in computational studies that use a supervised learning approach, with a "neutral" class that acts as a baseline state. Ekman further claimed that the facial expressions corresponding to these emotional states are universally recognizable [35] and even though later research established that facial morphology and culture do play a role in recognition, and subjects from Eastern and Western cultures do not perfectly interpret each other's facial expressions [57], the basic emotional expressions model formed the basis of a large number of works and systems for facial emotional expression analysis.

Partly motivated by the straightforward way of annotating emotional expressions, the basic emotions view also steered the AC community towards more categorical models, where at any moment, one of a small, discrete number of emotional states is assumed for each subject. While AC researchers are fully aware that this is an over-simplification and the true emotional state of a person is complex, there are many practical applications that can benefit from the estimation of an approximate affective state.

The alternatives to basic emotion categories are to allow overlaps between these categories to permit compound emotional states, such as "happily surprised" [32], or to use a continuous, dimensional model, where the emotion would be annotated as a real-valued vector [46]. The most popular choice for such a dimensional model is the 2-dimensional Valence-Arousal space, based on Russell's Circumplex model [81]. For this model, Russell estimated distances between emotion words and used multi-dimensional scaling (MDS) to project them to a 2D space with distances preserved as much as possible. The two dimensions that are created this way, when inspected, showed that valence (i.e. how positive or negative an emotion is) and arousal (i.e. the amount of energy in the emotion) are good labels to characterize the two dimensions. While Russell's work popularized such a characterization, the idea of mapping emotions to a multi-dimensional space goes back to Wundt [105], who proposed pleasantness versus unpleasantness and excitement versus depression as the first two dimensions of mapping feelings via introversion. This dimensional approach was used empirically for facial affect; Abelson and Sermat used MDS for facial expressions and found very similar axes, as early as 1962 [1]. Wundt initially proposed a third dimension (tension vs. relaxation), and later, projections to 3D space suggested that "dominance" can be the third factor, illustrating how much feeling of control is included in the particular emotion [82]. Consequently, most dimensional approaches in AC either use Valence-Arousal (VA) or Valence-Arousal-Dominance (VAD) as their representation of affect [111].

Coming back to computer systems that can recognize the affective state of a monitored person, examples of such systems include applications that can detect facial expressions and do inferences on positive affective states such as happiness and satisfaction, as well as negative affective states like frustration, sadness, or confusion. Similarly, body pose, voice, language, and other modalities can be used to make affect-related inferences about humans. Voice-based affect recognition initially also focused on the recognition of stress [87]. For all these modalities, machine learning approaches were used to create recognition systems. Initially, human actors portrayed emotional content to generate datasets that could be used in training such systems. Gradually, the community moved to "in-the-wild" scenarios, and more naturalistic data were annotated for training systems, which made it possible to observe humans in their living environments and infer their affective states.

In AAL systems, it is important both to monitor the state of the assisted individuals, as well as to recognize the timing of the signals for most effective interventions. Subsequently, AC finds several different application areas in this domain. In the next section, we provide an overview of the applications of AC on AAL.

9.3 Where Is AC Used in AAL?

AAL studies the development and utilization of smart devices, sensors, and computer systems that support the lives of the occupants of an environment enhanced by such technologies. AAL systems do not only sense the physical activities and behaviors of the users but also the affect, i.e., emotions, moods, and feelings. This section outlines the prominent types of AAL that specifically use AC.

Detecting affective signals using smart technologies differs from sensing non-affective behavior and activity. To examine the specific characteristics of AC for AAL, we try to answer the following questions in this and the next section:

- Which categories of AC in AAL are reported in the literature?
- What type of data and sensing technologies are used for detecting affective signals?
- What are the ethical, legal, and societal concerns specific to AC in AAL?

We use the taxonomy of AC [104] to explore the sensors utilized for detecting affective signals. This taxonomy categorizes AC based on the modalities supported by the underlying system. An AC system can rely on *text, audio, visual, physiological signals*, or a combination of these modalities. Text commonly represents the content of a speech or written messages, while audio covers a multitude of paralinguistic speech and sound features, such as prosody and signal frequency [109]. Visual affective signals vary from facial expressions to gestures and body language [64]. Finally, physiological signals include skin conductivity, heart rate variability, and electrical activity in the brain [84]. Data in each modality can be captured using different types of sensors (see [22, 24] in this volume), with varying degrees of intrusiveness and specific ethical, legal, and societal concerns.

A common initial step in computational approaches to affect analysis is the examination of informative signals such as facial expressions, verbal and non-verbal speech, gestures, physiological signals (such as heart rate and skin conductance), and mental states [99]. The technical literature in each of these areas is vast. We focus on the most common modalities and representative recent works here.

Face. Automatic facial affect analysis evolved significantly over the years, starting from work in the 90s that used image projections, multi-layer perceptrons and patch-based analysis [73] to deep neural networks trained on thousands of images in the 2020s [69]. The typical pipeline of face analysis starts with face detection in an image frame, followed by estimation of facial landmarks (such as the mouth and eye corners, and nose tip), facial registration (i.e., alignment of the face to a standardized template using the landmarks), feature extraction, and classification [85]. While end-to-end trained deep learning approaches, if trained on sufficient data, may short-circuit some of these tasks, widely used facial emotional expression analysis tools like OpenFace [8] still implement this pipeline. The wide-spread availability of face identity data makes it feasible to start training face analysis systems for an identity recognition task, and then use transfer learning to fine-tune the models for emotional expression analysis, with more limited data [31, 61].

In an AAL scenario, accurate facial analysis depends on the placement of the camera, which may be used for other tasks in parallel, such as fall detection [58]. Ceiling cameras typically do not have the ideal point of view to process emotions displayed on the face, and a static camera will only capture these when the subject faces the camera. Furthermore, when used in a setting with multiple people (including, for instance, caregivers), the system should be coupled with a face recognition module to correctly monitor and attribute affect for a single person. A more realistic scenario is to employ face analysis in a device that will have access to a frontal face view during interaction, such as a social assistive robot, or a smart mirror (see for instance [86] in this volume). Even smaller robots can provide support to older adults in AAL, such as for cleaning tasks or for simple emotional support, but most such scenarios do not require face or emotion analysis [83]. For more interactive tasks, such as a fitness coach for older adults, facial analysis can help detecting interaction quality [44, 45], as well as states such as frustration, confusion, or pain.

One marked advantage of monitoring affect via faces is that while the accuracy may be limited for single frames of analysis, long-term monitoring of the facial affect indeed provides a good indication of the overall affect for a person [30]. However, we note that the prevalence of facial emotional expression displays is not uniform over classes; the expression of "happiness" is typically much more common compared to more extreme emotions like "fear" or more subtle expressions like "disgust".

Text and Speech. The second major modality in behavior analysis is speech, which includes linguistic and paralinguistic information. The analysis of language is traditionally performed by transcribing speech and extracting, often manually, but also via simple text processing tools, certain characteristics of speech. Progress in text-based affective processing, coupled with the increased availability of automatic transcription tools makes language-based evaluation very attractive. English remains to be the language with the most advanced tools available, however, it is possible to create tools for under-studied languages by translating large affect-annotated dictionaries from English [48] or using tools/models trained in English after translation of the original texts into English [92]. While such approaches will not be perfect and some meaning will be lost in translation, the sheer volume of resources in English may result in a more accurate system compared to working in the original language, if its resources are too limited.

While multi-modality has been effectively used in categorical emotion recognition, in dimensional approaches, uni-modal systems may perform better for each task [92]. The literature suggests that acoustic features provide better discrimination for arousal and poorer discrimination for valence [88]. On the other hand, linguistic features are more discriminative in valence compared to arousal recognition [88, 92]. Developments in transformer-based acoustic models, including but not limited to WaV2Vec 2.0 [7] and HuBERT [54], which are pre-trained in a self-supervised manner, have recently revolutionized speech processing not only for automatic speech recognition (ASR) but also recognition of speaker states and traits. These are also successfully used in affective computing [76, 101]. Fine-tuning a WaV2Vec 2.0 model on a relatively large speech emotion corpus, Wagner et al. [101] achieved unprecedented performance on acoustics-based prediction of valence.

Having a major and long-term impact on life quality, depression (severity) prediction is one of the most intensely studied subjects in AC [25]. There are increasing efforts to use intelligent avatars that are capable of interacting with the users in their natural environment securely to estimate and monitor depression. One such effort resulted in collection of the E-DAIC depression corpus [26]. While acoustics-based depression (severity) prediction is popularly studied over a decade [3, 25, 51, 59, 60], interestingly, on this avatar-interaction corpus, the best-performing depression severity prediction methods are based on text modality [60, 68, 78, 96]. It may be the case that while interacting with an intelligent avatar, speakers may regulate their acoustics for optimal recognition of their spoken content and may lean to provide more linguistic information about their mental well-being, rather than reflecting their affective state to their voice. These findings have several implications for future data collection efforts and AC applications in AAL. First, it is possible to embed the intelligent avatar or a social robot with acoustics-based affect recognition functionality and make the user aware of it. Second, more emphasis can be placed on text-based depression severity recognition in these settings. There are commercial platforms (such as Silvercloud[3]) that are offering clinically validated mental health assistance tools based on text analysis and text interactions. As data accumulate in such platforms, their machine learning based capabilities will improve.

Wearable Sensors. AAL literature categorizes sensors into three types; *wearables*, *smart objects*, and *environmental sensors* [21]. Wearable sensors are characterized by being worn or carried by the user in some way. Examples include smartphones, smartwatches, and wristbands. Smart objects are everyday appliances that are equipped with sensors and processors. They can communicate and interact with each other and their users. For instance, sensors in furniture provide non-intrusive ways to monitor daily user activity. Environmental sensors operate in the physical environment, regardless of being interacted with by the user. Cameras and microphones are prominent examples of environmental sensors. Different types of sensors used by AAL systems offer varying degrees of risk to privacy and other ethical concerns. For instance, on the one hand, user consent is less of an issue with wearables and smart objects because their operation depends on being worn or actively interacted with by the user. On the other hand, environmental sensors tend to sense signals from whoever occupies the physical space, being the targeted users or not (Table 9.1).

Smart environments equipped with sensors provide a wealth of data that can be used to infer the behavior of persons to detect abnormalities or degradation of health [43]. One heavily studied scenario is distress situation detection, which relies on continuous monitoring of an individual using physiological or behavioral data to infer cases of distress [43]. Fall detection [62, 103] is a prime example, where sensors like accelerometers in smartphones or smartwatches [89] can trigger alerts (see [58] in this volume for a review). Cameras [90] and depth sensors offer alternative approaches, but raise privacy concerns. The use of ultra-wideband radars poses a viable alternative. They use radio signals that can penetrate walls and provide good precision. They capture essential information while maintaining some level of confidentiality [11].

Distress can also manifest in less obvious ways. Time spent outside [55], at home or in specific rooms [102], walking speed [6], and sleep quality [97] have all been linked to loneliness and depression. For instance, slowing gait velocity can indicate cognitive decline in the older adults [14].

Current AAL systems for activity and behavior monitoring face limitations in accuracy. They often struggle to identify complex activities beyond pre-defined ones [75]. Another important consideration is privacy. There is an inherent trade-off between the convenience offered by smart environments and the potential privacy concerns associated with constant monitoring. Developers of AAL systems must

---

[3] https://www.silvercloudhealth.com/, Accessed 27 September 2024.

Table 9.1 Examples of sensing technologies used in different combinations of AAL system types and the modalities of data utilized by the underlying AC component

		Wearables	Ambient
Audio and text	*Linguistic*	Microphone + speech to text	Microphone (+ASR) for text-based depression severity recognition [60, 68, 78, 96]
	Paralinguistic	Microphone	Microphone for speech-based depression (severity) prediction [3, 25, 51, 60]
Visual	*Facial expressions*	Wearable device for detecting non-verbal cues of the conversation partner [56]	Camera for facial expression [2, 61, 65, 106], stress [4, 41, 66, 98, 112] and depression recognition [39, 49, 52, 107]
	Gestures	Gloves, sleeves, suits	RGB and depth cameras for emotional gesture recognition [72]
	Body language	Motion trackers	Camera for posture and human activity based emotion recognition [13]; Doppler radar for gait analysis [80]
Physiological		Stress measurement of individuals [40, 94]; HR, Galvanic skin response (GSR) and temperature based emotion recognition [28]	Thermal Cameras for car driver's emotion recognition [63] and stress recognition [18, 42, 53]

consider alternative sensor technologies that provide the needed functionality while being less intrusive. For instance, a gait monitoring system utilizing Doppler radars enhances privacy and eliminates the inconvenience associated with wearable devices [80]. Nevertheless, ultimately, the decision of how much and what kind of data to share should lie with the individual who is impacted by the system, or a caregiver legally authorized to take such decisions [93].

9.4 Trust and Responsible Uses of AC in AAL

Ethical concerns for data science distinguish between issues related to data, algorithms, and practices [37]. Each of these correspond to several risks that should be taken into account. Data can be stolen or leaked, or misused for surveillance and control. Algorithms may be biased and favor one group over another, or may work poorly for some demographic, thereby increasing inequalities in the society. Erroneous estimation of affective states can have important consequences (e.g. missing relevant information and therefore delaying access to care, or creating intrusions into private life via false positives). Real-world practices of deploying AI and AC algorithms can create issues of power and control, or the loss of dignity [16].

Many ethics principles are proposed for guiding the use of technology, and AC research and practice are both shaped by these principles [27]. The general framework of principlism, laid out in the Belmont Report of 1979, stipulated respect for persons, beneficence, and justice [10]. Beneficence can be split into doing good (beneficence) and not doing harm (non-maleficence). Correct use of these principles creates trust in the user, and ensures sustainable usage of technologies. Consequently, fair restrictions imposed on AC technologies actually facilitate, rather than hamper the usage of these technologies by increasing trust.

There are many ways in which to consider these principles in designing AAL technology that contains affective elements. For instance, beneficence suggests that we design systems that help older adults to lead an independent, active, and happy life, while non-maleficence warns us about potential harms. Sometimes the latter is not immediately obvious; for example a robotic technology that controls the environment may facilitate an old person's life initially, but can cause laziness and muscle loss in the long run by promoting less activity [38]. For technology that senses emotions and affect, the way the information is used may create counter-intuitive or unexpected risks. For instance, if the system detects loneliness of the subject, and takes countermeasures, such as alerting family and friends, it may cause embarrassment or feelings of being a burden to others. In the SnowGlobe system, proposed by Visser et al. an interactive snow globe is placed at the home of an older adult subject, with its twin in the home of a close relative [100]. When the globe is manipulated, its twin will also register and display this (e.g. with a house covered in snow), and subtly alert the relative that they are being missed. A more direct technology, even if it is very accurate in detecting loneliness and informing relatives, may be harmful, if the true needs of the subjects are not taken into account.

In the literature of responsible affective computing, we see some principles to be more frequently pronounced compared to others [9, 71]. These include accountability, transparency (e.g., interpretability/explainability), privacy, and (algorithmic) fairness of the models, as well as the data they are trained with. Coping with these dimensions is mandatory for critical AI/ML applications, such as AC in AAL. Here, we define a task as critical if the decisions impact individuals or society. The motivations for developing responsible AI methods range from regulatory compliance to building trust, from scientific understanding of the causal relations to model auditing and debugging [20, 70]. We will briefly discuss the prominent responsible AI/AC principles here, and refer the reader to Chap. 11 ([16]) and [27] for more extensive discussions.

Accountability can be defined as the degree of transparency of a system's methods, internal decision processes and outcomes and the degree of communicating them to the users [9]. Accountability also implies the existence of regulatory mechanisms to protect people against unfair decisions taken by automated systems, and a means to hold the designers and operators of unfair systems accountable. Thus, these two ethical principles are connected.

Autonomy is related with human control and oversight, transparency, explainability, access to information, agency, consent, and privacy [15]. In AAL settings, it is particularly important to protect the dignity of the subjects. This can sometimes be very difficult, for instance when the subject does not fully possess the mental clarity to understand a technology and its implications. Legally, a guardian may provide consent in those cases, but this does not solve the ethical problems. Another issue is the substitution of human contact with some affective technology that is inadequate to provide human connection. This can lead to reduced care and increase in isolation.

Two concepts are linked to the ethics principles of accountability and autonomy. *Explainability* is the ability to relate the outcome of a machine learning model (i.e., its decision) to its input. Subsequently, it is more useful for the designers of AC systems, compared to users. Although frequently used interchangeably with explainability, *interpretability* refers to understanding the decision mechanism, rather than only understanding which part of the input (or feature subset) had the highest impact on a decision [79]. Interpretability can also be defined as the degree to which a human can understand the cause of a decision made by a model [29, 47]. An interpretable model should therefore be transparent (or simple enough to understand) and provide the means/methods of analyzing its decision-making mechanism without resorting to post-hoc methods. Moreover, to be understandable by humans, the input data/features must themselves be intelligible.

Fairness, in the context of AI, is defined as the absence of any bias regarding an individual or group's innate or learned characteristics (such as religion or gender) that are irrelevant in a given decision-making context. Thus, fairness is an "absence of any prejudice or favoritism toward an individual or group based on their inherent or acquired characteristics" [67]. Fair AC systems should for example sense affect of different demographics equally well. Many mathematical measures are proposed to quantify the fairness (or bias) of the algorithms [19, 33, 50, 110]. The main idea is to measure whether models output similar (if not the same) proportions of (dis)favoring outcomes (as in Demographic Parity [33]) or any other predictive performance measures (as in Equalized Odds [50]) across sensitive groups. Here, transparency via interpretable system design or explainability may help detect and mitigate bias [79]. If a model is biased, mitigation techniques, which can be broadly categorized into preprocessing, processing, and post-processing methods, can be applied.

In the scope of AC in AAL, recently there is increasing momentum in interpretable [36, 96], fair [17, 91], and privacy-preserving [12, 74, 108] methods. In most studies, we observe that the focus is on one aspect of responsible AI. For example, in [96] interpretability in depression severity prediction is sought via symptoms, and in [12] violence risk of inpatients is determined via federated learning to preserve privacy. There are also efforts to bridge the responsible AI themes, and to make more data available from older adults to enable development of systems with less demographic bias [88].

9.5 Legal Aspects and the AI Act

While a full treatment of legal and regulatory aspects of AC in AAL is not possible within the limited space of this chapter, we will provide some guidance for the regulatory approach of the European Union (EU), namely the AI Act, to shed light on the ethical considerations and specific challenges of AC and AAL. We refer the reader to Chap. 12 in this volume for a discussion of broader legal implications [23].

Passed in early 2024, the EU AI Act (Article 3(1)) defines an AI system as "a machine-based system designed to operate with varying levels of autonomy and that may exhibit adaptiveness after deployment and that, for explicit or implicit objectives, infers, from the input it receives, how to generate outputs such as predictions, content, recommendations, or decisions that can influence physical or virtual environments." As can be seen from the text, the autonomy of AI systems is seen as a risk, and adaptation during the operation of the system, while it may increase performance, can introduce non-anticipated elements into its behavior. This is particularly important for AC technologies, as affect can be idiosyncratic, and require a higher degree of personalization and adaptation.

The AI Act furthermore broadly groups AI applications into three risk categories: low-, high-, and unacceptable-risk, respectively. The deployment of systems that fall into the unacceptable-risk category is prohibited, while the high-risk applications must satisfy strict requirements. The AI Act has a territorial scope; meaning that even if the developers of an AI technology are established outside the borders of the EU, they are still subject to regulation provided that their services are used in the EU. Moreover, the AI Act affects not only development, but also scientific research. Despite the exemption of scientific research from the regulations, there is an undeniable indirect impact in the form of diminishing funding and hindering the transition from theory to practice. Therefore, the EU's AI Act and similar regulations prepared by other states are expected to pose significant legal challenges for both developers and researchers who operate in the domain of AC in AAL. On the other hand, as we mentioned earlier, having a strong regulatory framework will increase trust by the users, and positively impact the adoption of technological solutions.

AAL systems heavily depend on data collected by a vast variety of sensing technologies and machine learning techniques. For this reason, AAL systems will potentially be impacted by the AI Act regulations. In the remainder of this section, we will examine three concepts highlighted by the AI Act that are explicitly relevant to AAL and AC. These are the special status attributed to biometric data, emotion recognition practices, and sensing technologies in public spaces.

Biometric data. The AI Act provides the definition of "biometric data", as follows: *"Biometric data comprise personal data resulting from specific technical processing relating to the physical, physiological or behavioral characteristics of a natural person, which allow or confirm the unique identification of that natural person, such as facial images or dactyloscopic data"*. Examples include not only facial appearance but also eye movements, body shape, voice, prosody, gait, posture, heart rate, and blood pressure. Arguably, the definition of biometric data is broad enough to cover most types and modalities of data used in AC and AAL. Furthermore, the AI Act considers biometric data as a special category of personal data due to its sensitive nature, and therefore certain cases in which AI systems use biometric data are classified as high-risk.

Emotion recognition. The AI Act defines "emotion recognition systems" as AI systems designed to identify or infer the emotions or intentions of individuals based on their biometric data. This definition has two important points; the purpose of inferring emotions and intentions, and the use of biometric data for this purpose. The AI Act provides clarifications to these points as follows. The definition refers to emotions and intentions such as "happiness, sadness, anger, surprise, disgust, embarrassment, excitement, shame, contempt, satisfaction, and amusement", and excludes physical states (e.g., pain or fatigue) and "readily apparent expressions, gestures, or movements" unless they are used for inferring emotions. Such expressions, gestures, and movements are exemplified as facial expressions (e.g., frown, smile), movement of hands, arms, or head, and voice characteristics such as raised voice or whispering. Most use cases of emotion recognition systems are classified as high-risk. Moreover, deploying emotion recognition systems in situations related to education and the workplace is prohibited. However, use cases in which such systems are deployed strictly for medical and safety reasons are excluded by this prohibition.

Public spaces. According to the AI Act, "publicly accessible space" refers to *"any physical space that is accessible to an undetermined number of natural persons"* irrespective of being publicly or privately owned and the purpose for which the space is used. Examples of publicly accessible spaces include shops, cafes, restaurants, banks, swimming pools, gyms, stadiums, public transportation infrastructures and vehicles, cinemas, theatres, museums, public roads and squares, parks, and forests. The relevance of public spaces in the context of the EU AI Act is particularly concerning the use of AI systems for real-time remote biometric identification. These technologies have the potential to significantly intrude on individuals' rights and freedoms. Environmental sensors, particularly those deployed in public spaces, pose a higher risk to privacy due to the potential for collecting data on individuals without their knowledge or consent.

The specific impact of the AI Act on AAL depends on the type of the system and the underlying sensing technologies.

Wearables. As wearables often collect biometric data, the use of such systems will likely to be subject to restrictions and control, requiring stronger user consent policies, transparency in the use of the collected data, and robust data security protocols. Yet, user consent and data processing transparency challenges can be addressed easier than other types of AAL systems as the user of wearable systems is mostly a single individual.

Smart objects. Smart objects (or smart devices) can collect various types of data including voice recordings, which are considered biometric data, and environmental sounds. Smart objects might also embed video cameras. To address the risks to privacy posed by smart objects, new methods to seek informed user consent will be required.

Environmental sensors. Real-time biometric identification is subject to restrictions by the AI Act. Environmental sensors that utilize video recording technologies specifically in public spaces are likely to be impacted by these restrictions. In such settings, the use of motion sensors and Doppler radar-like sensors would pose less risks to privacy. However, user consent and transparency remain important challenges as any individual using public spaces will potentially be subject to data collection. The applications of AAL systems using environmental sensors for safety and healthcare are expected to be allowed, however, with restrictions.

9.6 Conclusions

A comprehensive understanding of the ethical, legal, societal, and technical concerns regarding AC for AAL is a multifaceted challenge. An ethically sound perspective on any technology seeks to balance the benefits of it against the potential harms. The regulatory AI frameworks that are being introduced now are about minimizing the latter, and the deep learning revolution of the last ten years is serving to improve the former. Furthermore, multimodality has entered the computational modeling in a major way, and it portends a boost into both accuracy and acceptability of AAL systems.

While the vision of affective computing did not change much in the last thirty years, safe commercial applications are already out there, and we have a good understanding of the risks of these technologies. The design and development of AC technologies for AAL should strictly adhere to legal and ethical requirements, as these technologies are considered critical by nature (classified as 'high-risk' by the EU AI Act). Designing an AC technology should consider not only the hardware, such as wearable or ambient sensors, but also how the data are collected, stored, represented, modeled, and communicated to a server or other humans. Thanks to increased awareness and legal developments, we observe growing research in the responsible AI/AC directions such as fairness, explainability/interpretability, and privacy which collectively contribute to the accountability of and trust in the developed systems.

Acknowledgements This publication is based upon work from COST Action GoodBrother—Network on Privacy-Aware Audio- and Video-Based Applications for Active and Assisted Living (CA19121), supported by COST (European Cooperation in Science and Technology). We thank Eftim Zdravevski and Pau Climent-Pérez for their constructive comments.

References

1. Abelson, R.P., Sermat, V.: Multidimensional scaling of facial expressions. J. Exp. Psychol. **63**(6), 546–554 (1962)
2. Adyapady, R.R., Annappa, B.: A comprehensive review of facial expression recognition techniques. Multimed. Syst. **29**(1), 73–103 (2023)
3. Almaghrabi, S.A., Clark, S.R., Baumert, M.: Bio-acoustic features of depression: a review. Biomed. Signal Process. Control **85**, 105,020 (2023). https://doi.org/10.1016/j.bspc.2023.105020
4. Almeida, J., Rodrigues, F.: Facial expression recognition system for stress detection with deep learning. In: In Proceedings of the 23rd International Conference on Enterprise Information Systems (ICEIS), vol. 1, pp. 256–263 (2021)
5. Auernhammer, J.: Human-centered AI: the role of human-centered design research in the development of AI. In: Synergy-DRS International Conference, pp. 11–14 (2020)
6. Austin, J., Dodge, H.H., Riley, T., Jacobs, P.G., Thielke, S., Kaye, J.: A smart-home system to unobtrusively and continuously assess loneliness in older adults. IEEE J. Trans. Eng. Health Med. **4**, 1–11 (2016)
7. Baevski, A., Zhou, Y., Mohamed, A., Auli, M.: wav2vec 2.0: A framework for self-supervised learning of speech representations. Adv. Neural Inf. Process. Syst. **33**, 12,449–12,460 (2020)
8. Baltrušaitis, T., Robinson, P., Morency, L.P.: Openface: an open source facial behavior analysis toolkit. In: 2016 IEEE Winter Conference on Applications of Computer Vision (WACV), pp. 1–10. IEEE (2016)
9. Batliner, A., Neumann, M., Burkhardt, F., Baird, A., Meyer Sarina Thang Vu, N., Schuller, B.W.: Ethical awareness in paralinguistics: a taxonomy of applications. Int. J. Human-Comput. Interact. **39**(9), 1904–1921 (2023). https://doi.org/10.1080/10447318.2022.2140385
10. Beauchamp, T.L., Childress, J.F.: Principles of Biomedical Ethics. Oxford University Press (1989)
11. Beaulieu, A., Thullier, F., Bouchard, K., Maître, J., Gaboury, S.: Ultra-wideband data as input of a combined EfficientNet and LSTM architecture for human activity recognition. J. Ambient Intell. Smart Environ. **14**(3), 157–172 (2022)
12. Borger, T., Mosteiro, P., Kaya, H., Rijcken, E., Salah, A.A., Scheepers, F., Spruit, M.: Federated learning for violence incident prediction in a simulated cross-institutional psychiatric setting. Expert Syst. Appl. **199**, 116,720 (2022). https://doi.org/10.1016/j.eswa.2022.116720. https://www.sciencedirect.com/science/article/pii/S0957417422001944
13. Calapatia, E., Suarez, M.: Using body posture, movement and human activity to predict emotions. In: Theory and Practice of Computation: Proceedings of Workshop on Computation: Theory and Practice WCTP2017, pp. 158–171. World Scientific (2019)
14. Camicioli, R., Howieson, D., Oken, B., Sexton, G., Kaye, J.: Motor slowing precedes cognitive impairment in the oldest old. Neurology **50**(5), 1496–1498 (1998)
15. Canca, C.: Operationalizing AI ethics principles. Commun. ACM **63**(12), 18–21 (2020)
16. Čartolovni, A., Dantas, C., Malešević, A., Ilgaz, A.: Ethical issues in AAL. In: Salah, A.A., Colonna, L., Florez-Revuelta, F. (eds.) Privacy-Aware Monitoring for Assisted Living. Springer, Cham (2025)
17. Cheong, J., Kuzucu, S., Kalkan, S., Gunes, H.: Towards gender fairness for mental health prediction. In: IJCAI, pp. 5932–5940 (2023)
18. Cho, Y., Julier, S.J., Bianchi-Berthouze, N.: Instant stress: detection of perceived mental stress through smartphone photoplethysmography and thermal imaging. JMIR Ment. Health **6**(4), e10,140 (2019). https://doi.org/10.2196/10140
19. Chouldechova, A., Roth, A.: A snapshot of the frontiers of fairness in machine learning. Commun. ACM **63**(5) (2020)
20. Choung, H., David, P., Ross, A.: Trust in AI and its role in the acceptance of AI technologies. Int. J. Human-Comput. Interact. **39**(9), 1727–1739 (2023). https://doi.org/10.1080/10447318.2022.2050543

21. Cicirelli, G., Marani, R., Petitti, A., Milella, A., D'Orazio, T.: Ambient assisted living: a review of technologies, methodologies and future perspectives for healthy aging of population. Sensors **21**(10), 3549 (2021)
22. Colantonio, S., et al.: A historical view of AAL. In: Salah, A.A., Colonna, L., Florez-Revuelta, F. (eds.) Privacy-Aware Monitoring for Assisted Living. Springer, Cham (2025)
23. Colonna, L., Riva, G.M.: The legal and regulatory issues in AAL: the case of smart mirrors. In: Salah, A.A., Colonna, L., Florez-Revuelta, F. (eds.) Privacy-Aware Monitoring for Assisted Living. Springer, Cham (2025)
24. Cristina, S., Počta, P., Zgank, A., Camilleri, K.P., Colantonio, S., Lambrinos, L.: Remote monitoring of vital signs. In: Salah, A.A., Colonna, L., Florez-Revuelta, F. (eds.) Privacy-Aware Monitoring for Assisted Living. Springer, Cham (2025)
25. Cummins, N., Scherer, S., Krajewski, J., Schnieder, S., Epps, J., Quatieri, T.F.: A review of depression and suicide risk assessment using speech analysis. Speech Commun. **71**, 10–49 (2015)
26. DeVault, D., Artstein, R., Benn, G., Dey, T., Fast, E., Gainer, A., Georgila, K., Gratch, J., Hartholt, A., Lhommet, M., et al.: Simsensei kiosk: a virtual human interviewer for healthcare decision support. In: Proceedings of the 2014 International Conference on Autonomous Agents and Multi-agent Systems, pp. 1061–1068 (2014)
27. Devillers, L., Cowie, R.: Ethical considerations on affective computing: an overview. Proc. IEEE **11**(10), 1445–1458 (2023)
28. Domínguez-Jiménez, J.A., Campo-Landines, K.C., Martínez-Santos, J.C., Delahoz, E.J., Contreras-Ortiz, S.H.: A machine learning model for emotion recognition from physiological signals. Biomed. Signal Process. Control **55**, 101,646 (2020)
29. Doshi-Velez, F., Kim, B.: Towards a rigorous science of interpretable machine learning. arXiv:1702.08608 (2017)
30. Doyran, M., Türkmen, B., Oktay, E.A., Halfon, S., Salah, A.A.: Video and text-based affect analysis of children in play therapy. In: 2019 International Conference on Multimodal Interaction, pp. 26–34 (2019)
31. Dresvyanskiy, D., Ryumina, E., Kaya, H., Markitantov, M., Karpov, A., Minker, W.: End-to-end modeling and transfer learning for audiovisual emotion recognition in-the-wild. Multimodal Technol. Interact. **6**(2) (2022). https://doi.org/10.3390/mti6020011
32. Du, S., Martinez, A.M.: Compound facial expressions of emotion: from basic research to clinical applications. Dialogues Clin. Neurosci. **17**(4), 443–455 (2015)
33. Dwork, C., Hardt, M., Pitassi, T., Reingold, O., Zemel, R.: Fairness through awareness. In: Proceedings of the 3rd Innovations in Theoretical Computer Science Conference, pp. 214–226 (2012)
34. Ekman, P.: An argument for basic emotions. Cognit. Emot. **6**(3–4), 169–200 (1992)
35. Ekman, P.: Facial expressions. In: Handbook of Cognition and Emotion **16**(301), e320 (1999)
36. Escalante, H.J., Kaya, H., Salah, A.A., Escalera, S., Gültürk, Y., Gülü, U., Baró, X., Guyon, I., Junior, J.C.S.J., Madadi, M., Ayache, S., Viegas, E., Gürpınar, F., Wicaksana, A.S., Liem, C.C.S., van Gerven, M.A.J., van Lier, R.: Modeling, recognizing, and explaining apparent personality from videos. IEEE Trans. Affect. Comput. **13**(2), 894–911 (2022). https://doi.org/10.1109/TAFFC.2020.2973984
37. Floridi, L., Taddeo, M.: What is data ethics? Phil. Trans. Royal Soc. A: Math. Phys. Eng. Sci. **374**(2083), 20160360 (2016)
38. Forlizzi, J., DiSalvo, C., Gemperle, F.: Assistive robotics and an ecology of elders living independently in their homes. Human-Comput. Interact. **19**(1–2), 25–59 (2004)
39. Gavrilescu, M., Vizireanu, N.: Predicting depression, anxiety, and stress levels from videos using the facial action coding system. Sensors **19**(17), 3693 (2019)
40. Giannakakis, G., Grigoriadis, D., Giannakaki, K., Simantiraki, O., Roniotis, A., Tsiknakis, M.: Review on psychological stress detection using biosignals. IEEE Trans. Affect. Comput. **13**(1), 440–460 (2022). https://doi.org/10.1109/TAFFC.2019.2927337
41. Giannakakis, G., Pediaditis, M., Manousos, D., Kazantzaki, E., Chiarugi, F., Simos, P., Marias, K., Tsiknakis, M.: Stress and anxiety detection using facial cues from videos. Biomed. Signal Process. Control **31**, 89–101 (2017). https://doi.org/10.1016/j.bspc.2016.06.020

42. Gioia, F., Pascali, M.A., Greco, A., Colantonio, S., Scilingo, E.P.: Discriminating stress from cognitive load using contactless thermal imaging devices. In: 43rd Annual International Conference of the IEEE Engineering in Medicine & Biology Society (EMBC), pp. 608–611 (2021). https://doi.org/10.1109/EMBC46164.2021.9630860
43. Gomez, C., Chessa, S., Fleury, A., Roussos, G., Preuveneers, D.: Internet of things for enabling smart environments: a technology-centric perspective. J. Ambient Intell. Smart Environ. **11**(1), 23–43 (2019)
44. Görer, B., Salah, A.A., Akın, H.L.: A robotic fitness coach for the elderly. In: Ambient Intelligence: 4th International Joint Conference, AmI 2013, Dublin, Ireland, December 3–5, 2013. Proceedings 4, pp. 124–139. Springer (2013)
45. Görer, B., Salah, A.A., Akın, H.L.: An autonomous robotic exercise tutor for elderly people. Auton. Robot. **41**, 657–678 (2017)
46. Gunes, H., Pantic, M.: Automatic, dimensional and continuous emotion recognition. Int. J. Synth. Emot. (IJSE) **1**(1), 68–99 (2010)
47. Haagen, T., Kaya, H., Snijder, J., Nierman, M., et al.: Autoxplain: towards automated interpretable model selection. In: xAI-2023 Late-Breaking Work, Demos and Doctoral Consortium Joint Proceedings, vol. 3554, pp. 18–23 (2023)
48. Halfon, S., Doyran, M., Türkmen, B., Oktay, E.A., Salah, A.A.: Multimodal affect analysis of psychodynamic play therapy. Psychother. Res. **31**(3), 313–328 (2020)
49. Harati, S., Crowell, A., Mayberg, H., Kong, J., Nemati, S.: Discriminating clinical phases of recovery from major depressive disorder using the dynamics of facial expression. In: 2016 38th Annual International Conference of the IEEE Engineering in Medicine and Biology Society (EMBC), pp. 2254–2257. IEEE (2016)
50. Hardt, M., Price, E., Srebro, N.: Equality of opportunity in supervised learning. In: Advances in Neural Information Processing Systems, vol. 29 (2016)
51. Hashim, N.W., Wilkes, M., Salomon, R., Meggs, J., France, D.J.: Evaluation of voice acoustics as predictors of clinical depression scores. J. Voice **31**(2), 256.e1-256.e6 (2017)
52. He, L., Guo, C., Tiwari, P., Su, R., Pandey, H.M., Dang, W.: DepNet: an automated industrial intelligent system using deep learning for video-based depression analysis. Int. J. Intell. Syst. **37**(7), 3815–3835 (2022)
53. Hong, K., Hong, S.: Real-time stress assessment using thermal imaging. Vis. Comput. **32**(11), 1369–1377 (2016)
54. Hsu, W.N., Bolte, B., Tsai, Y., Lakhotia, K., Salakhutdinov, R., Mohamed, A.: Hubert: self-supervised speech representation learning by masked prediction of hidden units. IEEE/ACM Trans. Audio, Speech, Lang. Process. **29**, 3451–3460 (2021)
55. Huynh, S., Tan, H.P., Lee, Y.: Towards unobtrusive mental well-being monitoring for independent-living elderly. In: Proceedings of the 4th International on Workshop on Physical Analytics, pp. 1–6 (2017)
56. Iren, D., Shingjergji, K., Böttger, F., Urlings, C., Osinga, J.M., Van De Goor, S., Bustowski, D., Passariello-Jansen, J., Klemke, R.: Augmented reality and affective computing for nonverbal interaction support of the visually impaired. In: 2023 IEEE Conference on Virtual Reality and 3D User Interfaces Abstracts and Workshops (VRW), pp. 360–363. IEEE (2023)
57. Jack, R.E., Blais, C., Scheepers, C., Schyns, P.G., Caldara, R.: Cultural confusions show that facial expressions are not universal. Curr. Biol. **19**(18), 1543–1548 (2009)
58. Lumetzberger, J., Ballester, I., Kampel, M.: Fall detection. In: Salah, A.A., Colonna, L., Florez-Revuelta, F. (eds.) Privacy-Aware Monitoring for Assisted Living. Springer, Cham (2025)
59. Kaya, H., Eyben, F., Salah, A.A., Schuller, B.: CCA based feature selection with application to continuous depression recognition from acoustic speech features. In: 2014 IEEE International Conference on Acoustics, Speech and Signal Processing (ICASSP), pp. 3729–3733. IEEE (2014)
60. Kaya, H., Fedotov, D., Dresvyanskiy, D., Doyran, M., Mamontov, D., Markitantov, M., Akdag Salah, A.A., Kavcar, E., Karpov, A., Salah, A.A.: Predicting depression and emotions in the cross-roads of cultures, para-linguistics, and non-linguistics. In: Proceedings of the 9th International on Audio/Visual Emotion Challenge and Workshop, pp. 27–35 (2019)

61. Kaya, H., Gürpınar, F., Salah, A.A.: Video-based emotion recognition in the wild using deep transfer learning and score fusion. Image Vis. Comput. **65**, 66–75 (2017)
62. Khan, S.S., Hoey, J.: Review of fall detection techniques: a data availability perspective. Med. Eng. Phys. **39**, 12–22 (2017)
63. Kolli, A., Fasih, A., Al Machot, F., Kyamakya, K.: Non-intrusive car driver's emotion recognition using thermal camera. In: Proceedings of the Joint INDS'11 & ISTET'11, pp. 1–5. IEEE (2011)
64. Leong, S.C., Tang, Y.M., Lai, C.H., Lee, C.: Facial expression and body gesture emotion recognition: a systematic review on the use of visual data in affective computing. Comput. Sci. Rev. **48**, 100,545 (2023)
65. Li, S., Deng, W.: Deep facial expression recognition: a survey. IEEE Trans. Affect. Comput. **13**(3), 1195–1215 (2020)
66. Maaoui, C., Bousefsaf, F., Pruski, A.: Automatic human stress detection based on webcam photoplethysmographic signals. J. Mech. Med. Biol. **16**(04), 1650,039 (2016)
67. Mehrabi, N., Morstatter, F., Saxena, N., Lerman, K., Galstyan, A.: A survey on bias and fairness in machine learning. ACM Comput. Surv. (CSUR) **54**(6), 1–35 (2021)
68. Milintsevich, K., Sirts, K., Dias, G.: Towards automatic text-based estimation of depression through symptom prediction. Brain Inform. **10**(1), 4 (2023)
69. Mollahosseini, A., Hasani, B., Mahoor, M.H.: AffectNet: a database for facial expression, valence, and arousal computing in the wild. IEEE Trans. Affect. Comput. **10**(1), 18–31 (2017)
70. Molnar, C.: Interpretable Machine Learning: A Guide For Making Black Box Models Explainable. Lulu.com (2022)
71. Nakao, Y., Strappelli, L., Stumpf, S., Naseer, A., Regoli, D., Del Gamba, G.: Towards responsible AI: a design space exploration of human-centered artificial intelligence user interfaces to investigate fairness. Int. J. Human-Comput. Interact. **39**(9), 1762–1788 (2023). https://doi.org/10.1080/10447318.2022.2067936
72. Noroozi, F., Corneanu, C.A., Kamińska, D., Sapiński, T., Escalera, S., Anbarjafari, G.: Survey on emotional body gesture recognition. IEEE Trans. Affect. Comput. **12**(2), 505–523 (2018)
73. Padgett, C., Cottrell, G.: Representing face images for emotion classification. In: Advances in Neural Information Processing Systems, vol. 9 (1996)
74. Pan, Y., Shang, Y., Shao, Z., Liu, T., Guo, G., Ding, H.: Integrating deep facial priors into landmarks for privacy preserving multimodal depression recognition. IEEE Trans. Affect. Comput. **15**(3), 828–836 (2024). https://doi.org/10.1109/TAFFC.2023.3296318
75. Patel, A., Shah, J.: Sensor-based activity recognition in the context of ambient assisted living systems: a review. J. Ambient Intell. Smart Environ. **11**(4), 301–322 (2019)
76. Pepino, L., Riera, P., Ferrer, L.: Emotion recognition from speech using wav2vec 2.0 embeddings. In: Proceedings of the Interspeech 2021, pp. 3400–3404 (2021). https://doi.org/10.21437/Interspeech.2021-703
77. Picard, R.W.: Affective Computing. MIT Press (2000)
78. Ray, A., Kumar, S., Reddy, R., Mukherjee, P., Garg, R.: Multi-level attention network using text, audio and video for depression prediction. In: Proceedings of the 9th International on Audio/Visual Emotion Challenge and Workshop, pp. 81–88 (2019)
79. Rudin, C.: Stop explaining black box machine learning models for high stakes decisions and use interpretable models instead. Nat. Mach. Intell. **1**(5), 206–215 (2019)
80. Rui, L., Chen, S., Ho, K., Rantz, M., Skubic, M.: Estimation of human walking speed by doppler radar for elderly care. J. Ambient Intell. Smart Environ. **9**(2), 181–191 (2017)
81. Russell, J.A.: A circumplex model of affect. J. Pers. Soc. Psychol. **39**(6), 1161 (1980)
82. Russell, J.A., Mehrabian, A.: Evidence for a three-factor theory of emotions. J. Res. Pers. **11**(3), 273–294 (1977)
83. Sadri, F.: Ambient intelligence: a survey. ACM Comput. Surv. (CSUR) **43**(4), 1–66 (2011)
84. Saganowski, S., Perz, B., Polak, A.G., Kazienko, P.: Emotion recognition for everyday life using physiological signals from wearables: a systematic literature review. IEEE Trans. Affect. Comput. **14**(3), 1876–1897 (2022)

85. Salah, A.A., Sebe, N., Gevers, T.: Communication and automatic interpretation of affect from facial expressions. In: Affective Computing and Interaction: Psychological, Cognitive and Neuroscientific Perspectives, pp. 157–183. IGI Global (2011)
86. Santofimia, M.J., del Toro, X., Bolaños, C., Dorado, J., Colantonio, S.: A smart mirror to your health: personalized virtual coaching for active and healthy ageing. In: Salah, A.A., Colonna, L., Florez-Revuelta, F. (eds.) Privacy-Aware Monitoring for Assisted Living. Springer, Cham (2025)
87. Schuller, B., Batliner, A., Steidl, S., Seppi, D.: Recognising realistic emotions and affect in speech: state of the art and lessons learnt from the first challenge. Speech Commun. **53**(9–10), 1062–1087 (2011)
88. Schuller, B.W., Batliner, A., Bergler, C., Messner, E.M., Hamilton, A., Amiriparian, S., Baird, A., Rizos, G., Schmitt, M., Stappen, L., Baumeister, H., MacIntyre, A.D., Hantke, S.: The INTERSPEECH 2020 computational paralinguistics challenge: elderly emotion. Breathing & masks. In: Proceedings of the Interspeech 2020, pp. 2042–2046 (2020). https://doi.org/10.21437/Interspeech.2020-0032
89. Şengül, G., Karakaya, M., Misra, S., Abayomi-Alli, O.O., Damaševičius, R.: Deep learning based fall detection using smartwatches for healthcare applications. Biomed. Signal Process. Control **71**, 103,242 (2022)
90. Shu, F., Shu, J.: An eight-camera fall detection system using human fall pattern recognition via machine learning by a low-cost android box. Sci. Rep. **11**(1), 2471 (2021)
91. Sogancioglu, G., Kaya, H., Salah, A.A.: The effects of gender bias in word embeddings on patient phenotyping in the mental health domain. In: 2023 11th International Conference on Affective Computing and Intelligent Interaction (ACII), pp. 1–8 (2023). https://doi.org/10.1109/ACII59096.2023.10388203
92. Sogancioglu, G., Verkholyak, O., Kaya, H., Fedotov, D., Cadée, T., Salah, A.A., Karpov, A.: Is everything fine, Grandma? Acoustic and linguistic modeling for robust elderly speech emotion recognition. In: Proceedings of the Interspeech 2020, pp. 2097–2101 (2020). https://doi.org/10.21437/Interspeech.2020-3160
93. Streitz, N., Charitos, D., Kaptein, M., Böhlen, M.: Grand challenges for ambient intelligence and implications for design contexts and smart societies. J. Ambient Intell. Smart Environ. **11**(1), 87–107 (2019)
94. Tomczak, M.T., Wojcikowski, M., Pankiewicz, B., Łubiński, J., Majchrowicz, J., Majchrowicz, M., Walasiewicz, A., Kiliński, T., Szczerska, M.: Stress monitoring system for individuals with autism spectrum disorders. IEEE Access **8**, 228,236–228,244 (2020)
95. Tracy, J.L., Randles, D.: Four models of basic emotions: a review of ekman and cordaro, izard, levenson, and panksepp and watt. Emot. Rev. **3**(4), 397–405 (2011)
96. Van Steijn, F., Sogancioglu, G., Kaya, H.: Text-based interpretable depression severity modeling via symptom predictions. In: Proceedings of the 2022 International Conference on Multimodal Interaction, pp. 139–147 (2022)
97. Veiga, A., Garcia, L., Parra, L., Lloret, J., Augele, V.: An IoT-based smart pillow for sleep quality monitoring in AAL environments. In: 2018 Third International Conference on Fog and Mobile Edge Computing (FMEC), pp. 175–180. IEEE (2018)
98. Viegas, C., Lau, S.H., Maxion, R., Hauptmann, A.: Towards independent stress detection: a dependent model using facial action units. In: 2018 International Conference on Content-Based Multimedia Indexing (CBMI), pp. 1–6 (2018). https://doi.org/10.1109/CBMI.2018.8516497
99. Vinciarelli, A., Pantic, M., Heylen, D., Pelachaud, C., Poggi, I., D'Errico, F., Schroeder, M.: Bridging the gap between social animal and unsocial machine: a survey of social signal processing. IEEE Trans. Affect. Comput. **3**(1), 69–87 (2012). https://doi.org/10.1109/T-AFFC.2011.27
100. Visser, T., Vastenburg, M.H., Keyson, D.V.: Designing to support social connectedness: the case of snowglobe. Int. J. Des. **5**(3) (2011)
101. Wagner, J., Triantafyllopoulos, A., Wierstorf, H., Schmitt, M., Burkhardt, F., Eyben, F., Schuller, B.W.: Dawn of the transformer era in speech emotion recognition: closing the valence gap. IEEE Trans. Pattern Anal. Mach. Intell. (2023)

102. Walsh, L., Kealy, A., Loane, J., Doyle, J., Bond, R.: Inferring health metrics from ambient smart home data. In: 2014 IEEE International Conference on Bioinformatics and Biomedicine (BIBM), pp. 27–32. IEEE (2014)
103. Wang, X., Ellul, J., Azzopardi, G.: Elderly fall detection systems: a literature survey. Front. Robot. AI **7**, 71 (2020)
104. Wang, Y., Song, W., Tao, W., Liotta, A., Yang, D., Li, X., Gao, S., Sun, Y., Ge, W., Zhang, W., et al.: A systematic review on affective computing: emotion models, databases, and recent advances. Inform. Fusion **83**, 19–52 (2022)
105. Wundt, W.: Grundriss der Psychologie [Fundamentals of Psychology], 15th ed. Engelmann, Leipzig (1896). http://psychclassics.yorku.ca/Wundt/Outlines/
106. Xefteris, S., Doulamis, N., Andronikou, V., Varvarigou, T., Cambourakis, G.: Behavioral biometrics in assisted living: a methodology for emotion recognition. Eng. Technol. Appl. Sci. Res. **6**(4), 1035–1044 (2016)
107. Xu, J., Gunes, H., Kusumam, K., Valstar, M., Song, S.: Two-stage temporal modelling framework for video-based depression recognition using graph representation. IEEE Trans. Affect. Comput. 1–18 (2024). https://doi.org/10.1109/TAFFC.2024.3415770
108. Xu, X., Peng, H., Bhuiyan, M., Hao, Z., Liu, L., Sun, L., He, L.: Privacy-preserving federated depression detection from multisource mobile health data. IEEE Trans. Industr. Inf. **18**(7), 4788–4797 (2022). https://doi.org/10.1109/TII.2021.3113708
109. Yildirim, H.E., Iren, D.: Informative speech features based on emotion classes and gender in explainable speech emotion recognition. In: 2023 11th International Conference on Affective Computing and Intelligent Interaction Workshops and Demos (ACIIW), pp. 1–8. IEEE (2023)
110. Zafar, M.B., Valera, I., Rogriguez, M.G., Gummadi, K.P.: Fairness constraints: mechanisms for fair classification. In: Artificial Intelligence and Statistics, pp. 962–970 (2017)
111. Zeng, Z., Pantic, M., Roisman, G., Huang, T.: A survey of affect recognition methods: audio, visual, and spontaneous expressions. IEEE Trans. Pattern Anal. Mach. Intell. **1**(31), 39–58 (2009)
112. Zhang, H., Feng, L., Li, N., Jin, Z., Cao, L.: Video-based stress detection through deep learning. Sensors **20**(19), 5552 (2020)

Open Access This chapter is licensed under the terms of the Creative Commons Attribution 4.0 International License (http://creativecommons.org/licenses/by/4.0/), which permits use, sharing, adaptation, distribution and reproduction in any medium or format, as long as you give appropriate credit to the original author(s) and the source, provide a link to the Creative Commons license and indicate if changes were made.

The images or other third party material in this chapter are included in the chapter's Creative Commons license, unless indicated otherwise in a credit line to the material. If material is not included in the chapter's Creative Commons license and your intended use is not permitted by statutory regulation or exceeds the permitted use, you will need to obtain permission directly from the copyright holder.

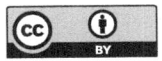

Chapter 10
A Smart Mirror to Your Health: Personalized Virtual Coaching for Active and Healthy Ageing

Maria J. Santofimia, Xavier del Toro, Cristina Bolaños, Javier Dorado, and Sara Colantonio

Abstract *"Sara"* represents a revolutionary approach in personalised care, embedded within a smart mirror to enable active and healthy ageing. This chapter examines the potential and developmental pathways of smart mirrors and their assistants, like Sara, highlighting their capacity to integrate advanced artificial intelligence and machine learning for personalised health solutions. Despite their promising capabilities, the application of smart mirrors in effective health monitoring and lifestyle management is still being developed. This chapter evaluates the essential technological advancements necessary for Sara to effectively address the needs of older adults, with an emphasis on personalisation, privacy, and user engagement. Moreover, the chapter explores how improvements in technology, such as increased accessibility and enhanced user interfaces, could promote broader adoption and continuous use among the ageing demographic. Through potential case studies and theoretical scenarios, this chapter demonstrates the potential role that fully developed smart mirrors

---

M. J. Santofimia (✉) · X. del Toro · J. Dorado
Technology and Information Systems, University of Castilla-La Mancha, Ciudad Real, Spain
e-mail: mariajose.santofimia@uclm.es

X. del Toro
e-mail: xavier.deltoro@uclm.es

J. Dorado
e-mail: javier.dorado@uclm.es

C. Bolaños
Computer Architecture and Networking Group, University of Castilla-La Mancha, Ciudad Real, Spain
e-mail: Cristina_Bolanos@uclm.es

S. Colantonio
Institute of Information Science and Technologies, National Research Council of Italy, Pisa, Italy
e-mail: sara.colantonio@isti.cnr.it

© The Author(s) 2025
A. A. Salah et al. (eds.), *Privacy-Aware Monitoring for Assisted Living*,
Intelligent Systems Reference Library 270,
https://doi.org/10.1007/978-3-031-84158-3_10

could play in supporting the health and well-being of older adults. The chapter concludes by exploring the future directions to transform smart mirrors from innovative concepts to essential health support tools.

Keywords Chatbots · Smart mirrors · Personalisation · Virtual assistants · Health support

10.1 Introduction

The integration of digital technologies into everyday health management is gaining attention because of their potential to provide healthcare professionals with a comprehensive view of an individual's health over time, rather than just the snapshots often captured during sporadic visits to the clinic. Continuous monitoring at home, under optimal conditions, can offer insight into trends and patterns that are critical to making informed medical decisions. In addition, these technologies have the potential to significantly improve access to healthcare services for individuals facing mobility challenges or living in remote areas, ensuring that essential healthcare support is more readily available [26]. According to [39] 56% of the rural populations lack access to essential healthcare services compared to 22% in urban areas. Telemedicine facilitates virtual consultations with urban-based specialists, reducing travel time and costs for rural patients [3].

These advancements are transforming how health and care services are delivered [1], enabling more proactive, personalised, and accessible care for individuals across diverse settings [32]. Driving this evolution are virtual assistants, particularly chatbots [5], which have rapidly gained importance in response to the ageing population and the challenges posed by the COVID-19 pandemic [40]. These AI-driven tools automate interactions and deliver benefits such as reduced service costs [15], increased customer satisfaction [22], and improved patient care by providing health literacy [33], managing chronic diseases, and even offering personalized lifestyle coaching [19]. However, despite extensive efforts and advances in this field, adoption by healthcare systems remains limited, highlighting a significant gap between innovation and practical implementation [42].

Several factors contribute to the slow adoption of chatbots in healthcare [21]. Although these tools offer substantial benefits, their interactions can often seem artificial, leading patients to prefer communication with human caregivers or healthcare professionals [7, 8]. Additionally, the use of hyper-realistic avatars can result in strange and awkward conversations, which further deters users [9]. The "uncanny valley" is a well-known effect, first observed in robotics, when a person's perception "abruptly shift from empathy to revulsion as it approached, but failed to attain, a lifelike appearance" [34]. Moreover, there is a critical need for chatbots to manage healthcare interactions with high reliability and empathy, as failures in these areas can lead to mistrust and reduced adoption rates [29]. To address these challenges, smart mirrors offer a unique advantage by incorporating anthropomorphic design elements that create a greater sense of connection and interaction for users. By allowing users to see both the chatbot avatar and their own reflection, smart mirrors make the virtual assistant feel more human-like [28]. This approach reduces the sense of artificiality and encourages more natural interactions, leading to better user satisfaction and engagement, which ultimately contributes to achieving positive outcomes like improved communication and adherence to health advice [35, 37].

The theory behind anthropomorphism is based on attributing human-like qualities to non-human entities, creating a sense of connection that can foster favourable responses from users [13, 18]. In the context of chatbot anthropomorphism, the style of conversation, particularly how chatbots communicate with users, plays a critical role in shaping the user's impression of the chatbot agent or avatar [45]. One important framework for understanding these impressions is Susan Fiske's warmth-competence model [14]. This model states that warmth (how friendly, kind, and trustworthy an entity is perceived to be) and competence (how skilled and effective they appear) are the two primary dimensions of social perception. The use of warm and competent conversational styles in chatbots is, therefore, vital for enhancing their perceived humanness, which directly influences user acceptance and engagement [38].

According to Fiske's model, warmth is often the first dimension evaluated when interacting with others, as it helps people determine whether the entity has good intentions. In the context of virtual assistants, this means that if users perceive the assistant as warm, they are more likely to trust its guidance and feel comfortable engaging with it. Competence, on the other hand, reflects the assistant's ability to effectively carry out tasks. When both warmth and competence are perceived positively, users are more likely to not only trust but also rely on the assistant for important tasks, such as health management. For virtual assistants like Sara, balancing these two dimensions, projecting empathy through warmth and demonstrating capability through competence, helps foster a stronger emotional connection with users, making them feel supported both emotionally and practically. This dynamic is essential in healthcare contexts, where trust and confidence in the assistant's abilities are crucial for ensuring sustained user engagement and adherence to health recommendations.

Smart mirrors can exploit this aspect by displaying avatars with human-like features and conversational styles, but simply mimicking human appearance is not enough to ensure warmth or competence. While human-like features can create an initial sense of familiarity, warmth and competence are conveyed through a more complex modulation of both visual and conversational skills. For example, warmth is often expressed through friendly, empathetic language, while competence is reflected through clear, professional communication and precise, reliable advice. Depending on the context, such as providing medical advice, a balance between warmth and professionalism must be achieved. For instance, delivering a message like "take your medicine" may benefit more from a tone of cool professionalism, which emphasizes competence and reliability, rather than a purely warm, personal style that could be perceived as less authoritative.

Beyond anthropomorphic aspects, the ability to express feelings through avatars in smart mirrors adds another layer of relevance for enhancing user interaction [36].

The human face plays an important role in communication, serving as an independent channel that aids in coordinating conversations in human–human interactions [43] and in providing non-verbal signals [25]. Facial expressions are universally recognized and play a crucial role in human communication, facilitating emotional expression and enhancing understanding between individuals. When integrated into human-computer interfaces, these expressions can significantly influence user engagement. However, merely incorporating facial expressions does not guarantee improved interaction. The work in [47] conducted a study that demonstrated how avatars with different facial expressions affected user responses in a questionnaire task. They found that participants interacting with a more "stern" or serious avatar, while spending more time and producing more accurate responses, rated their overall experience less positively compared to those interacting with a neutral avatar. This suggests that while avatars with expressive facial features can enhance task performance by increasing user engagement, they may also create discomfort or dissatisfaction if the expression is perceived as overly harsh or inappropriate for the context. Therefore, it is essential to carefully design the expressions of avatars to balance engagement with user comfort, ensuring that they match the intended emotional tone of the interaction.

Sara, the virtual assistant developed for the Miratar project [31], depicted in Fig. 10.1, represents the result of dedicated efforts to integrate an interactive, emotionally responsive avatar into a smart mirror system, explicitly designed to address active and healthy ageing. It has the ability to display a wide range of facial expressions, which extends beyond basic anthropomorphism and relates to the essential elements of human communication. Sara infers the emotional states of users by asking them how they feel, though it relies on self-reported responses, which may not always reflect the user's true emotional state. Her responses and facial expressions are then adjusted based on an analysis of their answers, enabling a more natural interaction. This makes Sara a key component of the smart mirror's interface.

The design of Sara is the product of research and development focused on creating an experience that mirrors the empathetic and understanding interactions characteristic of human caregivers. Having a realistic face, expressive eyes, and synchronised lip movement when speaking are not just technological feats, but are steps taken to make the interaction smoother and more natural.

It is not enough for a virtual assistant like Sara to simply have an anthropomorphic appearance. Ultimately, the assistant has to provide real assistance. This means that, in addition to talking and gesturing like a human, Sara has to be connected to a suite of services and even external and interconnected devices that offer a range of functionalities, designed to support active and healthy ageing. To achieve this, Sara is linked to a set of digital services that operate within the smart mirror, allowing her to interact with various interconnected devices. These devices might include medical devices like blood pressure monitors, scales, and other health-related tools, as well as non-medical devices such as home sensors or activity bands. By accessing this broad network of information, Sara can deliver more personalised and actionable guidance.

10 A Smart Mirror to Your Health: Personalized Virtual Coaching …

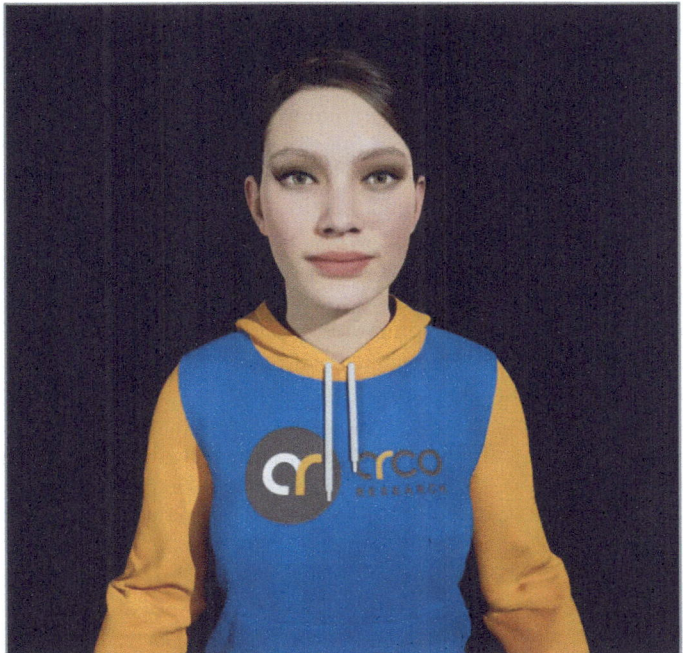

Fig. 10.1 Sara, the virtual assistant in our smart mirror system

This book chapter explores the evolving role of smart mirrors in healthcare and well-being, focusing on the use case of Sara, the virtual assistant. The following sections are structured to provide a comprehensive view of smart mirrors in healthcare.

10.2 Smart Mirrors in Health and Well Being

A smart mirror is a specialised type of mirror that, in addition to reflecting images, integrates digital technology to offer interactive features and display information. The concept started developing in the late 1990s and early 2000s [4], with inspiration drawn from science fiction movies like "Minority Report". The first documented smart mirror was built by Michael Teeuw in 2014, using a Raspberry Pi 2 [44]. His project, named MagicMirror, laid the foundation for subsequent do-it-yourself smart mirror projects and gave rise to the MagicMirror community.[1] At a more commercial level, Toshiba presented its own smart mirror concept at the Consumer Electronics

---
[1] MagicMirror² open source modular smart mirror platform. https://magicmirror.builders/, Accessed 27 September 2024.

Show in 2014, showcasing reflective screens that could display general information like weather and news, as well as personal data from connected devices.

Bianco et al. [4] categorise smart mirrors based on the purposes they serve, highlighting that these devices are no longer limited to displaying basic information, but now include a variety of specialised functions depending on their intended use. According to this work, smart mirrors can be grouped into four categories: general purpose, medical, fashion, and hotel applications, respectively. Chaparro et al. [6] identify other categories, including fitness, social network, home security or automation (active assisted living), in their review. Nonetheless, considering the various applications of smart mirrors, a more refined categorisation can be achieved by distinguishing between those that primarily provide visual information and those that actively interact with the environment, the user, or both. This categorisation addresses the fact that some smart mirrors are designed solely to display information, such as news, weather, and calendar events, while others can influence the surroundings or guide the user through personalised coaching and other interventions. This can include interaction with connected devices, sensors, or AI-driven coaching mechanisms to encourage specific behaviors or achieve health-related outcomes.

Smart mirrors in the second category provide added value to health monitoring at home by connecting to various medical devices and tracking real-time health data such as heart rate, blood pressure, and blood glucose levels. Bianco et al. [4] provide a comprehensive list of the features and technologies employed for medical purposes, such as face detection, face recognition, eye tracking, speech recognition, and augmented reality. These mirrors can monitor weight fluctuations and even analyze sleep patterns (by tracking the first and last interaction of the user with the mirror during the day), offering insights for maintaining or improving health, or pulling information from a health application on the user's mobile phone and displaying this information. Some advanced smart mirrors employ facial recognition technology to detect changes in skin color or signs of fatigue, providing early warnings for potential health issues. This is the case of the Wize Mirror proposed in the SEMEOTICONS project [2, 11] or other works such as [4, 6, 30, 41, 48]. The SHAPES project[2] (Smart and Healthy Ageing through People Engaging in Supportive Systems) proposed a smart mirror that had functionalities like call service, fall detection, physical activity monitoring, voice assistant, calendar reminders, home monitoring, and basic security via login services [6]. The integration possibilities across services is an advantage of mirror platforms.

The use of smart mirrors in health-related applications, particularly for active and healthy ageing, has gained significant attention as a way to provide continuous, around-the-clock care for older adults. This technology offers an opportunity to move healthcare and support services away from conventional institutional settings, promoting the process of deinstitutionalization that many welfare state models are striving for. This shift can reduce the need for hospital or clinic visits for routine tasks such as blood pressure monitoring, diet assessment, or physical therapy. Yet,

---

[2] https://shapes2020.eu, Accessed 27 September 2024.

the smart mirror depends on additional services (such as ambient sensors or mobile phones) to gather information about the subjects, and possibly from the caregivers.

Despite the clear advantages of smart mirrors, several challenges could hinder their broader adoption. The limitations outlined in the study [12] include concerns about the fixed location of smart mirrors, which might require multiple units for comprehensive sensing and displaying coverage, as well as the difficulty of setting up and using them, particularly for older adults or individuals with disabilities. Additionally, there is a fear of redundancy, as many users already have a range of devices (most notably, smartphones and smart watches) that offer similar functionalities, and a potential lack of portability could make smart mirrors impractical.

Another significant barrier is the lack of trust in data sharing, with users expressing concerns about privacy, data security, and the risk of feeling surveyed. This lack of trust might deter users from incorporating smart mirrors into their homes, especially if they worry about how shared data might be used or misused. The more services are integrated within the smart mirror system, the more extensive the data storage requirements will get. If, however, it is just used as a hub to display information coming from other services, the additional security requirements may be minimized.

To ensure that smart mirrors become widely adopted and as ubiquitous in homes as other common appliances, these challenges must be addressed. This includes making smart mirrors more accessible and user-friendly, ensuring user control over data sharing, and emphasising portability to reduce redundancy and improve practicality. Addressing these issues is critical if smart mirrors are to play a key role in supporting health and well-being among older adults. Achieving this goal requires a careful and user-centred approach that considers these limitations and finds ways to mitigate them, ultimately gaining the trust and acceptance of users.

10.3 Sara: Designing a Personal Health Companion

Modern interaction mechanisms predominantly rely on touch screens, which are not well-suited to the needs of older adults [16]. These interfaces, designed primarily for younger generations, often prove challenging due to the physiological changes that come with age. Older adults typically have a lower skin conductivity, which can hinder the ability to register touch accurately on a capacitive screen. This reduced conductivity is influenced by factors such as colder finger temperatures, decreased moisture levels, and the natural thickening and hardening of the skin that occurs with age [27]. These changes make touch-based interactions unreliable, leading to frustration and difficulty in navigating digital devices. On the other hand, voice assistants like Apple Siri[3] and Amazon Alexa,[4] designed to facilitate intuitive interactions via voice commands, often struggle to accurately interpret the speech of older adults.

---

[3] https://www.apple.com/siri/, Accessed 27 September 2024.

[4] https://www.alexa.com/, Accessed 27 September 2024.

This is due to several ageing or health conditions that lead to motor speech disorders such as dysarthria [49], where neuromuscular control issues impair speech clarity and intelligibility [23]. As a result, voice assistants have trouble understanding commands from older adults due to altered pronunciation and intonation. This leads to frequent misinterpretation or failure to recognise instructions. Another issue is accents and deviations from the norm in the speech of the elderly. In many rural areas, the local dialect may be quite different than the mainstream language. (See e.g. [20].) Older adults also report using the voice assistants for a limited number of tasks, and with always the same voice commands, which they have confirmed as working before [46].

Despite significant advancements in technology, it is evident that current solutions often fail to meet the expectations and needs of older adults, leading to low adoption rates among this demographic. To address this gap, it is essential to identify and incorporate specific requirements for a virtual assistant designed for smart mirrors, especially those aimed at promoting active and healthy ageing. Such requirements include a user-friendly interface that accommodates reduced tactile sensitivity and vision issues, ensuring intuitive interaction through voice commands and clear visual feedback. Moreover, the virtual assistant must prioritize user privacy and data security to foster trust, providing transparent control over shared information. Emotional needs should also be considered, enabling the virtual assistant to deliver empathetic companionship while reducing social isolation by facilitating connections with family, friends, and caregivers. Additionally, it should offer personalized coaching and advice tailored to individual health goals, daily routines, and preferences. By addressing these challenges, a well-designed virtual assistant can greatly enhance older adults' engagement, improving their quality of life while ensuring that smart mirrors become invaluable tools for health and wellbeing.

Sara, designed as a personal assistant specifically for the smart mirror being developed by the University of Castilla-La Mancha, incorporates key features that align with the identified requirements for supporting active and healthy ageing [31]. The user interface has been designed to be user friendly. Sara employs a simple and intuitive interface. Nevertheless, the primary interaction relies on straightforward voice commands, ensuring that users can interact hands-free. The technological readiness level of the Automatic Speech Recognition (ASR) system is not sufficiently high for Sara to work *"in the wild"*. This means that the system has been trained to answer to specific user commands.

As a companion, Sara is empathetic and engaging. She checks in on the user every morning, asking how they feel to asses their emotional state. Using natural language processing, she analyses their speech to categorise their mood as positive, neutral, or negative. Based on this analysis, she responds accordingly. For example, if the person seems down, Sara might suggest calling a relative, like a son, to lift his/her spirits and encourage social connection. This proactive approach is intended to reduce the risk of social isolation while ensuring that users feel understood and supported. Sara also facilitates seamless video calls with family, friends, and caregivers to support these essential relationships.

10 A Smart Mirror to Your Health: Personalized Virtual Coaching ...

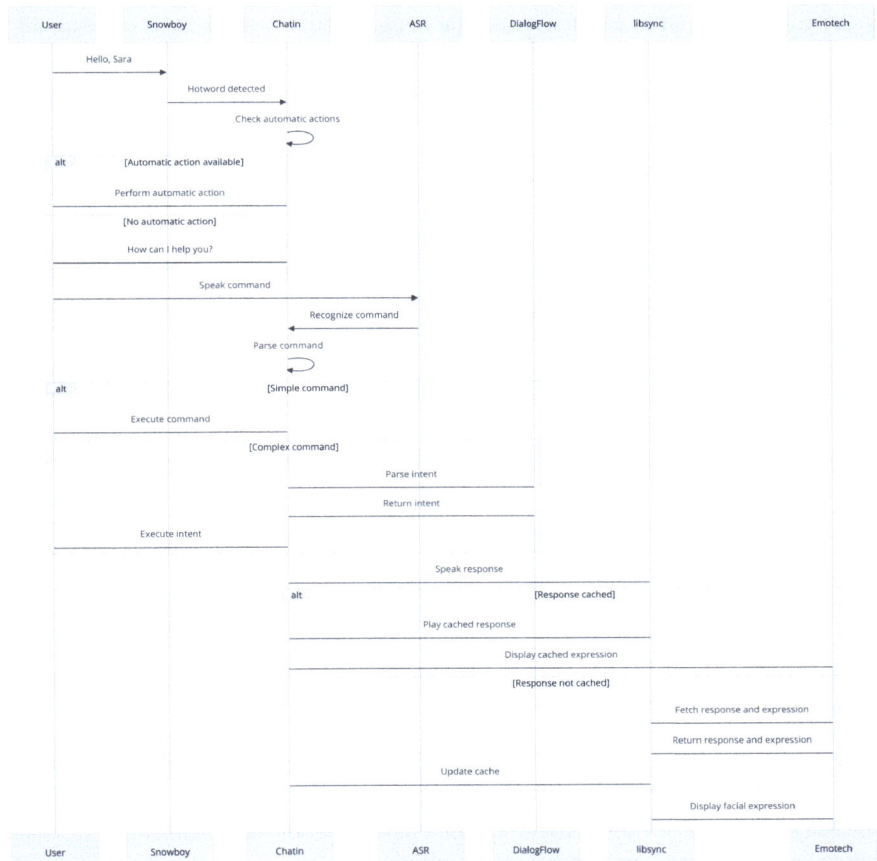

Fig. 10.2 Workflow for virtual assistant

Figure 10.2 depicts the workflow of the virtual assistant developed under the Miratar project [31]. The virtual assistant Sara is activated when the user says the hotword "*Hello, Sara*", detected by KITT.AI's Snowboy service [24], part of the chatin service.[5] Upon activation, chatin checks for automatic actions to perform based on pre-configured triggers. If no automatic actions are found, Sara asks the user how she can help. The user then speaks the command, which is processed by an automatic speech recognition (ASR) service. If the command matches a simple predefined command, chatin executes it. For more complex commands, chatin

---

[5] The KITT.AI products (Snowboy, NLU, and Chatflow) were discontinued as of December 31st, 2020. However, other similar services are available for as building blocks.

uses Google's DialogFlow [10] to parse the intent and then executes the corresponding action. `chatin` then connects to a lip synchronisation service to make the avatar speak the response.

10.4 Case Studies: Impact on Active and Healthy Ageing

This section explores three detailed use cases designed to assess the effectiveness of a virtual assistant integrated into a smart mirror platform. Through these case studies, this chapter aims to demonstrate how personalised digital assistance can support day-to-day health management, improve quality of life, and ensure continued engagement in personal health. Each use case will illustrate different aspects of the virtual assistant's functionality, from monitoring chronic conditions to facilitating wellness activities, highlighting the pivotal role such technologies can play in modern older adult's care frameworks.

10.4.1 Use Case 1: Personalised Risk Prediction and Prevention

This scenario focuses on empowering individuals at risk of frailty and multimorbidity, such as older adults with chronic conditions or lifestyle risk factors, to manage their health proactively. The virtual assistant, integrated into the smart mirror platform, plays a central role by facilitating the tracking and monitoring of health indicators using wearable devices, providing personalized recommendations for lifestyle changes, and delivering preventive interventions.

John, a 65-year-old man with diabetes and high blood pressure, represents the target user persona for this use case. Every morning, Sarah reminds John to wear his smartwatch and to check his blood pressure and glucose level using the devices he has near the mirror. Devices such as the continuous glucose monitor or the smartwatch are crucial as they continuously gather data and feed them to the smart mirror when they are nearby it. The virtual assistant interacts with John through voice commands and text-based communication, providing him with real-time updates on his blood pressure and blood glucose levels and suggesting modifications to his diet, exercise routines, and medication management.

The effectiveness of this use case is measured by several key performance indicators, including the accuracy of the machine learning models used for risk prediction, the user experience provided by the avatar, and the overall impact on John's quality of life. Technical tasks involved in this use case include the development of these predictive models, the integration of wearable and medical devices with the smart mirror platform, and the enhancement of the virtual assistant's conversational capabilities.

This use case not only showcases the practical application of a virtual assistant in managing chronic health conditions, but also demonstrates the potential of smart health platforms to enhance the autonomy and activity levels of older adults.

10.4.2 Use Case 2: Integrated Care Platform and Virtual Assistant

This use case focuses on AI models for frailty and multi-morbidity risk prediction, prevention, and personalised interventions. This conceptual case study involves Emma, a 70-year-old woman with osteoarthritis and hypertension, who leverages the smart mirror platform to manage her health and maintain an active lifestyle despite her chronic conditions.

Emma's daily routine is significantly affected by joint pain, driving her need to find exercises that are both effective and gentle on her joints. The virtual assistant on her smart mirror plays a pivotal role in her health management by providing personalized exercise recommendations. Through the Phyx.io system[6] running on the smart mirror platform, Emma interacts with the virtual assistant, which gathers information on her mobility level, existing limitations, and exercise preferences to tailor its advice effectively.

The core of this use case is the integration of advanced AI algorithms that analyse Emma's input to generate customised exercise plans. These plans include low-impact activities such as gentle stretching, range-of-motion exercises, and water-based activities like swimming or aqua aerobics. The exercise suggestions emphasise gradual progression to ensure safety and effectiveness, aligned with Emma's specific health needs and conditions.

Expert geriatricians contribute to the platform by providing evidence-based exercise guidelines and insights on managing osteoarthritis through physical activity. Their expertise ensures that the virtual assistant's recommendations are medically sound and suitable for Emma's age and physical capabilities.

10.4.3 Use Case 3: Health Literacy and Self-management

This use case aims to empower individuals like Maria, an 80-year-old with hypertension and osteoarthritis, through health education and tailored exercise programs that promote self-management and sustainable behavioural change. The goal is to enhance Maria's ability to manage her conditions effectively, using the smart mirror.

---

[6] Phyx.io is a comprehensive physical activity monitoring platform specifically devoted to support remote rehabilitation, developed under the SHAPES project. https://shapes2020.eu/2023/02/13/phyx-io-a-physical-rehabilitation-platform-for-older-adults/, Accessed 27 September 2024.

Maria engages with a virtual assistant to access customised exercise routines that accommodate her physical limitations and help manage her joint pain. This system provides her with interactive guidance on performing exercises correctly, ensuring her safety and maximising the effectiveness of her workouts. There are prototype systems for exercise coaching the elderly (e.g. [17]), and they provide both corrective and motivational feedback. However, an autonomous system misses out the social aspects of fitness exercises with a real coach or a group of older adults, and the subjects may find it hard to get motivated by such systems.

The healthcare professionals involved, experts in geriatrics and physical therapy, provide the platform with evidence-based exercise programs and detailed instructions on exercise safety specifically designed for older adults with similar health profiles to Maria's. These programs focus on improving joint flexibility and managing pain, crucial for enhancing Maria's mobility and quality of life.

Technical aspects of the use case involve the virtual assistant uses natural language processing to communicate with Maria, guiding her through exercise sessions. The platform also features display capabilities that visually demonstrate exercise techniques, making it easier for Maria to follow along. Once should be careful to leverage multimodality, as older adults may have impaired perception in one or more modalities.

Maria's interaction with the platform is monitored to track her progress and ensure she is engaging with the exercise programs as recommended. The virtual assistant prompts Maria to report her pain levels before and after exercise sessions, using this data to adjust the exercise recommendations as needed to optimise her comfort and health outcomes.

This use case focuses on evaluating the effectiveness of these tailored exercise programs. It measures her adherence to the regimen, her reported pain levels, and the overall impact on her joint flexibility and mobility. Feedback from Maria and other participants is collected to refine the platform's offerings and ensure they meet the users' needs effectively.

This use case illustrates how integrated digital health platforms can support older adults in managing chronic conditions more independently and effectively, promoting better health outcomes and enabling older adults like Maria to lead more active, fulfilling lives.

10.5 Conclusion and Future Work

While the potential of virtual assistants embedded in smart mirrors has been clearly demonstrated through the technological details and use cases explored in this chapter, the widespread adoption of such technology remains a vision not yet fully realised. Key technological and socio-economic challenges must be addressed to bridge the gap between the current capabilities of these devices and their full potential in healthcare and personal wellness settings.

One critical area requiring further advancement is the development of artificial intelligence models that can reliably perform early detection of health risks. Current models show promise in analysing vast amounts of health data to identify potential health issues before they become critical. But will a smart mirror system have access to such a broad range of information, and will it be able to integrate all these sources into a coherent outlook? While enhancing the accuracy and predictive power of these models is essential for them to become a practical tool in preventive health care, data compatibility and protection issues also need to be addressed.

Improvements in ASR technology are also important for spoken interfaces. The effectiveness of smart mirrors greatly depends on their ability to understand and process user commands accurately, which is currently limited, especially in understanding diverse accents and dialects or the altered speech patterns associated with many ageing-related conditions [20]. Advanced ASR systems that can more effectively decode the speech of the older adults or those with speech impairments will make smart mirrors more accessible and functional for a broader user base.

Another significant consideration is cost. Ensuring that smart mirrors are affordable is essential for their widespread adoption. Strategies to keep costs down could include streamlined manufacturing processes, use of cost-effective materials, and potentially, subsidies from healthcare providers or government health initiatives.

Moreover, the integration of smart mirrors into the wider health and social care systems requires rigorous evaluation of their impact on health outcomes and cost-effectiveness. Decision-makers need robust data to justify investments in this technology. Therefore, extensive studies and pilot programs are necessary to demonstrate the benefits of smart mirrors in terms of improving health outcomes, enhancing patient engagement, and reducing overall healthcare costs.

By addressing these challenges, enhancing AI capabilities, improving ASR technology, ensuring affordability, and rigorously evaluating health impact smart mirrors can transition from innovative prototypes to essential tools in health and social care ecosystems. The successful integration of smart mirrors would mark a significant step forward in making healthcare more accessible, personalised, and proactive, aligning with broader public health goals and improving quality of life for users across diverse populations.

Acknowledgements This publication is based upon work from COST Action GoodBrother—Network on Privacy-Aware Audio- and Video-Based Applications for Active and Assisted Living (CA19121), supported by COST (European Cooperation in Science and Technology).

References

1. Albahri, A., Alwan, J.K., Taha, Z.K., Ismail, S.F., Hamid, R.A., Zaidan, A., Albahri, O., Zaidan, B., Alamoodi, A., Alsalem, M.: IoT-based telemedicine for disease prevention and health promotion: state-of-the-art. J. Netw. Comput. Appl. **173**, 102,873 (2021). https://doi.org/10.1016/j.jnca.2020.102873

2. Andreu, Y., Chiarugi, F., Colantonio, S., Giannakakis, G., Giorgi, D., Henriquez, P., Kazantzaki, E., Manousos, D., Marias, K., Matuszewski, B.J., Pascali, M.A., Pediaditis, M., Raccichini, G., Tsiknakis, M.: Wize mirror—a smart, multisensory cardio-metabolic risk monitoring system. Comput. Vis. Image Underst. **148**, 3–22 (2016). https://doi.org/10.1016/j.cviu.2016.03.018
3. Bhaskar, S., Bradley, S., Chattu, V.K., Adisesh, A., Nurtazina, A., Kyrykbayeva, S., Sakhamuri, S., Yaya, S., Sunil, T., Thomas, P., et al.: Telemedicine across the globe-position paper from the covid-19 pandemic health system resilience program (reprogram) international consortium (part 1). Front. Public Health **8**, 556,720 (2020)
4. Bianco, S., Celona, L., Ciocca, G., Marelli, D., Napoletano, P., Yu, S., Schettini, R.: A smart mirror for emotion monitoring in home environments. Sensors **21**(22) (2021). https://doi.org/10.3390/s21227453
5. Casheekar, A., Lahiri, A., Rath, K., Prabhakar, K.S., Srinivasan, K.: A contemporary review on chatbots, AI-powered virtual conversational agents, ChatGPT: applications, open challenges and future research directions. Comput. Sci. Rev. **52**, 100,632 (2024). https://doi.org/10.1016/j.cosrev.2024.100632
6. Chaparro, J.D., Ruiz, J.F.B., Romero, M.J.S., Peño, C.B., Irurtia, L.U., Perea, M.G., Garcia, X.d.T., Molina, F.J.V., Grigoleit, S., Lopez, J.C.: The shapes smart mirror approach for independent living, healthy and active ageing. Sensors **21**(23) (2021). https://doi.org/10.3390/s21237938
7. Chaves, A.P., Egbert, J., Hocking, T., Doerry, E., Gerosa, M.A.: Chatbots language design: the influence of language variation on user experience with tourist assistant chatbots. ACM Trans. Comput. Human Interact. **29**(2), 1–38 (2022)
8. Chaves, A.P., Gerosa, M.A.: How should my chatbot interact? A survey on social characteristics in human-chatbot interaction design. Int. J. Human Comput. Interact. **37**(8), 729–758 (2021)
9. Ciechanowski, L., Przegalinska, A., Magnuski, M., Gloor, P.: In the shades of the uncanny valley: an experimental study of human-chatbot interaction. Futur. Gener. Comput. Syst. **92**, 539–548 (2019)
10. Cloud, G.: Dialogflow. https://cloud.google.com/dialogflow (2024). Accessed 27 May 2024
11. Colantonio, S., Coppini, G., Germanese, D., Giorgi, D., Magrini, M., Marraccini, P., Martinelli, M., Morales, M.A., Pascali, M.A., Raccichini, G., et al.: A smart mirror to promote a healthy lifestyle. Biosys. Eng. **138**, 33–43 (2015)
12. Dowthwaite, L., Cruz, G.R., Pena, A.R., Pepper, C., Jäger, N., Barnard, P., Hughes, A.M., Nair, R.D., Crepaz-Keay, D., Cobb, S., Lang, A., Benford, S.: Examining the use of autonomous systems for home health support using a smart mirror. Healthcare **11**(19) (2023)
13. Epley, N., Waytz, A., Cacioppo, J.T.: On seeing human: a three-factor theory of anthropomorphism. Psychol. Rev. **114**(4), 864 (2007)
14. Fiske, S.T., Cuddy, A.J., Glick, P.: Universal dimensions of social cognition: warmth and competence. Trends Cogn. Sci. **11**(2), 77–83 (2007)
15. Følstad, A., Skjuve, M.: Chatbots for customer service: user experience and motivation. In: Proceedings of the 1st International Conference on Conversational User Interfaces, pp. 1–9 (2019)
16. Gao, Q., Sun, Q.: Examining the usability of touch screen gestures for older and younger adults. Hum. Factors **57**(5), 835–863 (2015)
17. Görer, B., Salah, A.A., Akın, H.L.: An autonomous robotic exercise tutor for elderly people. Auton. Robot. **41**, 657–678 (2017)
18. Guthrie, S.E.: Faces in the Clouds: A New Theory of Religion. Oxford University Press (1995)
19. Haque, A., Chowdhury, M.N.U.R., Soliman, H.: Transforming chronic disease management with chatbots: key use cases for personalized and cost-effective care. In: 2023 Sixth International Symposium on Computer, Consumer and Control (IS3C), pp. 367–370. IEEE (2023)
20. Holliday, N.: Siri, you've changed! acoustic properties and racialized judgments of voice assistants. Front. Commun. **8**, 1 116,955 (2023)
21. Janson, A.: How to leverage anthropomorphism for chatbot service interfaces: the interplay of communication style and personification. Comput. Human Behav. **149**, 107,954 (2023). https://doi.org/10.1016/j.chb.2023.107954

22. Jiang, H., Cheng, Y., Yang, J., Gao, S.: AI-powered chatbot communication with customers: dialogic interactions, satisfaction, engagement, and customer behavior. Comput. Human Behav. **134**, 107,329 (2022)
23. Kent, R.D., Kim, Y.J.: Toward an acoustic typology of motor speech disorders. Clin. Linguist. Phonet. **17**(6), 427–445 (2003)
24. Kitt.AI: Snowboy hotword detection. https://github.com/Kitt-AI/snowboy (2017). Accessed 27 May 2024
25. Knapp, M.L., Hall, J.A., Horgan, T.G.: Nonverbal Communication in Human Interaction, vol. 1. Holt, Rinehart and Winston New York (1978)
26. Lestari, H.M., Miranda, A.V., Fuady, A.: Barriers to telemedicine adoption among rural communities in developing countries: a systematic review and proposed framework. Clin. Epidemiol. Glob. Health **28**, 101,684 (2024). https://doi.org/10.1016/j.cegh.2024.101684
27. Li, B., Gerling, G.J.: Individual differences impacting skin deformation and tactile discrimination with compliant elastic surfaces. In: 2021 IEEE World Haptics Conference (WHC), pp. 721–726. IEEE (2021)
28. Liu, K., Tao, D.: The roles of trust, personalization, loss of privacy, and anthropomorphism in public acceptance of smart healthcare services. Comput. Human Behav. **127**, 107,026 (2022). https://doi.org/10.1016/j.chb.2021.107026
29. Luger, E., Sellen, A.: "Like having a really bad PA" the gulf between user expectation and experience of conversational agents. In: Proceedings of the 2016 CHI Conference on Human Factors in Computing Systems, pp. 5286–5297 (2016)
30. Miotto, R., Danieletto, M., Scelza, J.R., Kidd, B.A., Dudley, J.T.: Reflecting health: smart mirrors for personalized medicine. NPJ Digit. Med. **1**(1), 62 (2018)
31. MIRATAR Project: Miratar project (ted2021-132149b-c41). Funded by MCIN/AEI/10.13039/501100011033 with funds from NextGenerationEU (2021)
32. Mohammadpour, M., Heidari, Z., Mirghorbani, M., Hashemi, H.: Smartphones, tele-ophthalmology, and vision 2020. Int. J. Ophthalmol. **10**(12), 1909 (2017)
33. Mokmin, N.A.M., Ibrahim, N.A.: The evaluation of chatbot as a tool for health literacy education among undergraduate students. Educ. Inf. Technol. **26**(5), 6033–6049 (2021)
34. Mori, M., MacDorman, K.F., Kageki, N.: The uncanny valley [from the field]. IEEE Robot. Autom. Mag. **19**(2), 98–100 (2012)
35. Munnukka, J., Talvitie-Lamberg, K., Maity, D.: Anthropomorphism and social presence in human–virtual service assistant interactions: the role of dialog length and attitudes. Comput. Human Behav. **135**, 107,343 (2022)
36. Nasoz, F., Lisetti, C.L.: Maui avatars: mirroring the user's sensed emotions via expressive multi-ethnic facial avatars. J. Vis. Lang. Comput. **17**(5), 430–444 (2006). https://doi.org/10.1016/j.jvlc.2006.05.001
37. Pfeuffer, N., Benlian, A., Gimpel, H., Hinz, O.: Anthropomorphic information systems. Bus. Inf. Syst. Eng. **61**, 523–533 (2019)
38. Roy, R., Naidoo, V.: Enhancing chatbot effectiveness: the role of anthropomorphic conversational styles and time orientation. J. Bus. Res. **126**, 23–34 (2021). https://doi.org/10.1016/j.jbusres.2020.12.051
39. Scheil-Adlung, X.: Global evidence on inequities in rural health protection: new data on rural deficits in health coverage for 174 countries. Technical report, International Labour Organization (2015)
40. Schillaci, C.E., de Cosmo, L.M., Piper, L., Nicotra, M., Guido, G.: Anthropomorphic chatbots' for future healthcare services: effects of personality, gender, and roles on source credibility, user satisfaction, and intention to use. Technol. Forecast. Soc. Change **199**, 123,025 (2024). https://doi.org/10.1016/j.techfore.2023.123025
41. Silapasuphakornwong, P., Uehira, K.: Smart mirror for elderly emotion monitoring. In: 2021 IEEE 3rd Global Conference on Life Sciences and Technologies (LifeTech), pp. 356–359 (2021). https://doi.org/10.1109/LifeTech52111.2021.9391829
42. Srivastava, B.: Did chatbots miss their "Apollo moment"? Potential, gaps, and lessons from using collaboration assistants during covid-19. Patterns **2**(8), 100,308 (2021). https://doi.org/10.1016/j.patter.2021.100308

43. Takeuchi, A., Nagao, K.: Communicative facial displays as a new conversational modality. In: Proceedings of the INTERACT'93 and CHI'93 Conference on Human Factors in Computing Systems, pp. 187–193 (1993)
44. Teeuw, M.: Magicmirror (2014). https://michaelteeuw.nl/. Accessed on 23 April 2024
45. Thomas, P., Czerwinski, M., McDuff, D., Craswell, N., Mark, G.: Style and alignment in information-seeking conversation. In: Proceedings of the 2018 Conference on Human Information Interaction and Retrieval, pp. 42–51 (2018)
46. Trajkova, M., Martin-Hammond, A.: "Alexa is a toy": exploring older adults' reasons for using, limiting, and abandoning echo. In: Proceedings of the 2020 CHI Conference on Human Factors in Computing Systems, pp. 1–13 (2020)
47. Walker, J.H., Sproull, L., Subramani, R.: Using a human face in an interface. In: Proceedings of the SIGCHI Conference on Human Factors in Computing Systems, pp. 85–91 (1994)
48. Yu, H., Bae, J., Choi, J., Kim, H.: Lux: smart mirror with sentiment analysis for mental comfort. Sensors **21**(9) (2021). https://doi.org/10.3390/s21093092
49. Yılmaz, E., Mitra, V., Sivaraman, G., Franco, H.: Articulatory and bottleneck features for speaker-independent ASR of dysarthric speech. Comput. Speech Lang. **58**, 319–334 (2019). https://doi.org/10.1016/j.csl.2019.05.002

Open Access This chapter is licensed under the terms of the Creative Commons Attribution 4.0 International License (http://creativecommons.org/licenses/by/4.0/), which permits use, sharing, adaptation, distribution and reproduction in any medium or format, as long as you give appropriate credit to the original author(s) and the source, provide a link to the Creative Commons license and indicate if changes were made.

The images or other third party material in this chapter are included in the chapter's Creative Commons license, unless indicated otherwise in a credit line to the material. If material is not included in the chapter's Creative Commons license and your intended use is not permitted by statutory regulation or exceeds the permitted use, you will need to obtain permission directly from the copyright holder.

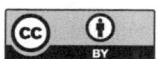

Part III
Trustworthy AAL

Chapter 11
Ethical Issues in AAL

Anto Čartolovni, Carina Dantas, Anamaria Malešević, and Aysegül Ilgaz

Abstract This chapter introduces the reader to the main ethical issues underlying designing, developing, and implementing AAL (Active Assisted Living) technologies created to assist the older population. The nature of AAL technologies, including audio and video-based monitoring, often raises a sense of mistrust or invokes the fear of constant surveillance. However, the full operation of these technologies is not always easy to be understood by non-experts, hindering the performance of quick assessments and impacting the informed consent given and obtained by individual users. Moreover, the primary discussion on the use of AAL technologies often focuses on an ethical trade-off between the privacy of the users and the need to closely monitor and improve their safety, overlooking other valuable nuances from the discussion. A comprehensive framework is needed to assess the risks and benefits of deploying AAL technologies. This framework should integrate ethical principles, stakeholder perspectives, and a risk-benefit analysis to guide decision-making processes and promote responsible deployment. Additionally, there is a need to focus on the utility of AAL devices to provide proper functionality to the user and independence to function socially without constant intervention from caregivers. To ensure an inclusive approach, multi-stakeholder engagement methods with quadruple-helix

---

A. Čartolovni (✉) · A. Malešević
Digital Healthcare Ethics Laboratory (Digit-HeaL), Catholic University of Croatia, Zagreb, Croatia
e-mail: anto.cartolovni@unicath.hr

A. Malešević
e-mail: anamaria.malesevic@unicath.hr

C. Dantas
SHINE 2Europe, Coimbra, Portugal
e-mail: carinadantas@shine2.eu

ICBAS, University of Porto, Porto, Portugal

A. Ilgaz
Department of Public Health Nursing, Akdeniz University, Antalya, Turkey
e-mail: ailgaz@akdeniz.edu.tr

participation can gather perceptions, challenges, risks, barriers, and enablers for a comprehensive and continuous dialogue.

Keywords Active Assisted Living (AAL) · Ethics issues · Risk & benefit analysis · Ethical principles · Stakeholder engagement · Quadruple-helix model

11.1 Introduction

Active assisted living technologies are greatly needed but still unavailable worldwide. Depending on the country's socioeconomic status, at least one in ten individuals require assistive technologies, with this percentage ranging from 10 to 69%. Access to these technologies varies widely, from 3 to 90% [50]. AAL encompasses any technology designed to help older adults adapt to the mental and physical changes that come with aging. The goal is to improve their quality of life and reduce the burden on caregivers. AAL includes hardware, software, and human-machine technology that assists people in their daily lives, including work, despite environmental or physical and cognitive limitations [38]. AAL involves using structured knowledge, abilities, processes, and systems to preserve or enhance an individual's autonomy, functioning, and overall quality of life and well-being [18]. "The values, needs, and expectations of society" as well as "respect for human dignity, freedom, democracy, equality, the rule of law, and human rights, including the rights of persons belonging to minorities" are important considerations for AAL technology [40]. The widespread use of these devices also brings ethical problems in individuals' personal lives [38, 49, 50].

The majority of older people prefer to age in their own homes rather than receiving care in an institution [2]. However, this choice brings up medical and social care costs. AAL techniques can ensure that caregivers feel supported in their caregiving duties and help older adults maintain their autonomy in their homes. Ultimately, this may improve the well-being of older people and their caregivers [13].

Age-related issues require creative and adaptable processes early in life. Incorporating AAL into the living space of older adults may represent an adaptive process that allows compensation and optimization of daily activities to enable autonomous aging, possibly in personal and social domains [16]. Therefore, the compensation and optimization process would differ in an older adult's home or care facility environment.

For instance, while many authors argue that monitoring and surveillance are the same, we believe there are terminological and semantic distinctions between surveillance and monitoring. These differences extend to the ethical issues that arise in the context of AAL, such as depending on in which contexts AAL has been implemented, whether it is an older adult's home or care facility environment. These AAL technologies provide clear examples of how the disparity between monitoring and surveillance becomes apparent, particularly when the level of intrusiveness varies compared to other surveillance technologies, assuming that ethical principles are already integrated into their design and development.

AAL technologies are often seen as intrusive because they may invade private aspects of individuals' lives. When applied in caring contexts, they may lead to potential stigmatization due to their association with certain health conditions such as dementia, dependency, and disability [9, 39].

To ensure AAL's ethical development and deployment, it is important to consider the associated risks and benefits. This involves focusing on underlying ethics issues such as informed consent, data management and access and equal access and distributive justice. Each of these issues will be explored in the following sections.

11.2 Informed Consent

One of the main issues in AAL is the matter of obtaining informed consent concerning the level of obtrusiveness and autonomy, primarily because these technologies have a tendency to "fade into the background" [12, 34]. The consent must be freely given and independent, not just a superficial agreement on the ethical trade-off between privacy and the end user's safety. However, it should support privacy-protecting measures and provide users with clear information. This process involves safeguarding users' safety, as well as upholding and promoting their autonomy [19, 24]. When utilizing AAL technologies in patients with cognitive impairment, including those with dementia, it is recommended that surrogates have a clear understanding of the technology's capabilities and the patient's preferences in order to make decisions accordingly [23]. It is also emphasized that any previously expressed wishes or decisions by the patient should take precedence [49].

The involvement of artificial intelligence (AI) does not make these systems static but highly dynamic. Allowing its use now may not necessarily provide sufficient approval in the future, as the functions and capabilities of these technologies may evolve. The inclusion of AI components in assistive systems increases the ethical importance as it blurs the boundaries of personal autonomy [49]. The technological complexity of various AAL solutions can make it challenging for individuals and their surrogate decision-makers, such as caregivers, to fully understand the implications of their consent. Therefore, all older persons using tracking devices must regularly confirm their agreement because artificial intelligence, including the programming of their gadgets, is constantly evolving [47]. It has been suggested that advance directives could help resolve challenges in obtaining consent from older individuals with dementia. It is important to note that understanding older adults' decisions about AAL use before their cognitive impairment advances could be a clinically effective and ethically sound way to empower them and honor their future autonomy [49].

In this area, it is important to consider the concept of dynamic consent in various contexts, as recently suggested in the biomedical field e.g. biobanking [32, 46]. While implied consent is assumed and preferred in many surveillance contexts, in the AAL context, it should be specific and clear about the technologies used, their purposes, the data collected, and how individual privacy will be protected. Therefore, dynamic consent, which can be modified and updated as AAL technologies become more advanced and complex, might be an appropriate solution for end users.

11.3 Data Management and Access

Data management is an important ethics issue when using AAL technologies to ensure data security and the transmission of this data to third-party services [49]. Reports indicate a higher risk that data collected and processed by AALs may be used for malicious purposes, posing a threat to the user or other parties. Data security standards should be upheld for devices that can access and handle users' personal and medical information, such as tracking and tracing devices [25].

It is important to ensure data sharing that respects people's rights to privacy and autonomy, as well as access to data. Reports indicate that to protect privacy, data collection should be limited to what is necessary for clinical purposes [22], as also emphasized in the data minimization principle of the EU Regulation 2016/679.[1] It is also important to provide clearer conditions for data access and storage in order to give individuals using AAL technologies more control over their personal data and where it will be stored [49]. Medical experts have stated that data transfer should occur within a closed system to protect people's privacy. They also emphasized the importance of obtaining the consent of data owners before sharing relevant information with outside parties, such as medical practitioners [5, 49].

11.4 Equal Access and Distributive Justice

The emerging ethical issue with novel technologies is access, which relates to the affordability of these technologies and the costs of research and development. This is because they often involve expensive equipment and specialized software [1, 3]. In a study of healthcare professionals, participants felt that social inequality is not a new problem, but that AAL technologies may become more affordable over time and widely used across all socioeconomic levels. In other words, although AAL solutions are likely to create socioeconomic inequalities between upper- and lower-middle-class older adults, these inequalities are expected to diminish over time [49]. The implementation of welfare strategies is believed to provide fair access to AAL technologies and accelerate their adoption across all socioeconomic levels. It is important to note that health insurance funds do not typically cover such technologies in most

---

[1] The data minimization principle is expressed in Article 5(1)(c) of the GDPR and Article 4(1)(c) of Regulation (EU) 2018/1725, which provide that personal data must be "adequate, relevant and limited to what is necessary in relation to the purposes for which they are processed".

countries. As a result, users are often responsible for the costs, leading to widening health inequities and leaving the most vulnerable individuals behind. Many older adults prefer to age in place, rather than in residential care facilities. There is an argument for the broader adoption of these technologies through the inclusion of social insurance policies, either fully or partially, under basic health insurance [25, 49].

The ultimate goal should be to ensure that everyone has equal access to AAL technologies. However, in the meantime, fair distribution of these technologies should be prioritized. Implementing AAL-friendly practices in public nursing homes and offering government-sponsored incentives for the advancement of technology development are two strategies that could help reduce inequality. Additionally, it is important to support user-centered research involving patients and caregivers in order to further reduce disparities [7, 25]. Therefore, equal access to AAL technologies and distributive justice require more attention at the design stage [15].

11.5 Ethical Principles in AAL

As AAL technologies become more prevalent in aging care, ethical issues associated with their use increasingly come to the forefront. Focusing on ethical issues in the use of AAL technologies requires fulfilling fundamental ethical principles in the design and development of next-generation personalized AAL devices. Kitchener and Anderson (2011) have identified five ethical principles to guide the implementation of AAL technologies, including autonomy, beneficence, non-maleficence, justice and fidelity [28].

11.5.1 Autonomy

The principle of autonomy states that people's lives should not be interfered with, allowing them to live as they choose, while respecting their rights and tendencies. In essence, autonomy is the right and power that individuals have to fully decide how their lives will unfold [36, 38]. All people have inherent and unconditional value and therefore should have the power to make rational decisions and moral choices [36, 38]. In the context of AAL technologies, autonomy means ensuring that assistive devices designed for older adults' care do not interfere with the individual's will [43].

AAL technologies contribute to increased autonomy [11]. In the development and application of these technologies, autonomy is often equated with independence [20]. However, despite their relationship, the principles of autonomy and non-interference are distinct from one another [38]. AAL technologies should be beneficial and appropriate, but they shouldn't compel users to give up their independence. Encouraging individuals to take responsibility for their choices is a big part of ensuring this independence.

To minimize the risks associated with AAL technologies and maximize their benefits, more ethical supervision and control are necessary. In a study addressing ethical issues in the use of AAL technologies, healthcare professionals highlighted concerns about socially assistive robots, such as human-shaped or pet-shaped ones, potentially misleading older adults with dementia into perceiving them as real people or pets [49]. The participants expressed fear that older people with dementia may not exhibit negative behaviors while using these technologies, and stated that this deception goes against professional ethics and is related to human dignity. Involving users in decision-making processes on a regular basis and not disregarding them will also ensure that AAL solutions are seen as empowering, and consequently, an important instrument for fostering users' autonomy and independence [25].

11.5.2 Beneficence

Beneficence is the action of doing good and benefiting others, while also considering the potential positive and negative consequences of an action [28]. The principle of beneficence is the physician's obligation to act for the benefit of the patient. It supports a number of moral rules to protect and defend the rights of others, prevent harm, eliminate harmful situations, and help and save disabled people and those in dangerous situations. By aiding patients and advancing their well-being, the idea also demands preventing harm from occurring [48]. AAL solutions that benefit the individual are practices that prevent harm and maintain or improve their physical, cognitive, emotional, and social well-being [25]. Any application must be made only for the benefit of the individual to whom it belongs, according to the notion of AAL applications' benefits. According to the beneficence principle, healthcare providers have an obligation to continue until they are unable to support the patient's residual physical and mental capacities through any other AAL intervention. Here, the emphasis is on how far a person may advance in terms of their autonomy and dignity [38].

The concepts of beneficence and non-maleficence (see the next section) in the context of AAL necessitate careful consideration of striking a balance between potential hazards or distress and therapeutic, helpful, or psychosocial benefit [26, 31]. It's important to regularly evaluate the preferences and experiences of AAL users to ensure their best interests. As an illness progresses, people's experiences with these technologies may change, and over time, their ability to express their preferences and experiences may also change [25].

11.5.3 Non-maleficence

Non-maleficence means never harming users, including avoiding actions that risk harming others. Non-maleficence upholds a number of moral precepts, including the following: do not murder, inflict agony or suffering, disable, offend, or deprive others of life's blessings [48]. The ethical principle of non-maleficence presents a challenge as harm is not solely physical [38]. The use of AAL applications may have psychological costs, such as feelings of being under surveillance [35], confusion or emotional distress, that are associated with harm because users may feel that their limitations are their own fault. In this context, AAL practices should only be recommended if patients are not compelled to use them and don't experience any harm, including distress, from having their will, judgment, self-confidence, integrity, and preferences disregarded [21, 43].

11.5.4 Justice

Justice encompasses issues of fairness across individual, interpersonal, organizational, and social realms [28]. The concept of justice involves the obligation to treat people equally, respect their rights, and acknowledge diversity and individual differences, including the freedom to make questionable decisions. This means upholding justice in social, organizational, interpersonal, and individual contexts [38]. The concepts of justice adhered to by healthcare systems vary across nations, as do the requirements that arise from distinct social structures and cultural backgrounds in each nation [25].

Many people consider healthcare as a public good and one that should not be solely driven by the market. With the increasing shortage of healthcare workers due to demographic aging, technology is seen as a cost-effective alternative. This situation presents a promising future for the development of advanced technology in the care of older adults, which could lead to a highly competitive and profitable market [42]. The development of assistive technologies implies various levels of savings, not only in production and distribution costs, but also potentially higher costs for long-term management and sustainable operation. Moreover, these economic dimensions also need to be considered in technological care, as part of an economic system that shifts care responsibilities from the state to the individual and the family [17, 27]. Justice issues in this context extend beyond equal treatment and fair resource distribution [6, 10], as the widespread use of AAL solutions could have significant effects on healthcare workers, the labor market, social relations, and the environment.

11.5.5 Fidelity

The definition of fidelity is being obedient, devoted, truthful, and reliable [28]. The fidelity principle encompasses the concepts of fidelity, truthfulness, and genuineness of shared commitments. It emphasizes the importance of users being able to trust technology and have faith in human-machine interactions. It also warns against compromising users' willingness to engage with technology, even if it appears to improve their current psychological and physical well-being [38]. Although hidden AAL technologies may be inherently good, they may violate user trust by not being easily noticeable [31]. Established relationships between AAL technology and users build trust, affecting healthcare services' possible efficacy. More detailed insights about transformed caring relationships and trust can be found in Lutz et al. [30] in this volume. Growing ethical concerns result from elements including hacking incidents,[2] spying, feeling vulnerable, and declining confidence in authorities and professionals [47].

The principles of AAL systems may be easy to understand in theory, but putting them into practice can be challenging. It's important to recognize that these principles can sometimes conflict with each other and may be interpreted differently. The AAL Guidelines for Ethics, Data Privacy, and Security, developed by the AAL Program [14], can be a valuable resource for those involved in designing, developing, and deploying AAL technologies. These guidelines provide a structured approach to navigate ethical dilemmas and aim to help stakeholders make morally informed decisions throughout the technology development lifecycle, based on principles such as beneficence, autonomy, and justice.

11.6 Stakeholder Engagement in AAL Development and Deployment

To enhance the analysis of ethical principles, it is important to consider perspectives from all stakeholders involved in the design, development, deployment, and regulation of AAL technologies. This includes input from end-users, such as older adults and people with impairments and disabilities, as they can provide valuable insights into their preferences, values, and needs. Additionally, caregivers and family members can offer insights into the practical implications of AAL technologies for those they care for, which is instrumental for ensuring the trustworthy adoption of available solutions. Furthermore, developers and technology providers play a key role as they must recognize and address the ethical responsibilities inherent in the design and implementation of AAL technologies under their responsibility. Regulatory bodies

---

[2] Having AAL technology installed may increase the risks for phantom hacker scams. See for instance https://www.fbi.gov/contact-us/field-offices/phoenix/news/press-releases/the-phantom-hacker-fbi-phoenix-warns-public-of-new-financial-scam, Accessed 19 September 2024.

and policymakers, who establish the legal frameworks governing the ethical use of AAL technologies, should be engaged, as they are the main potential protectors of individuals' rights.

Therefore, to strengthen an inclusive approach, it is critical to bring together the quadruple helix of actors. It integrates academia, industry, government, and civil society, fostering collaboration and innovation, while also promoting acceptance and increasing the effectiveness of solutions tailored to the needs of older adults [41].

Traditional models of stakeholder engagement typically involve a three-way relationship among academia, industry, and government. However, these models often neglect the viewpoints and concerns of end-users and the wider civil society. Stemming from the Triple Helix model of university-industry-government collaboration [29], the Quadruple Helix introduces a fourth dimension by including civil society, which represents the interests and values of citizens. The increasing production of AAL technologies in transdisciplinary, economic, and social contexts indicates that society must be considered when developing a Quadruple Helix model [41]. This approach emphasizes the importance of co-creation and participatory decision-making, leveraging the collective knowledge and diverse expertise of stakeholders to foster innovation and societal progress. This model is very useful for the design of AAL technologies, promoting knowledge production and exchange [8].

The Quadruple Helix approach can bring several benefits to the development and deployment of AAL technologies. By integrating the perspectives of end-users and civil society organizations, this approach increases the likelihood that the developed technologies address real-world needs, encompass users' preferences, are culturally sensitive, and are ethically sound. Collaboration among different stakeholders through ongoing discussions can uncover perceptions, challenges, risks, obstacles, and facilitators [33].

Engaging all stakeholders in the co-creation of solutions will enhance acceptance and adoption. When end-users actively participate, rather than being passive recipients, they are more likely to use and embrace the technologies, leading to better outcomes and sustained engagement. Additionally, the Quadruple Helix model encourages cross-sectoral knowledge exchange, facilitating the identification of innovative solutions that improve healthcare access, social inclusion, and economic empowerment, with long-term societal benefits [4].

11.7 Human Dignity as a Guiding Path and Overarching Concept

There is a widely held belief that AAL solutions should complement, but not replace, human-provided care, which is linked to moral obligations, particularly the principles of beneficence and non-maleficence [44, 45]. This belief is based on ethical values, particularly the notion that the human touch and empathy are unavoidable aspects of effective and morally acceptable care. The concept that AAL technologies cannot and should not replace care is linked to moral obligations, particularly the principles of beneficence and non-maleficence [44, 45]. The expansion of scientific knowledge may create conflicts between the need to minimize potential hazards and provide healthcare services [31]. Dealing with these conflicts can be quite challenging. Human dignity should receive great care when designing and implementing AAL technologies. The dignity of individuals should take precedence over any social, care, or research issue [37].

AAL solutions cannot and should not replace care, but their proper implementation can actually encourage and improve human-provided care rather than threaten it [5, 44, 49]. It is believed that successful AAL solutions can alleviate healthcare professionals, particularly nurses, from administrative and physical tasks, enabling them to dedicate more time to providing social and emotional support to patients.

11.8 Conclusions

The analysis provided in this chapter focuses on ethical principles and concepts such as autonomy, privacy, beneficence, justice, and dignity. It also takes into account diverse stakeholder perspectives, including those of end-users, caregivers, developers, and policymakers. By combining ethical principles and stakeholder perspectives, we can assess risks and benefits to systematically evaluate the ethical deployment of specific Active Assisted Living (AAL) technologies. The potential risks of AAL technologies, including privacy, security, and autonomy concerns, need to be carefully identified and assessed. Simultaneously, the expected benefits, such as increased independence, safety, and well-being, should be thoroughly evaluated. Finally, a comprehensive risk-benefit analysis should be conducted to assess the ethical justification of AAL deployment and ensure alignment with key ethical principles.

Acknowledgements This publication is based upon work from COST Action GoodBrother—Network on Privacy-Aware Audio- and Video-Based Applications for Active and Assisted Living (CA19121), supported by COST (European Cooperation in Science and Technology). Anamaria Malešević and Anto Čartolovni were also supported for this work by the Hrvatska zaklada za znanost (Croatian Science Foundation (CSF)) [grant number UIP-2019-04-3212] "(New) Ethical and Social Challenges of Digital Technologies in the Healthcare Domain". The funder had no role in the design of this study and its execution, analyses, interpretation of the data, or decision to submit results.

References

1. Abe, Y., Ito, M., Abumi, K., Kotani, Y., Sudo, H., Minami, A.: A novel cost-effective computer-assisted imaging technology for accurate placement of thoracic pedicle screws: technical note. J. Neurosurg. Spine **15**(5), 479–485 (2011). https://doi.org/10.3171/2011.6.SPINE10721

2. Aclan, R., George, S., Block, H., Lane, R., Laver, K.: Middle aged and older adult's perspectives of their own home environment: a review of qualitative studies and meta-synthesis. BMC Geriatr. **23**(1), 707 (2023). https://doi.org/10.1186/s12877-023-04279-1
3. Ahmad, F.K.: Use of assistive technology in inclusive education: making room for diverse learning needs. Transcience **6**(2), 62–77 (2015). https://www2.hu-berlin.de/transcience/Vol6_No2_62_77.pdf
4. Ahonen, L., Hämäläinen, T.: CLIQ: a practical approach to the quadruple helix and more open innovation. In: MacGregor, S.P., Carleton, T. (eds.) Sustaining Innovation: Collaboration Models for a Complex World, pp. 15–29. Springer (2012). https://doi.org/10.1007/978-1-4614-2077-4_2
5. Al-Shaqi, R., Mourshed, M., Rezgui, Y.: Progress in ambient assisted systems for independent living by the elderly. SpringerPlus **5**(1), 624 (2016). https://doi.org/10.1186/s40064-016-2272-8
6. Austin, V., Holloway, C.: Assistive Technology (AT), for What? Societies **12**(6), 169 (2022). https://doi.org/10.3390/soc12060601
7. Beauregard, L.K., Miller, E.A.: Federal incentives to reform long-term care under the affordable care act: state adoption of the balancing incentive program, 2011–2014. J. Gerontol. Ser. B **77**(1), 191–200 (2022). https://doi.org/10.1093/geronb/gbab031
8. Carayannis, E.G., Rakhmatullin, R.: The quadruple/quintuple innovation helixes and smart specialisation strategies for sustainable and inclusive growth in Europe and beyond. J. Knowl. Econ. **5**(2), 212–239 (2014). https://doi.org/10.1007/s13132-014-0185-8
9. Chen, K.: Why do older people love and hate assistive technology?—an emotional experience perspective. Ergonomics **63**(12), 1463–1474 (2020). https://doi.org/10.1080/00140139.2020.1808714
10. Cook, A.M.: Ethical issues related to the use/non-use of assistive technologies. Dev. Disabil. Bull. **37**(1), 127–152 (2009)
11. Coret Gorgonio, F.J., Bou Pérez, J., Alcantud Marín, F.: Location and orientation technologies based on Wi-Fi systems for people with disabilities in indoor environment. In: Active and Assisted Living: Technologies and Applications, pp. 261–280 (2016)
12. Courtney, K.L., Demiris, G., Hensel, B.K.: Obtrusiveness of information-based assistive technologies as perceived by older adults in residential care facilities: a secondary analysis. Med. Inform. Internet Med. **32**(3), 241–249 (2007). https://doi.org/10.1080/14639230701447735
13. Daniel, K.M., Cason, C.L., Ferrell, S.: Emerging technologies to enhance the safety of older people in their homes. Geriatr. Nurs. **30**(6), 384–389 (2009). https://doi.org/10.1016/j.gerinurse.2009.08.010
14. Dantas, C., Hoonedoorn, P., Kryspin-Exner, I., Stuckelberger, A., Tijink, D.: AAL Guidelines for ethics, data privacy and security. Technical Report. Active and Assisted Living Programme (2022). https://www.aal-europe.eu/aal-guidelines-for-ethics-data-privacy-and-security/
15. Duquenoy, P., Thimbleby, H.W.: Justice and design. In: IFIP TC13 International Conference on Human-Computer Interaction (1999)
16. Fiocco, A.J., Yaffe, K.: Defining successful aging: the importance of including cognitive function over time. Arch. Neurol. **67**(7), 876–880 (2020). https://doi.org/10.1001/archneurol.2010.130
17. Folbre, N.: Nursebots to the rescue? Immigration, automation, and care. Globalizations **3**, 349–360 (2006). https://doi.org/10.1080/14747730600870217
18. Garçon, L., Khasnabis, C., Walker, L., Nakatani, Y., Lapitan, J., Borg, J., Ross, A., Velazquez Berumen, A.: Medical and assistive health technology: meeting the needs of aging populations. Gerontologist S293–S302 (2016). https://doi.org/10.1093/geront/gnw005
19. Gesualdo, F., Daverio, M., Palazzani, L., Dimitriou, D., Diez-Domingo, J., Fons-Martinez, J., Jackson, S., Vignally, P., Rizzo, C., Tozzi, A.E.: Digital tools in the informed consent process: a systematic review. BMC Med. Ethics **22**(1), 18 (2021). https://doi.org/10.1186/s12910-021-00585-8
20. Güldenpfennig, F., Mayer, P., Panek, P., Fitzpatrick, G.: An autonomy-perspective on the design of assistive technology experiences of people with multiple sclerosis. In: Proceedings of the

2019 CHI Conference on Human Factors in Computing Systems, CHI'19, pp. 1–14. Association for Computing Machinery, New York, NY, USA (2019). https://doi.org/10.1145/3290605.3300357
21. Hammel, J.: Technology and the environment: supportive resource or barrier for people with developmental disabilities? Nurs. Clin. North Am. **38**(2), 331–349 (2003). https://doi.org/10.1016/S0029-6465(02)00053-1
22. Health Information Quality and Authority: Guidance on a Human Rights-based Approach in Health and Social Care Services|HIQA. Technical report (2019). https://www.hiqa.ie/reports-and-publications/guide/guidance-human-rights-based-approach-health-and-social-care-services
23. Hofmann, B.: Ethical challenges with welfare technology: a review of the literature. Sci. Eng. Ethics **19**(2), 389–406 (2013). https://doi.org/10.1007/s11948-011-9348-1
24. Ienca, M., Fosch-Villaronga, E.: Privacy and security issues in assistive technologies for dementia: the case of ambient assisted living, wearables, and service robotics. In: Jotterand, F., Ienca, M., Wangmo, T., Elger, B.S. (eds.) Intelligent Assistive Technologies for Dementia: Clinical, Ethical, Social, and Regulatory Implications. Oxford University Press (2019). https://doi.org/10.1093/med/9780190459802.003.0013
25. Ienca, M., Jotterand, F., Vică, C., Elger, B.: Social and assistive robotics in dementia care: ethical recommendations for research and practice. Int. J. Soc. Robot. 565–573 (2016). https://doi.org/10.1007/s12369-016-0366-7
26. Jahn, W.T.: The 4 basic ethical principles that apply to forensic activities are respect for autonomy, beneficence, nonmaleficence, and justice. J. Chiropractic Med. **10**(3), 225–226 (2011). https://doi.org/10.1016/j.jcm.2011.08.004
27. Kenner, A.: Securing the elderly body: dementia, surveillance, and the politics of "aging in place". Surveill. Soc. **5**, 252–269 (2008). https://doi.org/10.24908/ss.v5i3.3423
28. Kitchener, K.S., Anderson, S.K.: Foundations of ethical practice, research, and teaching in psychology and counseling. Routledge (2011). https://doi.org/10.4324/9780203893838
29. Leydesdorff, L., Etzkowitz, H.: The triple helix as a model for innovation studies. Sci. Public Policy **25**(3), 195–203 (1998). https://doi.org/10.1093/spp/25.3.195
30. Lutz, C., Miguel, C., Mujirishvili, T., Perez-Vega, R., Fedosov, A.: Social and societal issues in AAL. In: Salah, A.A., Colonna, L., Florez-Revuelta, F. (eds.) Privacy-Aware Monitoring for Assisted Living. Springer, Cham (2025)
31. Macklin, R.: Bioethics, vulnerability, and protection. Bioethics 472–486 (2003). https://doi.org/10.1111/1467-8519.00362
32. Mamo, N., Martin, G.M., Desira, M., Ellul, B., Ebejer, J.P.: Dwarna: a blockchain solution for dynamic consent in biobanking. Eur. J. Hum. Genet. **28**(5), 609–626 (2020). https://doi.org/10.1038/s41431-019-0560-9
33. Marinelli, E., Perianez Forte, I.: Smart specialisation at work: the entrepreneurial discovery as a continuous process—S3 Working Paper Series No. 12/2017 (2017). https://publications.jrc.ec.europa.eu/repository/handle/JRC108571
34. Mittelstadt, B.: Ethics of the health-related Internet of Things: a narrative review. Ethics Inform. Technol. **19**(3), 157–175. British Lib (2017). https://doi.org/10.1007/s10676-017-9426-4
35. Mortenson, W.B., Sixsmith, A., Beringer, R.: No place like home? Surveillance and what home means in old age. Can. J. Aging/La Revue canadienne du vieillissement **35**(1), 103–114 (2016)
36. Motloba, P.: Understanding of the principle of autonomy (Part 1). SADJ **73**(6), 418–420 (2018)
37. Novitzky, P.: Ethics of ambient assisted living technologies for persons with dementia. Ph.D. thesis, Dublin City University (2016)
38. Panico, F., Cordasco, G., Vogel, C., Trojano, L., Esposito, A.: Ethical issues in assistive ambient living technologies for ageing well. Multimedia Tools Appl. **79**(47), 36077–36089 (2020). https://doi.org/10.1007/s11042-020-09313-7
39. Parette, P., Scherer, M.: Assistive technology use and stigma. Educ. Train. Dev. Disabil. **39**, 217–226 (2004)

40. Participants and organisers of the conference "Science, Innovation and Society: Achieving Responsible Research and Innovation": Rome declaration on responsible research and innovation in Europe. Technical report (2014). https://digital-strategy.ec.europa.eu/en/library/rome-declaration-responsible-research-and-innovation-europe
41. Roman, M., Varga, H., Cvijanovic, V., Reid, A.: Quadruple helix models for sustainable regional innovation: engaging and facilitating civil society participation. Economies **8**(2), 48 (2020). https://doi.org/10.3390/economies8020048
42. Schicktanz, S., Schweda, M.: Aging 4.0? Rethinking the ethical framing of technology-assisted eldercare. Hist. Philos. Life Sci. **43**(3), 93 (2021). https://doi.org/10.1007/s40656-021-00447-x
43. Schülke, A.M., Plischke, H., Kohls, N.B.: Ambient Assistive Technologies (AAT): sociotechnology as a powerful tool for facing the inevitable sociodemographic challenges? Philos., Ethics, Humanit. Med. **5**(1), 8 (2010). https://doi.org/10.1186/1747-5341-5-8
44. Sharkey, A., Sharkey, N.: Granny and the robots: ethical issues in robot care for the elderly. Ethics Inform. Technol. **14**(1), 27–40 (2012). https://doi.org/10.1007/s10676-010-9234-6
45. Sparrow, R.: Robots in aged care: a dystopian future? AI Soc. **31**(4), 445–454 (2016). https://doi.org/10.1007/s00146-015-0625-4
46. Teare, H., Prictor, M., Kaye, J.: Reflections on dynamic consent in biomedical research: the story so far. Eur. J. Hum. Genet. **29**(4), 649–656 (2021). https://doi.org/10.1038/s41431-020-00771-z
47. Trothen, T.J.: Intelligent assistive technology ethics for aging adults: spiritual impacts as a necessary consideration. Religions **13**(5), 452 (2022). https://doi.org/10.3390/rel13050452
48. Varkey, B.: Principles of clinical ethics and their application to practice. Med. Principles Pract. **30**(1), 17–28 (2020). https://doi.org/10.1159/000509119
49. Wangmo, T., Lipps, M., Kressig, R.W., Ienca, M.: Ethical concerns with the use of intelligent assistive technology: findings from a qualitative study with professional stakeholders. BMC Med. Ethics **20**(1), 98 (2019). https://doi.org/10.1186/s12910-019-0437-z
50. World Health Organization and United Nations Children's Fund: Global report on assistive technology. World Health Organization (2022). https://www.who.int/publications/i/item/9789240049451

Open Access This chapter is licensed under the terms of the Creative Commons Attribution 4.0 International License (http://creativecommons.org/licenses/by/4.0/), which permits use, sharing, adaptation, distribution and reproduction in any medium or format, as long as you give appropriate credit to the original author(s) and the source, provide a link to the Creative Commons license and indicate if changes were made.

The images or other third party material in this chapter are included in the chapter's Creative Commons license, unless indicated otherwise in a credit line to the material. If material is not included in the chapter's Creative Commons license and your intended use is not permitted by statutory regulation or exceeds the permitted use, you will need to obtain permission directly from the copyright holder.

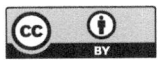

Chapter 12
Smart Mirrors and Data Protection Regulation

Liane Colonna and Gianluigi M. Riva

Abstract Smart mirrors have the potential to significantly enhance the quality of life for older adults by supporting their health, well-being, and social connectivity. However, they also introduce substantial legal and regulatory challenges, particularly in the realm of data protection. This paper aims to examine these challenges and contribute to the interdisciplinary discourse on smart mirrors, facilitating the integration of legal and technological considerations. At the outset, the paper provides an overview of smart mirrors to understand the technological foundation for which the law applies. It then explores various data protection concerns raised by smart mirrors, such as issues related to consent and transparency, security vulnerabilities, and the potential misuse of personal information. Next, the paper presents a taxonomy of key factors that influence how data protection rules apply to smart mirrors, such the physical location of the smart mirror, the context in which it is used (e.g., private home, public facility, healthcare environment), the status of the user (e.g., adult, minor, patient), the status of the service provider (e.g., manufacturer, third-party service), the involvement of any intermediaries in data processing, and the nature and sensitivity of the data being gathered (e.g., biometric data, personal health information). The paper concludes with an examination of the role of data protection by design (DPbD) in this context, highlighting the importance of incorporating regulatory compliance into smart mirrors from the beginning of its development and deployment.

Keywords Smart mirrors · Data protection by design · AI Act · GDPR · Active assisted living (AAL)

L. Colonna (✉)
Stockholm University, Stockholm, Sweden
e-mail: Liane.Colonna@juridicum.su.se

G. M. Riva
Bocconi University, Milan, Italy
e-mail: gianluigi.riva@unibocconi.it

12.1 Introduction

Imagine the situation where a senior citizen living alone decides to install in her private home a smart mirror equipped with features like voice commands and health monitoring to assist her to live at home longer and more independently. Initially, the woman enjoyed the convenience offered by her newly installed smart mirror, and since it was purchased through a well-known company, she also trusted the device. One day, however, the woman began noticing unusual activities. First, she started to suspect the mirror's camera was activated without her consent, although she was not certain because she suffered from memory loss and thought maybe she was just confused. Several days later, the smart mirror started displaying inappropriate and intrusive messages, making her feel uncomfortable and violated in her own home. Later, she was sexually propositioned and physically threatened causing her to become terrified and deeply traumatized. This was made possible by the failure to implement fundamental privacy and security measures, which allowed hackers to gain control over her smart mirror.[1]

This scenario highlights that while smart mirrors, like other technologies and devices, can contribute to improving the overall quality of life for older individuals, supporting their health, well-being, and connectivity with the broader community, they nevertheless present serious legal and regulatory challenges, together with other potential design and interactive issues. This chapter seeks to explore these challenges from the perspective of data protection. The main goal of the chapter is to contribute to the interdisciplinary discourse around smart mirrors, facilitating the deeper integration of law and technology in this context.

First, this chapter will provide an overview of smart mirrors to understand the technological foundation for which the law applies. Second, it will explore various data protection concerns associated with smart mirrors, including issues related to consent and transparency, security vulnerabilities, and the potential misuse of personal information. Next, it will provide a description of the how data protection rules might apply to smart mirrors, offering a taxonomy of key factors to consider. Section 12.6 specifically explores the role of data protection by design (DPbD), emphasizing the critical importance of incorporating regulatory compliance from the outset in the development and deployment of smart mirrors.

---

[1] Press Release, FTC Says Ring Employees Illegally Surveilled Customers, Failed to Stop Hackers from Taking Control of Users' Cameras, FTC Press Release (31 March 2023), https://www.ftc.gov/news-events/news/press-releases/2023/05/ftc-says-ring-employees-illegally-surveilled-customers-failed-stop-hackers-taking-control-users, Accessed 15 July 2024; Federal Trade Commission v. Ring LLC, Complaint for permanent injunction and other relief (31 May 2023), https://www.ftc.gov/system/files/ftc_gov/pdf/complaint_ring.pdf, Accessed 19 September 2024.

12.2 Smart Mirrors

Smart mirrors are sophisticated electronic devices equipped with several advanced features [12, 42]. They are Internet-connected and capable of interoperability with other Internet of Things (IoT) devices, enhancing their functionality and integration into smart ecosystems. Key components of smart mirrors include cameras, microphones, and interactive screens. These components allow for a range of functionalities, from facial recognition to touch or gesture-based interactions. Moreover, smart mirrors can serve as platforms for various applications, providing users with a customizable and interactive experience. The ability to enable vocal interaction adds another layer of convenience and utility, making smart mirrors a versatile tool in modern smart homes and environments.

Smart mirrors can offer numerous benefits for older individuals by incorporating technology into a familiar object found in almost every household. First, they can be used to support health monitoring such as by tracking an individual's vital signs like heart rate, blood pressure and temperature, potentially leading to personalized care [32]. They can also display medication reminders, ensuring that older individuals take their prescribed medications on time [12]. They can support fitness and wellness, by, for example, offering guided workout routines, exercise programs as well as advice about nutrition. Another application of a smart mirror in the active assisted living (AAL) context includes posture correction. Furthermore, smart mirrors with built-in cameras and communication features can enable video calls, allowing older individuals to stay connected with family and friends. This can reduce feelings of isolation and provide social interaction [42]. Integrated with calendars, smart mirrors can provide reminders for doctor's appointments, social events, and other important dates [14]. Smart mirrors equipped with voice recognition technology can assist and guide older individuals in controlling other smart home devices, or searching for information without the need for complex interfaces [14, 28]. Integrated with emergency alert systems, smart mirrors can quickly send notifications or alerts to caregivers or emergency services in case of falls or health emergencies. Finally, emotion recognition can analyze facial expressions to determine the older person's mood and then provide personalized feedback or suggestions based on the detected emotions [53].

Smart mirrors incorporate various technologies to function effectively and to offer the applications described above. The specific features and functionalities of a smart mirror may vary depending on the manufacturer, model, and operating system, but some of the key technologies commonly used include (1) built-in touchscreen displays, allowing users to interact with the mirror's interface (2) cameras and sensors which in many cases enable facial recognition for personalized user experiences (3) microphones and voice recognition (4) Wi-Fi and Bluetooth (5) health monitoring sensors like heart rate monitors and (6) machine learning and other types of AI, allowing the mirror to identify users and personalize their experience [12, 32, 42] (see further [49]). Importantly, technology in the context of smart mirrors is advancing rapidly and as such, there may be potential to integrate Augmented Reality (AR) technology to enable smart mirrors to offer more immersive and interactive experiences [21]. It is also possible that the customization and personalization involved with smart mirrors will increase as well as their integration with other smart home devices [28].

12.3 Smart Mirror Characteristics

Smart mirrors may be likened to smartphones and other smart devices because they incorporate similar technologies and features. However, it is essential to recognize that there are certain peculiarities that characterize smart mirrors as a standalone technology. Unlike smartphones, smart mirrors are typically fixed to a wall and, despite being movable, cannot be classified as mobile or wearable devices. Smart mirrors generally lack sensors such as gyroscopes and accelerometers but may be equipped with passive sensors to detect motion and temperature.

While a smart speaker might also be considered comparable to a smart mirror, they primarily rely on vocal interaction and lack the interactive screens that characterize smart mirrors. It is also worth noting that smart speakers can potentially connect to and control smart mirror interfaces, requiring a shift in the legal focus from the device itself to the type of interaction it facilitates [37], specifically the interactive service provided by, typically, a private entity (i.e. the service provider) via the AI assistant. This shift underscores the importance of addressing the technical and ontological specifics of these technologies in evolving legal frameworks [39].

Another technology that smart mirrors can be compared with concerns security cameras. This is because smart mirrors share with security cameras the capability to capture dynamic images of the environment and the people within it. However, a pivotal difference lies in their intended purpose, which influences their design and placement. Security cameras are designed primarily for security purposes, meant to capture specific types of images in designated locations and conditions, and are subject to particular data protection limitations[2] [44]. Furthermore, security cameras are often deployed in multiple units and are typically movable, whereas the camera embedded in a smart mirror is generally a single, fixed component. Nevertheless, it is conceivable that smart mirrors could be equipped with multiple movable cameras or connected to other cameras positioned around a room.

Mobile devices, such as smartphones and smartwatches, are personal devices that typically rely on a one-to-one interaction and data processing paradigm with the owner. In contrast, smart mirrors are designed to interact with multiple individuals and can potentially capture third parties who are not directly engaged in the interaction, such as minors or guests present in the room.[3] Moreover, smartphones and

---

[2] EDPB Guidelines 3/2019 on processing of personal data through video devices. Version 2.0 Adopted on 29 January 2020.

[3] It must be noted that also security cameras may potentially record third parties within the room where they are installed. However, typically, video-surveillance systems are intended for perimetral

similar mobile devices necessitate direct user interaction, whereas smart mirrors can facilitate indirect interaction through intermediaries, such as doctors delivering treatments via the mirror. Unlike smart speakers, which rely solely on vocal interaction, smart mirrors offer both audio and video interaction.

Smart mirrors can further be compared to smart TVs, laptops, and tablet devices, such as Apple iPad. However, they differ from smart TVs, which involve passive interaction where live programs or videos are shown without direct user interaction, with the user simply selecting content via a remote or vocal interface. Tablets and laptops share similarities with smart mirrors due to their touch-screen interaction (in the case of tablets) and general functionality. Yet, neither laptops nor tablets function as interactive, mirror-like cameras (although they potentially could). Additionally, laptops and tablets are personal, movable devices, unlike the stationary nature of smart mirrors.

The unique features of smart mirrors—multi-user interaction, direct interaction, potential for capturing bystanders, ambient-sensitive, and combined audio-visual interface—highlight their distinctiveness from other smart devices. These characteristics necessitate a nuanced approach to their technical, legal, and ethical considerations, ensuring that the frameworks governing their use address the specificities of these innovative technologies. Nevertheless, it is important to consider that as IoT environments become fully developed, these differences may diminish. Smart mirrors will likely become terminal devices within a large, unified, interconnected user interface, allowing users to govern and interact seamlessly with the intelligent environment and connected smart devices.

12.4 Data Protection Concerns Raised by Smart Mirrors

The deployment of smart mirrors gives rise to a myriad of legal concerns, primarily stemming from the extensive collection, processing, and sharing of various types of data by these interconnected devices [49]. A central challenge associated with IoT devices like smart mirrors revolves around privacy issues [32]. A related legal concern is data security, where the interconnected nature of a smart mirror amplifies the risk of data breaches. The inclusion of AI in these devices adds further complexity to the legal landscape, giving rise to concerns regarding the transparency of certain AI algorithms deployed in smart mirrors and the potential incorporation of bias into these devices. This is evident in the various regulations that apply to these items,

---

and external activities and they are not allowed, for instance, for workers monitoring (which implies domestic workers), or guests surveillance (e.g. in a rented room) ([44], pp. 111 and following).

including the GDPR,[4] the AI Act,[5] and the Cyber Resilience Act,[6] among others. These regulations must be considered in combination when addressing issues arising from interactions with smart mirrors, although the focus of this article is mainly on the GDPR.

More precisely, privacy challenges associated with smart mirror technologies stem from their ability to passively collect extensive personal information, including detailed full-body video, voice recordings, health data, biometric information, user preferences, and behavioral patterns [32, 43, 54]. Due to their specific characteristics, smart mirrors differ from other technologies in their ability to collect extensive audio-video biometric and behavioral patterns, habits, and unique movements. This capability significantly raises the level of privacy concerns associated with their use. Like with other smart technologies, individuals often do not fully understand the extent of data collection by smart mirrors, as it is difficult to convey the surveillance capabilities of these versatile devices in a way that clearly communicates their power [31]. This is particularly true for those users, such as older adults, that typically are less prone to have a basic digital education. This data collection, which may be seen as inherently invasive, can even potentially alter how an individual's identity is perceived externally without their full knowledge and consent [54]. This process can disrupt the individual's ability to construct their own narrative about their personal identity, as the information used to analyze them may be inaccessible or aggregated in ways that do not align with their own self-view. Moreover, service providers or third parties may exploit this data for purposes like targeted marketing or discriminatory practices [54]. For example, insurance companies might use health data collected by smart mirrors to adjust premiums based on perceived health risks, or employers could analyze personal habits to make hiring or promotion decisions.

Allen discusses how IoT technologies like smart mirrors raise serious surveillance concerns due to their invasive and constant monitoring capabilities, which she terms "pernicious surveillance" [2]. She further highlights the issue of "pernicious memory," where these technologies create a persistent and potentially never-ending record of an individual's life. This perpetual data collection can lead to significant privacy infringements, as it captures and stores detailed personal information over time, making it possible to reconstruct and scrutinize a person's activities, behaviors, and preferences long after the events have occurred. However, Allen wrote at a time when these technologies were merely theoretical, and the first smartphone had just

---

[4] Regulation (EU) 2016/679 of the European Parliament and of the Council of 27 April 2016 on the protection of natural persons with regard to the processing of personal data and on the free movement of such data, and repealing directive 95/46/EC (General Data Protection Regulation, 'GDPR') (2016) OJ L 119.

[5] Regulation (EU) 2024/1689 of the European Parliament and of the Council of 13 June 2024 laying down harmonized rules on artificial intelligence and amending Regulations (EC) No 300/2008, (EU) No 167/2013, (EU) No 168/2013, (EU) 2018/858, (EU) 2018/1139 and (EU) 2019/2144 and Directives 2014/90/EU, (EU) 2016/797 and (EU) 2020/1828 (AI Act)(2024) OJ L 1689.

[6] Proposal for a Regulation of the European Parliament and of the Council on horizontal cybersecurity requirements for products with digital elements and amending Regulation (EU) 2019/1020, COM (2022) 454 final (CRA).

been introduced. Therefore, it must be kept in mind how much current IoT technological advancements may surpass Allen's concerns, leading to further and much more invasive intrusions into individuals' privacy [6].

As explained above, smart mirrors may utilize AI algorithms such as for facial recognition [28], raising the potential for unfair treatment based on individual characteristics or group affiliations [13, 25, 29]. At this point, it is well understood that an AI algorithm, trained on historical data, may unintentionally reflect biases present in the training data, potentially enhancing racism, sexism, ableism, and create other injustices (see e.g. [4, 9, 57]). For instance, if the training data is predominantly biased towards a specific demographic group (e.g., young, white, female users), the smart mirror may disproportionately recommend content, or even medical treatments, that align with those characteristics (rather than e.g. older, black, male users). This danger is like those posed by other technologies. However, the specific characteristics of smart mirrors enable them to potentially become the primary terminal device in an IoT environment. Their capacity for direct user interaction, combined with various audio-video interactive features, significantly increases their potential for invasiveness.

Additionally, smart mirrors, if powered by complex AI algorithms, may lack transparency and explainability, making it challenging for users to understand how they work. Under Nicholson Price's definition, "black-box medicine" is "the use of opaque computational models to make decisions related to health care" [34]. While "black-box medicine" offers tremendous opportunities in terms of prognostics, diagnostics, and treatment recommendations, it raises serious legal concerns connected to matters like privacy and accountability [33]. Explainable AI is a developing field that centers around offering methods and approaches for comprehending algorithms that operate as black boxes [1]. However, there remains much work to do, particularly in terms of understanding complex models and how to make difficult tradeoffs between explainability and model performance [41].

While the black-box concept is shared by many smart devices running AI systems, smart mirrors differ significantly from other "black-box" technologies due to their purpose and architecture, which function as a sort of "stargate" where AI tools and results, users (particularly patients), service providers, and intermediaries (such as doctors and practitioners) converge. Intermediaries play a role in interpreting the algorithm's results and applying the correct outcomes for the user. For instance, when a doctor interprets diagnostic results derived from an algorithmic analysis of a patient's behavioral data, they should not simply validate the algorithm's output. Instead, they should compare these results with other empirical medical data to formulate a comprehensive final diagnosis. Therefore, the architecture of smart mirrors should be designed to empower interpreters to understand and adjust the algorithm's results to meet the user's specific needs and characteristics, rather than simply accepting AI outputs. This interpretative process cannot rely solely on profiling, which is based on statistical methods rather than causal ones. Hence, the digital competence of interpreters is a critical element in the design process, particularly within the so-called black box.

Felzmann et al. explain that there is an urgent need for both prospective and retrospective transparency within the context of AI-based technologies like smart mirrors [18]. Prospective transparency informs users at the outset about data processing and how the system generally reaches decisions, serving as an accountability mechanism, while retrospective transparency provides post hoc explanations and rationales for specific decisions, detailing the data processing steps involved.

For smart mirrors, achieving prospective transparency is necessary, for example, to clearly inform bystanders who may also be captured by the sensing technology, ensuring they understand how their data is being collected and used [18]. Moreover, this aligns with the mandatory informative requirements set out by binding legal requirements explained more below. However, informational duties should not devolve into another legalistic list of elements that users agree to without reading. Instead, they should be designed in a user-friendly and comprehensible manner, guiding users step by step—even on demand—regardless of their literacy background or level of digital education. This approach should help users understand the complexity of data collection, including why the system needs specific data for specific processes, how the data is collected, stored, and secured, the duration of data retention and the reasons behind it, who has access to the data and why, and other relevant details. Achieving retrospective transparency is also necessary for auditing purposes, enabling users and regulators to understand and trust the decision-making processes of these systems [17, 18]. Implementing these solutions by design will empower users to exercise their right to access information on demand, in real-time, and without the need for offline intermediaries.[7]

There is a further concern about the role of automated individual decision making where there is no human involvement [7]. Smart mirrors used in AAL may incorporate AI algorithms for health monitoring or diagnostic purposes, and if these algorithms are not sufficiently accurate or reliable, there is a risk of providing incorrect health assessments or diagnoses (see more generally [26]. This issue has implications beyond liability. Here, there are additional concerns about what it means to take users, caregivers, doctors and other relevant stakeholders "out of the loop" where it concerns decisions about health and wellbeing [7].

As mentioned above, professional intermediaries must be empowered to critically assess the output of AI before acting on the results, especially in the healthcare context. An effective human-in-the-loop protocol requires intermediaries to evaluate algorithmic results based on the methods and criteria used, the training database, and the specific correlations considered. Achieving this level of granular transparency requires that AI systems be designed to allow retrospective investigations into the decision-making process, akin to a layered blockchain [38].

While smart mirrors can be used in hospitals, care facilities or in public spaces like gyms, many smart mirrors are designed to be used in the home, traditionally an area designated with a very high level of legal protection [5, 11]. Crabtree and

---

[7] Typically, the request should be sent to the data controller, who then provides a first reply within a reasonable time frame (usually laid out by national regulators), according to Article 15 of the GDPR.

Rodden have discussed the intricate nature of the home as a social space characterized by diverse practices and routines [15, 50]. In their work, they emphasize that situating computing within this context necessitates deep consideration about what is "appropriate." For smart mirrors, this means manufacturers or service providers must carefully design the device's features with the specific environment in mind. For instance, a smart mirror installed in a bathroom can capture more intimate images than one placed in a sitting room, whereas a smart mirror in a sitting room might record more private conversations. Therefore, the type, quality, and quantity of sensitive data that the device can collect must undergo scrutiny. In practice, this involves conducting an in-depth data protection impact assessment (DPIA) to consider these aspects thoroughly and aim to minimize data processing.[8]

Data deletion in the context of smart mirrors presents another challenge, as the intricacies of AI systems and the ways in which data intertwines within them make this a Herculean task. Ginart et al. explain [20], "For many standard ML models, the only way to completely remove an individual's data is to retrain the whole model from scratch on the remaining data, which is often not computationally practical." To address these challenges, sophisticated techniques such as machine unlearning, which can be broadly described as "removing the influences of training data from a trained model" are essential [27].

The topic of machine unlearning falls within the ambit of black box issues already highlighted, particularly considering the rights that data subjects have to control their data. The complexity of the problem increases when a data subject's request pertains to specific types of data or particular personal information. Data controllers must be able to address these requests and design their systems accordingly. Failure to comply with these legitimate requests infringes on data subjects' rights and violates the law.[9] Therefore, IoT devices, and smart mirrors in particular, should be enabled—by design—to allow users to access and selectively delete their data directly on the interactive platform, similar to how a browser allows users to erase their browsing history. These considerations are especially relevant for smart mirrors used for health purposes, because they process highly sensitive information that requires high levels of privacy protection.[10]

The use of smart mirrors with weak security features can lead to a range of concerns, including device hacking, spying, and harassment.[11] Smart mirrors can provide real-time information about what is happening in the home as well as archived

---

[8] According to the combined reading of Article 35 and 25 of the GDPR, and in line with the EDPS Recommendation 01/2019 on the draft list of the European Data Protection Supervisor regarding the processing operations subject to the requirement of a data protection impact assessment (Article 39.4 of Regulation (EU) 2018/1725), European Data Protection Board.

[9] EDPB (2020) EDPB Guidelines 5/2019 on the criteria of the Right to be Forgotten in the search engines cases under the GDPR—Version 2.0 (part 1). European Data Protection Board.

[10] EDPS (2015) EDPS Opinion 1/2015 Mobile Health, Reconciling technological innovation with data protection.

[11] Federal Trade Commission (FTC) v. Ring LLC, Complaint for permanent injunction and other relief (31 May 2023), https://www.ftc.gov/system/files/ftc_gov/pdf/complaint_ring.pdf; see also [24], discussing numerous incidents of video device hacking.

footage which is very attractive information for cybercriminals [24]. Hackers may be able to speak directly through the microphone to the occupants in the home. This could lead to verbal assaults and threats. As explained above, smart mirrors used in the AAL context might also present risks to the physical safety of their users such as when, for example, they lead to an incorrect diagnosis or incorrect administration of medicine [26].

It is important to emphasize the sensitivity of the data collected by smart mirrors and the risks associated with the theft or misuse of this data. When breaches occur in databases holding biometric data, the impact on an individual's life can be extensive [60]. In contrast to passwords or social security numbers that can be changed after a breach, there is almost no recourse for addressing a breach involving biometric data which is "unique and unchangeable" [47]. Stolen facial data, for instance, could be exploited by individuals with malicious intent to impersonate someone, even years after the initial breach [45].

In addition to threats to individuals, there are also threats to the public that can arise when smart mirrors are "poorly designed or operated with indifference to security" [30]. For example, critical infrastructure can become vulnerable to attacks if it is connected through a shared network to a compromised smart mirror [26, 30]. In other words, the proliferation of IoT devices like smart mirrors expands the attack surface of critical infrastructure, representing new entry points for cyber attackers to exploit vulnerabilities and gain unauthorized access.

12.5 Data Protection Regulation and Smart Mirrors

12.5.1 An Overview of the GDPR

An old legal maxim states, "ubi societas, ibi jus"—where there is society, there is law. This Latin maxim can be nowadays updated into something like "where there is personal data, there is the GDPR." This is to state that smart mirrors almost always involve the application of the GDPR as any technological device that processes (collects, stores, accesses, analyses, deletes, and, however, somehow uses) personal data will generally fall within its scope.

Smart mirrors, along with all digital devices, collecting personal data must have a clear and legitimate purpose for processing.[12] Manufacturers should specify the intended uses of the data and obtain a legal ground for each processing activity.[13] Data controllers should design smart mirrors in a way that avoids excessive data collection and does not store data longer than necessary.[14] Moreover, smart mirrors should have mechanisms to delete or anonymize data when it is no longer needed for the specified purpose.[15] If the smart mirror processes special categories of personal

---

[12] GDPR Article 5.
[13] GDPR Article 5, Article 6.
[14] GDPR Article 5.
[15] GDPR Article 5, Article 25.

data (e.g., biometric data for facial recognition), it is necessary to obtain explicit consent from users, unless one of the other exceptions in Article 9 applies.

An important issue arises here concerning minors and individuals who have diminished mental or decision-making capacity, even if temporary (often older adults or disabled). This concern also extends to those who lack appropriate digital education.[16] These factors can hinder an individual's full comprehension of personal data processing concepts (including sensitive data) and the potential consequences of data processing abuses. The validity and effectiveness of such consent are still widely debated, necessitating the evaluation of alternative legal bases for data processing [3]. One approach could be to practically support the patient's consent with relatives' consent. However, this scenario is not explicitly addressed by the GDPR and may not be considered valid under the regulation. This underscores the need for careful consideration and potentially new frameworks to protect these vulnerable populations while complying with legal standards.

On the other hand, manufacturers of smart mirrors are obligated to provide users with transparent information about the processing of their personal data such as details about the types of data collected, the purposes of processing, and the identity of the data controller.[17] Smart mirrors must have robust security measures to prevent unauthorized access, disclosure, alteration, or destruction of data.[18] Importantly, users have the right to access their personal data processed by smart mirrors and if the data is inaccurate or incomplete, individuals can request rectification.[19]

If smart mirrors use algorithms or automated decision-making processes that significantly affect individuals, users have the right to know the logic behind such processes and to contest the decision, at least if certain conditions are met.[20] If personal data is transferred outside the EU/EEA, smart mirror manufacturers must ensure compliance with GDPR provisions related to international data transfers, such as using standard contractual clauses or relying on other appropriate safeguards.[21] Finally, smart mirror manufacturers need to adopt a privacy-by-design approach, integrating data protection measures into the development process which will be discussed more below.[22]

---

[16] EDPS (2018) EDPS Opinion No. 3/2018 on online manipulation and personal data. European Data Protection Supervisor.
[17] GDPR, Article 13.
[18] GDPR, Article 32.
[19] GDPR, Article 15.
[20] GDPR, Article 22.
[21] GDPR, Chapter V.
[22] GDPR, Article 25.

12.5.2 Key Factors in Applying the GDPR to Smart Mirrors

While it is generally expected that the GDPR may apply within the context of smart mirrors, the existing literature has not yet sufficiently explored how smart mirrors differ from other technologies and, what implications this has for the application of the GDPR. This evaluation is necessary to assess whether specific technological differences necessitate the application of distinct data protection rules to identify any regulatory gaps that need addressing.

As explained above, the cameras in smart mirrors differ ontologically from security cameras. Unlike security cameras, which are passive, the video component in smart mirrors is active and designed for interactive use by the user. Moreover, smart mirrors may integrate additional visual elements, such as infrared, heat vision, and augmented reality filters. Nonetheless, the central element that distinguishes smart mirrors from cameras and the other devices is the technological and interactive purpose for which they are designed and adopted, which, in turn, affects the data processing they perform.

Indeed, smart mirrors can be adopted for a variety of purposes, ranging from e-health treatments to fitness, clothing, and cosmetics, among others. These purposes influence the specific interactions with users and the data processing involved, including the types of data processed or potentially accessible. For example, a smart mirror positioned in the user's private sitting room for general health monitoring, as per the introductory case described, involves a different purpose and type of data processing than a smart mirror positioned in a gym for guiding physical exercises. Similarly, a smart mirror installed in a hospital for therapeutic support—whether psychological or physical—has different implications for the data involved and the patients' privacy. Here, it is important to observe that the intended use affects the device's privacy and data protection implications, as much as the actual place in which it is installed. That is, it is the specific combination of the intended use and space that determines the specific data protection regime for smart mirrors, as well as the peculiarities concerning users' privacy.

We observe that the legal status of the user also plays a key role in determining the general legal rules applicable. Indeed, whether the user is a patient, an employee, or a consumer creates an enormous difference in how the law may be applied. Additional granular aspects of the user's legal status include age and mental capabilities. These attributes impact key issues like, as mentioned, the validity of consent and the nature of contractual relationships. For example, minors and individuals with diminished mental capacities require special considerations regarding informed consent and the enforceability of agreements [19]. Similarly, the legal and ethical responsibilities towards older users might differ significantly from those towards younger adults. These aspects should be considered carefully within the preliminary auditing process concerning the data protection impact assessment and the subsequent design implementation process.

To add complexity, whether the service provider is a hospital, a research institute, a professional (e.g. a psychiatrist), or a commercial entity makes a difference in the application of the law. In other words, the status of the data controller—and, overall, of the legal parties involved—play a significant role in determining the type of applicable regime both in terms of privacy, data protection and general legal implications. For example, the legal requirements for a healthcare service provided by a university laboratory for research purposes will require the application of different legal rules from a healthcare service provided by a hospital for caring purposes [59]. The difference, for instance, concerns the type and scope of the informed consent,[23] as well as the regime for the secondary usage of the personal data.[24] Furthermore, if one of these services involves the intermediation of a third party such as a general practitioner then this relationship will imply the application of specific deontological duties of patient-doctor confidentiality [56]. These duties must be reflected in the doctor's responsibility for professional secrecy, as well as in the end-to-end cryptographic design of the communication transmission, data transfer, secure storage, and accessibility (no other individuals than the users and the doctor, or those with a proxy, could log in these data).

As described earlier, it appears that smart mirrors entail specific technological, interactive and data processing peculiarities that differentiate this device/platform from other smart devices. Therefore, the elements that characterize smart mirrors and that could make a difference in defining the specific legal and data protection regime to be applied, can be classified as following: location, use context, user status, service provider status, the existence of intermediaries, and the nature of the data gathering (e.g. biometric). Each will be explained below.

First, location concerns the general environment in which the smart mirror is located. This can be public, publicly accessible (commercial), or private. Public locations include any place open to the wider public, such as public offices, squares, airports, train stations, or hospitals. Currently, this remains a theoretical example, but it is conceivable that in the near future, public spaces will be equipped with interactive smart mirrors for various services. These could include providing tourist information within smart cities or offering check-in support in hospitals [22].

Publicly accessible (commercial) locations include shops, clubs, and private entities open to the public, such as restaurants, or specific public services, like hospitals. Within these environments, further sub-classifications apply based on the specific site where the smart mirror is located. These sub-classifications include open environments, such as hotel halls, gyms, or rooms in restaurants, where everyone who enters is captured without the possibility to avoid it; temporary private environments, such as hotel rooms or shop changing rooms, where people access privately for a specific purpose and for a limited time; and sensitive environments, such as locker rooms in gyms and clubs, or medical or professional rooms, where users enter for the specific purpose of receiving a primary service, such as medical treatment or psychological support. In these cases, smart mirrors provide a secondary service that supports the professional activity, like assisting with physical rehabilitation.

---

[23] That must not be confused with the data protection consent (GDPR Articles 6(1)a and 7).
[24] See Article 89 of the GDPR.

Private locations include homes or other personal spaces. In these environments, smart mirrors provide a service that has been requested or agreed upon by the user. Like publicly accessible environments, private environments may be sub-classified according to the specific location where the smart mirror is placed. Accessible environments, such as kitchens or sitting rooms, may inadvertently capture third parties (e.g., guests or cohabitants), while more confidential environments, such as bathrooms, bedrooms, or walk-in closets, are where users typically perform intimate and particularly sensitive activities. Depending on the situation, these environments may also be subject to third-party passages.

Due to these characteristics, private environments present a two-fold legal and data protection relationship. The primary relationship exists between the user and the service provider. Additionally, a further relationship may involve intermediaries within the service offered via the smart mirror (e.g., live or remote professional support for psychological therapies). Any third-party (e.g. supporting psychiatrics, cloud service, professional trainer) that performs data gathering on behalf or in account of the data controller represents either a contractual relationship between the data controller and the third party (data processor), and a secondary relationship between the user and the third party concerning the duty of transparency and potential direct civil liability ([44], p. 119, 20).

Second, the use context refers to the specific objective for which the device is placed and utilized, which affects the data processing purposes. This encompasses the particular function the smart mirror is intended to serve, whether for personal use, commercial applications, or public services. Use context directly affects the data protection and legal regime, despite the location, although the latter may constitute a relevant legal criterion. For instance, smart mirrors for medical support should follow the same legal regime (medical devices) regardless of whether they are in a private environment or in a publicly accessible one [35]. On the other hand, smart mirrors designed for a specific purpose or providing a specific service (e.g. cosmetic filters, food advice) may differ as per the legal regime they involve depending on the location (private home or shop), and the service itself (authorizations, duty of disclosure, hygienic-sanitary standards and duties, etc.).

Third, user status concerns the individual interacting with the smart mirror. They may hold different legal statuses, depending on the situation. For instance, the individual may be both a user, data subject, and potentially also a patient. The individual may also be the owner of the device, a minor, or a person with diminished mental conditions. In other cases, the individual may be a consumer, a third party, a professional or even an employee. These legal statuses may overlap in a complex scenario, depending on the situation, the location, and purpose of the smart mirror.

Fourth, service provider status involves determining whether the entity is the manufacturer, the data controller, or a combination of these roles. The service provider may operate as a private entity, a public entity or under a public-private partnership to supply public services. Each of these scenarios brings distinct legal and ethical considerations, depending on the specific situation. For instance, a research lab providing the service to selected patients in the context of a blind psychological experiment (where subjects do not know precisely the purposes of their involvement and of the data processing), may undergo different regimes[25] than a research lab providing the service for testing an e-health service for research purposes only.[26]

Intermediaries are entities or individuals that participate in the provision of the service. This category may be divided into first, direct intermediaries such as a doctor, a professional, a researcher or a practitioner that interacts with the platform or the providing services, in real-time or ex-post, physically or remotely, to assist, support, guide, or else help the user in using the service. Second, indirect intermediaries: those subjects, such as cloud service providers, cybersecurity service providers, technical or administrative maintenance professionals, that may interact with the service or access somehow the user's personal data. Third, auxiliaries: those individuals, such as nursing and cleaning staff, assistants, technicians, and so on, that may assist, directly or indirectly, the intermediaries. From a data protection perspective, the intermediaries can be assumed to be data processors, although they may be considered data joint-controllers whereas they jointly define the purposes of the data processing.[27]

Finally, specific data gathering considerations depend on the nature, location, and purpose of the smart mirrors. The data processing involved may encompass a wide range of personal information, which can be categorized into various types, such as health data, psychological data, facial recognition information, biometric data, metadata, IoT data (metadata and non-personal data), and third-party data. Each category carries its own set of privacy and security implications—or combination with other specific regulation, as per biometric data with the AI Act, and non personal data, with the Data Act—, requiring careful handling to ensure compliance with relevant regulations and to protect user privacy.

12.6 The Role of "Data Protection by Design" in the Smart-Mirror Context

Data Protection by Design (DPbD) refers to an approach that integrates legal and regulatory considerations into the design and development process of products or systems, such as smart mirrors, from the outset [11, 48]. By adopting a DPbD approach, data controllers ensure that smart mirrors comply with legal and regulatory requirements, mitigate risks, protect user rights, and promote the responsible and ethical use of technology [48]. This proactive, future-oriented legal strategy aims not to halt

---

[25] Also depending on the national regulation and the internal ethical policy on human involvement in experiments.

[26] E.g. the exceptions provided by Article 89 of the GDPR.

[27] Article 29 Data Protection Working Party (2017) WP29 Guidelines on consent under Regulation 2016/679 as last Revised and Adopted on 10 April 2018. EU; Guidelines 07/2020 on the concepts of controller and processor in the GDPR: Version 1.0, at 18, EURO. DATA PROTECTION BD. (Sept. 2, 2020); See also [51], at 271, 277 ("If the parties do not pursue the same objectives ("purpose"), or do not rely upon the same means for achieving their respective objectives, their relationship is likely to be one of 'separate controllers' rather than 'joint controllers'.").

data processing but to enhance and shape it in socially desirable ways [40]. DPbD has its roots in the concepts of Privacy Enhancing Technologies (PETs) and Privacy by Design (PbD).[28] PETs encompass a range of technology-driven solutions aimed at bolstering the protection of personal data within information and communication technologies (ICT), with encryption being a classic example.[29] While PETs focus solely on technological measures (and have been recently criticized [10]), DPbD extends to include organizational practices designed to meet legal requirements, such as conducting DPIAs.

The introduction of the GDPR transformed PbD from a theoretical framework into a binding legal mandate known as Data Protection by Design (DPbD), as explicitly stipulated in Article 25 (see more generally [23]). This provision mandates that systems be designed from the outset to adhere to data protection principles, thereby minimizing data collection and mitigating potential privacy risks. Article 25 can be considered the "backbone" of the GDPR since a breach of any GDPR provision, such as one of the core principles in Article 5, can simultaneously constitute a violation of Article 25, thereby incurring significant penalties [46].

On the one hand, DPbD is reflected in a binding, black-letter law (the GDPR) that carries the threat of sanctions. Yet, the EU allows the regulated entities to meet the legal requirements through introducing various architectural components that either constrain or guide human behavior [16]. Here, it is important to recognize the growing importance of co-regulation in this context, as regulatory bodies and industry stakeholders collaboratively establish and enforce standards to ensure compliance and protect user privacy.[30] Arguably, a more advanced form of regulation is emerging within the realm of cutting-edge technologies like smart mirrors. This regulatory approach balances the need for legal stability with the necessity to adapt, evolve, and respond swiftly to an increasingly digital environment [55]. This dynamic form of regulation ensures that legal frameworks remain robust yet flexible, capable of addressing the rapid advancements and challenges posed by modern technological innovations [55].

From a practical perspective, DPbD strategies may include risk management, implementing strong data encryption and anonymization methods to safeguard sensitive information, establishing clear protocols for data access, storage, and sharing,

---

[28] EU Agency for Cybersecurity, Privacy by Design, https://www.enisa.europa.eu/publications/privacy-and-data-protection-by-design, Accessed 15 July 2024; [58].

[29] See [52]; Commission of the European Communities. Communication from the Commission to the European Parliament and the Council on Promoting Data Protection by Privacy Enhancing Technologies (PETs). COM 2007 228 Final 2007. Available online: https://eurlex.europa.eu/legal-content/EN/LSU/?uri=CELEX%3A52007DC0228.

[30] See [8] explaining, "Coregulation refers to a degree of legislative underpinning of codes or standards, e.g. legislative delegation of power to industry to regulate and enforce codes, expecting or requiring industry to have a code but having back-stop legislative power to impose one, prescribing industry codes as voluntary or mandatory in legislation, legislation setting minimum standards which industry can improve upon, or enforcing undertakings to comply with a code.".

and ensuring transparent communication about data collection practices.[31] Obtaining explicit and genuinely informed user consent—ensuring that the information provided is fully understandable—is also essential. Additionally, selecting the most appropriate and protective legal basis for the user, and maintaining transparency throughout the process, are important for building trust and in ensuring that users are fully aware of how their data will be used [18].

New methodological approaches to addressing the specific challenges of visual privacy within the context of AAL are ongoing [31, 36, 58]. For example, Siddharth Ravi et al. have conducted a comprehensive review of the state of the art in visual privacy protection techniques, specifically tailored for AAL [36]. Their work introduces a novel taxonomy for classifying these methods, providing a structured framework to better understand and address the diverse privacy concerns inherent in video-based monitoring systems used in AAL environments. This taxonomy not only categorizes existing techniques but also highlights areas for further research and development, paving the way for more robust and effective privacy protection strategies [36].

Ultimately, it is recommended that smart mirror developers and service providers consider the full range of issues mentioned above to assess potential threats, legal, ethical, and practical implications, as well as users' needs and vulnerabilities. This assessment should consider the intended purpose, location, type of user, and intermediaries involved. Additionally, given the unique features of smart mirrors, including AI systems, IoT interconnections, and various stakeholders interacting with users, any DPIA should also include a Fundamental Human Rights Impact Assessment (FHRIA) and a preliminary ethics audit. These assessments should evaluate the potential short- and long-term effects on specific user categories, such as patients, older adults, and disabled individuals.

12.7 Conclusion

Smart mirrors offer numerous benefits in the context of active assisted living, such as providing personalized reminders, health monitoring, real-time alerts, and facilitating social connectivity to enhance safety, independence, and engagement. While these devices offer substantial benefits, they also introduce a plethora of legal and regulatory challenges that necessitate careful examination. This chapter has explored these challenges with a particular focus on data protection, providing an overview of data protection concerns surrounding smart mirrors as well as the relevant legal framework, and highlighting the peculiarities that smart mirrors involve.

To understand how laws like the GDPR apply to smart mirrors, it is essential to classify the key elements that define these devices. These elements include the physical location of the smart mirror, the context in which it is used (e.g., private home, public facility, healthcare environment), the status of the user (e.g., adult, minor, patient), the status of the service provider (e.g., manufacturer, third-party service),

---

[31] GDPR, Recital 78; see also [48, 58].

the involvement of any intermediaries in data processing, and the nature and sensitivity of the data being gathered (e.g., biometric data, personal health information). Each of these factors plays an important role in determining the applicable legal requirements and ensuring compliance with privacy and data protection regulations.

It is also critically important to integrate legal considerations into the design and development of these technologies to ensure compliance with privacy and data protection laws from the outset. Key steps include conducting thorough data protection impact assessments to identify potential risks to users' privacy, implementing robust data encryption and anonymization techniques to protect sensitive information, and establishing clear protocols for data access, storage, and sharing. Additionally, obtaining explicit user consent and providing transparent information about data collection practices are essential to build trust and ensure users are fully informed about how their data will be used. By proactively addressing these legal considerations, developers can create smart mirrors that not only offer innovative features but also safeguard users' privacy and comply with regulations such as the GDPR and the continuously evolving EU acquis.[32]

Acknowledgments and Drafting Notes Liane Colonna's contribution to this work was partially supported by the Wallenberg AI, Autonomous Systems v—Humanities and Society (WASP-HS) funded by the Marianne and Marcus Wallenberg Foundation and the Marcus and Amalia Wallenberg Foundation. Liane Colonna took care of the "Introduction" and "Conclusion", the sections "Smart Mirrors" and "The role of 'data protection by design' in the smart-mirror context", and overall edited the chapter. Gianluigi M. Riva took care of the sections "Data protection regulation and smart mirrors" and "Key factors in applying the GDPR to smart mirrors". Both authors equally contributed to the sections "Smart mirrors", "Smart mirrors characteristics", and "Data protection concerns raised by smart mirrors".

References

1. Ali, S., Abuhmed, T., El-Sappagh, S., Muhammad, K., Alonso-Moral, J.M., Confalonieri, R., Guidotti, R., Del Ser, J., Díaz-Rodríguez, N., Herrera, F.: Explainable artificial intelligence (XAI): what we know and what is left to attain trustworthy artificial intelligence. Inform. Fusion **99**, 101,805 (2023)
2. Allen, A.L.: Dredging up the past: lifelogging, memory, and surveillance. Univ. Chicago Law Rev. **75**, 47 (2008)
3. Ambrosini, D.L., Hirsch, C.H., Hategan, A.: Ethics, mental health law, and aging. In: Geriatric Psychiatry: A Case-Based Textbook, pp. 233–251. Springer (2024)
4. Aronson, J.D.: Computer vision and machine learning for human rights video analysis: case studies, possibilities, concerns, and limitations. Law Soc. Inq. **43**(4), 1188–1209 (2018)
5. Balos, B.: A man's home is his castle: how the law shelters domestic violence and sexual harassment. Saint Louis Univ. Public Law Rev. **23**, 77 (2004)
6. Bianco, S., Celona, L., Ciocca, G., Marelli, D., Napoletano, P., Yu, S., Schettini, R.: A smart mirror for emotion monitoring in home environments. Sensors **21**(22), 7453 (2021)

---

[32] The European Union (EU) acquis is the collection of common rights and obligations that constitute the body of EU law, and is incorporated into the legal systems of EU Member States.

7. Binns, R.: Human judgment in algorithmic loops: individual justice and automated decision-making. Regul. Gov. **16**(1), 197–211 (2022)
8. Black, J.: Decentring regulation: understanding the role of regulation and self-regulation in a 'post-regulatory' world. Curr. Leg. Probl. **54**(1), 103–146 (2001)
9. Buolamwini, J., Gebru, T.: Gender shades: intersectional accuracy disparities in commercial gender classification. In: Conference on Fairness, Accountability and Transparency, pp. 77–91. PMLR (2018)
10. Calvi, A., Malgieri, G., Kotzinos, D.: The unfair side of privacy enhancing technologies: addressing the trade-offs between pets and fairness. In: ACM Conference on Fairness, Accountability, and Transparency, pp. 2047–2059 (2024)
11. Cavoukian, A., Mihailidis, A., Boger, J.: Sensors and in-home collection of health data: A privacy by design approach. Technical report, Information and Privacy Commissioner (2010)
12. Chaparro, J.D., Ruiz, J.F.B., Romero, M.J.S., Peño, C.B., Irurtia, L.U., Perea, M.G., Garcia, X.d.T., Molina, F.J.V., Grigoleit, S., Lopez, J.C.: The shapes smart mirror approach for independent living, healthy and active ageing. Sensors **21**(23), 7938 (2021)
13. Cofone, I.N.: Algorithmic discrimination is an information problem. Hastings Law J. **70**, 1389 (2018)
14. Colantonio, S., Coppini, G., Germanese, D., Giorgi, D., Magrini, M., Marraccini, P., Martinelli, M., Morales, M.A., Pascali, M.A., Raccichini, G., et al.: A smart mirror to promote a healthy lifestyle. Biosys. Eng. **138**, 33–43 (2015)
15. Crabtree, A., Rodden, T.: Domestic routines and design for the home. Comput. Support. Coop. Work **13**(2), 191–220 (2004)
16. Diver, L.: Digisprudence: the affordance of legitimacy in code-as-law. Ph.D. thesis, Doctoral thesis, University of Edinburgh (2019)
17. Felzmann, H., Fosch-Villaronga, E., Lutz, C., Tamò-Larrieux, A.: Towards transparency by design for artificial intelligence. Sci. Eng. Ethics **26**(6), 3333–3361 (2020)
18. Felzmann, H., Villaronga, E.F., Lutz, C., Tamò-Larrieux, A.: Transparency you can trust: transparency requirements for artificial intelligence between legal norms and contextual concerns. Big Data Soc. **6**(1), 2053951719860,542 (2019)
19. Gatt, L., Montanari, R., Caggiano, I.A.: Consent to the processing of personal data: a legal and behavioural analysis insights into the effectiveness of data protection law. Eur. J. Privacy L. Tech. 1 (2018)
20. Ginart, A., Guan, M., Valiant, G., Zou, J.Y.: Making AI forget you: data deletion in machine learning. Adv. Neural Inf. Process. Syst. **32** (2019)
21. Heim, H.: Smart mirrors: augmented, but not yet reality. In: Digital Fashion Innovations, pp. 125–143. CRC Press (2023)
22. Hussain, F.: Internet of everything. In: Hussain, F. (ed.) Internet of Things: Building Blocks and Business Models, pp. 1–11. Springer International Publishing, Cham (2017)
23. Jasmontaite, L., Kamara, I., Zanfir-Fortuna, G., Leucci, S.: Data protection by design and by default: framing guiding principles into legal obligations in the GDPR. Eur. Data Prot. L. Rev. **4**, 168 (2018)
24. Johnson, G.: Consumer in a coalmine: Lax security of IoT video devices puts corporations before users. Arizona Law J. Emerg. Technol. **5**, 1 (2021)
25. Käde, L., von Maltzan, S.: Towards a demystification of the black box-explainable AI and legal ramifications. J. Internet Law **23**, 1–27 (2019)
26. Kirtley, J.E., Memmel, S.: Rewriting the "book of the machine": regulatory and liability issues for the internet of things. Minn. J. Law Sci. Technol. **19**, 455 (2018)
27. Liu, K.Z.: Machine Unlearning in 2024 (2024, May). Ken Ziyu Liu—Stanford Computer Science. https://ai.stanford.edu/~kzliu/blog/unlearning. Accessed 15 July 2024
28. Lu, B.Y., Liu, J., Wang, Z., Li, H., He, J., Wen, X., Chen, P., Chen, J., Lai, W., Huang, C.: Smart mirror activated by user's face recognition with simulation of artificial intelligence classifier. In: 25th International Conference on Advanced Communication Technology (ICACT), pp. 23–27. IEEE (2023)

29. Manheim, K., Kaplan, L.: Artificial intelligence: risks to privacy and democracy. Yale J. Law Technol. **21**, 106 (2019)
30. Metzger, R.S.: Security and the internet of things: the role of the federal government to reconcile opportunity and risk. Scitech Lawyer **14**(3), 4–13 (2018)
31. Mihaildis, A., Colonna, L.: A methodological approach to privacy by design within the context of lifelogging technologies. Rutgers Comput. Tech. LJ **46**, 1 (2020)
32. Miotto, R., Danieletto, M., Scelza, J.R., Kidd, B.A., Dudley, J.T.: Reflecting health: smart mirrors for personalized medicine. NPJ Digit. Med. **1**(1), 62 (2018)
33. Price, I., Nicholson, W.: Artificial intelligence in health care: applications and legal issues. Scitech Lawyer; Chicago **14**(1), 10–13 (2017)
34. Price, W., Nicholson, I.: Regulating black-box medicine. Mich. Law Rev. **116**, 421 (2017)
35. Qazvini, A., Ramazani, J.: The nature and effects of the additional conditions. Relig. Res. **17**(3), 997–1024 (2021)
36. Ravi, S., Climent-Pérez, P., Florez-Revuelta, F.: A review on visual privacy preservation techniques for active and assisted living. Multimed. Tools Appl. **83**(5), 14715–14755 (2024)
37. Riva, G.M.: Fantastic interfaces and where to regulate them: three provocative privacy reflections on truth, deception and what lies between. In: Digital Transformation of Collaboration: Proceedings of the 9th International COINs Conference, pp. 217–230. Springer (2020)
38. Riva, G.M.: What happens in blockchain stays in blockchain. A legal solution to conflicts between digital ledgers and privacy rights. Front. Blockchain **3**, 36 (2020). https://doi.org/10.3389/fbloc.2020.00036
39. Riva, G.M., Barry, M.: The lord of the (speaking) rings: an interdisciplinary fellowship to deal with 7 legal issues. In: Proceedings of the 2nd Conference on Conversational User Interfaces, pp. 1–3 (2020)
40. Rommetveit, K., Van Dijk, N.: Privacy engineering and the techno-regulatory imaginary. Soc. Stud. Sci. **52**(6), 853–877 (2022)
41. Rotenberg, M.: Artificial intelligence and the right to algorithmic transparency. In: The Cambridge Handbook of Information Technology, Life Sciences and Human Rights (Cambridge Law Handbooks), pp. 153–165 (2022)
42. Santofimia, M.J., Villanueva, F.J., Dorado, J., Rubio, A., Fernández-Bermejo, J., Llumiguano, H., del Toro, X., Wiratunga, N., Lopez, J.C.: Miratar: A virtual caregiver for active and healthy ageing. In: International Conference on Image Analysis and Processing, pp. 49–58. Springer (2022)
43. Sayegh, M.: Mirror, Mirror On The Wall. Forbes (2021, 23 March). https://www.forbes.com/sites/emilsayegh/2021/03/23/mirror-mirror-on-the-wall/. Accessed 15 July 2024
44. Soffientini, M.: Gli adempimenti privacy per i sistemi di videosorveglianza. Giuffrè Francis Lefebvre, Milano (2023)
45. Solove, D.J., Citron, D.K.: Risk and anxiety: a theory of data-breach harms. Texas Law Rev. **96**, 737 (2017)
46. Stalla-Bourdillon, S., Rossi, A., Zanfir-Fortuna, G.: Data protection by process: how to operationalize data protection by design for machine learning. In: V1.0. Immuta & Future of Privacy Forum White Paper (2019)
47. Stewart, L.: Big data discrimination: maintaining protection of individual privacy without disincentivizing businesses' use of biometric data to enhance security. Boston Coll. Law Rev. **60**, 349 (2019)
48. Tamò-Larrieux, A.: Designing for Privacy and Its Legal Framework. Springer (2018)
49. Tschider, C.A.: Regulating the internet of things: discrimination, privacy, and cybersecurity in the artificial intelligence age. Denver Law Rev. **87**, 92–97 (2018)
50. Urquhart, L., Rodden, T.: New directions in information technology law: learning from human-computer interaction. Int. Rev. Law Comput. Technol. **31**(2), 150–169 (2017)
51. Van Alsenoy, B.: Liability under EU data protection law: from directive 95/46 to the general data protection regulation. J. Intell. Prop. Info. Tech. Elec. Com. L. **7**, 271 (2016)
52. Van Blarkom, G., Borking, J.J., Olk, J.E.: Handbook of privacy and privacy-enhancing technologies. Privacy Incorporated Software Agent (PISA) Consortium, The Hague **198**, 14 (2003)

53. Von Hollen, S., Reeh, B.: Smart mirror devices: for smart home and business. In: Innovations for Community Services: 18th International Conference, I4CS 2018, Žilina, Slovakia, June 18–20, 2018, Proceedings, pp. 194–204. Springer (2018)
54. Wachter, S.: Normative challenges of identification in the internet of things: privacy, profiling, discrimination, and the GDPR. Comput. Law Secur. Rev. **34**(3), 436–449 (2018)
55. Wahlgren, P.: From Lex Scripta to law 4.0. Scand. Stud. Law **65: 50 years of Law and IT**, 159–174 (2018)
56. Warren, C., Laslett, B.: Privacy and secrecy: a conceptual comparison. J. Soc. Issues **33**(3), 43–51 (1977)
57. West, S.M., Whittaker, M., Crawford, K.: Discriminating systems. AI Now pp. 1–33 (2019)
58. Wiese Schartum, D.: Making privacy by design operative. Int. J. Law Inf. Technol. **24**(2), 151–175 (2016)
59. Wiewiorówski, W.: A preliminary opinion on data protection and scientific research. European Data Protection Supervisor: Brussels, Belgium (2020)
60. Wright, E.: The future of facial recognition is not fully known: developing privacy and security regulatory mechanisms for facial recognition in the retail sector. Fordham Intell. Prop. Med. Entertain. Law J. **29**, 611 (2018)

Open Access This chapter is licensed under the terms of the Creative Commons Attribution 4.0 International License (http://creativecommons.org/licenses/by/4.0/), which permits use, sharing, adaptation, distribution and reproduction in any medium or format, as long as you give appropriate credit to the original author(s) and the source, provide a link to the Creative Commons license and indicate if changes were made.

The images or other third party material in this chapter are included in the chapter's Creative Commons license, unless indicated otherwise in a credit line to the material. If material is not included in the chapter's Creative Commons license and your intended use is not permitted by statutory regulation or exceeds the permitted use, you will need to obtain permission directly from the copyright holder.

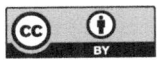

Chapter 13
Social and Societal Issues in AAL

Christoph Lutz, Cristina Miguel, Tamara Mujirishvili, Rodrigo Perez-Vega, and Anton Fedosov

Abstract Active Assisted Living (AAL) systems use advanced technology to help older, impaired, or frail people live independently and stay active in society. These systems rely on automated data monitoring in home or care environments, processing video, image, audio, environmental, and motion data through artificial intelligence (AI), particularly machine learning. Thus, AAL systems offer considerable opportunities for efficient health monitoring, increased autonomy, and enhanced quality of life for older adults. However, AAL technologies also present ethical, legal, and social challenges, particularly around privacy due to the sensitive nature of the data collected and the vulnerability of the populations served. Beyond privacy, the broader social implications of AAL must be considered, including the potential reshaping of care relationships and work within the sector. This chapter provides an in-depth overview of the social and societal issues surrounding AAL, offering a comprehensive literature review that highlights the challenges in implementing these systems in everyday life. Specifically, the chapter discusses cultural differences, biases, the normalization of surveillance, the reshaping of care work and relationships, and matters of trust and adoption, alongside the opportunities AAL technology offers for prolonged independent living.

C. Lutz (✉)
BI Norwegian Business School, Department of Communication and Culture, Oslo, Norway
e-mail: christoph.lutz@bi.no

C. Miguel · R. Perez-Vega
University of Reading, Henley Business School, Reading, UK
e-mail: r.perezvega@henley.ac.uk

T. Mujirishvili
Department of Computer Technology, University of Alicante, Alicante, Spain
e-mail: tamar@gcloud.ua.es

A. Fedosov
Institute for Interactive Technologies, University of Applied Sciences and Arts Northwestern Switzerland, Windisch, Switzerland
e-mail: anton.fedosov@fhnw.ch

Keywords Active assisted living (AAL) · Society · Trust · Bias · Dataveillance · Cultural adaptation · Care work · Digital inequality

13.1 Introduction

Active Assisted Living (AAL) systems have emerged as a response to the aging populations in many countries and the corresponding increase in demand for long-term care [3]. These systems leverage sophisticated technology such as machine vision and natural language processing (NLP) to create environments that support older adults, individuals with disabilities, and those with chronic illnesses in maintaining their independence and quality of life. One example of AAL technology is the use of smart home sensors to monitor the daily activities and health status of older adults. For instance, the final evaluation report of the European Active and Assisted Living Research and Development Programme (AAL2) highlighted how integrated AAL systems "actively contributed to developing a positive perspective on ageing instead of considering ageing as a social and economic problem" [35, p. 41]. However, this deployment also brings to light significant potential for social issues, for example privacy infringements and caregivers' need for new skills to manage and interpret the data generated by these systems.

The rise of AAL technologies represents both a technological innovation and a societal challenge. While these systems promise enhanced autonomy and health monitoring for older adults, they also raise ethical, legal and social concerns (see [19, 29] in this volume). For instance, the pervasive data collection inherent in AAL systems can lead to a sense of constant surveillance among users, potentially impacting their sense of privacy and autonomy. Furthermore, the introduction of AAL technologies into caregiving environments can alter traditional care relationships, leading to shifts in roles and responsibilities among caregivers, patients, and their families. Addressing these issues requires a multidisciplinary approach that considers not only the technological aspects of AAL but also the broader social, cultural, and ethical implications.

The goal of this chapter is to provide a non-exhaustive overview of key social and societal issues in AAL technologies. We developed this overview of issues based on our involvement in the GoodBrother COST Action,[1] our own research on this and adjacent topics such as social robots [40, 64], smart speakers [63], and other AI systems and emerging technologies as well as constructive conversations in the author team, with the editors and with the authors of the chapters on legal issues and ethical issues in this volume. Our objective is to highlight the multifaceted nature of these issues, drawing attention to the complex interplay between technology, society, and individual users. We aim to foster a deeper understanding of how AAL systems impact various stakeholders and to promote informed discussions on how to address these challenges effectively.

---

[1] https://goodbrother.eu/, last accessed 02.09.24.

The chapter is structured into five sections, each describing a relevant social or societal issue, in addition to the Introduction and Conclusion. In the first section, we will review aspects of cultural adaptation and cross-cultural differences in readiness and openness towards AAL systems. While some cultures tend to be more ready to embrace AAL, others are more reluctant. We elaborate on how and why such cultural differences occur. In the second section, we will spotlight the important issue of bias, discussing how AAL technologies can have biases embedded that disadvantage certain population groups such as ethnic or gender minorities. In the third section, we address the issue of dataveillance, power asymmetries between different stakeholders in the AAL eco-system, and associated concerns about the normalization of surveillance. In the fourth section, a perspective on the roles of those involved in care services is taken, as their practices, responsibilities and expectations might be shifting due to AAL technologies. Thus, we reflect on changing roles, including de-skilling or re-skilling. In the fifth section, we look at trust in AAL systems and barriers to adoption. Finally, the conclusion provides a quick summary and sets forth an outlook for future research interested in the social and societal issues in AAL technologies.

13.2 Cultural Adaptation and Differences

The way technologies are perceived and adopted can vary based on several factors. Although a significant amount of research has focused on elements directly related to the use of the technology, such as how useful and easy to use the technology can be [7, 45] there is also strong evidence that these perceptions can also be determined by different cultural values [99]. For instance, one of the largest studies that examined how new technologies like self-driving cars elicit attitudinal and moral questions of users around the world [6] found that geographical and cultural proximity can lead to large groups of territories to converge on shared preferences and attitudes towards this technology. There is increasing evidence that AAL technologies are also influenced by cultural norms, values, and beliefs, affecting their perception and adoption. For instance, research has shown that the acceptance of AAL technologies is influenced by factors such as perceived motives, barriers (e.g. invasion of privacy, concerns about personal data, attitudes towards the replacement of human care), benefits (e.g. reducing dependency on others, increased autonomy, enabling fast reactions of emergency services), individual care preferences, and the properties of the technology itself [100, 102]. However, other studies have also highlighted the importance of cultural differences when designing and implementing assistive technologies. For instance, a study comparing German and Turkish participants found that cultural influences significantly affect the acceptance of video-based assistive technology in private environments, with Turkish users having more positive perceptions of the benefits that these technologies bring [100]. Similarly, research on older adults in continuing care retirement communities emphasized the need to understand cultural perspectives to enhance the quality of life and safety through smart home technologies [30]. In a similar vein, the work of Chung et al. highlights that even where cultural similarities exist within diasporas, the views on the roles that different stakeholders have towards enabling older users to use these technologies change between apparent similar groups, as it would be the case of Korean and Korean American older adults [25].

The acceptance of assistive technologies can vary widely across different cultures. For example, a study on the acceptance of a socially assistive robot by older adults showed positive attitudes towards the technology among a group of older adults [61]. Attitudes towards the use of AAL technologies might not only be determined by cultural values, but also by drivers that affect specific populations. For instance, [73] found in their feasibility study of older adults in Puerto Rico that the use of these technologies would be particularly embraced by the population due to the prevalence of disabilities among this population for independent living. Furthermore, the cultural context can impact the design and implementation of assistive technologies. A framework has been proposed to outline how culture influences perceptions and expectations of individuals with disabilities, leading to implications for assistive technology design [13]. Understanding the cultural nuances and preferences of older adults is important for the successful adoption of assistive smart home technologies [50].

In summary, while factors like perceived usability and utility are considered important to the adoption of these types of technologies, cultural norms and beliefs, together with macro-level factors (e.g. lifestyle affecting the prevalence of certain morbidities) can also shape attitudes towards AAL technologies, and should be considered when designing interventions to help with the adoption of these technologies. It is worthwhile noting that while shared attitudinal elements between cultural diasporas can be maintained through the use of communication technology [84], elements of cultural assimilation will end up shaping attitudes in the long run [9].

13.3 Socio-Cultural, Ethnic and Linguistic Biases

As AAL technologies become more integrated into healthcare and personal use, it is necessary to recognize and address the biases they may perpetuate. Biases can disproportionately affect ethnic and gender minorities, leading to unequal access to and outcomes from these technologies and the digital divide in healthcare [60]. Bias in AAL technologies primarily stems from the data used in their development, the design of the technologies themselves, and the societal norms and values embedded by the designers [68].

Like other artificial intelligence (AI) systems, AAL technologies often suffer from biases that can affect their performance across different ethnic and gender groups. The design of the majority of algorithms ignores the sex and gender dimension and its contribution to health and disease differences among individuals, resulting in flawed results and mistakes as well as discriminatory outcomes [26]. Moreover, medical devices that monitor health parameters may not be as accurate for all types of skin tones [37, 52], due to variations in physiology and skin reflectivity that were not adequately considered in their design. Biases are not limited to skin tone. Human factors and cultural practices can also contribute to the performance of health technologies [21]. For example, Choy et al. demonstrate how certain cultural and ethnic groups might need to change their customs (e.g. change their hairstyle by removing cornrows or braids) to join the research studies, which may result in lower participation of certain groups during data collection [24]. This can lead to biases in the development of the technologies, ending up with misdiagnosis or delayed treatments for certain groups. In line with this, Kim et al. demonstrated that facial emotional expression recognition systems are most effective at identifying emotional expressions in images of young adults, and their accuracy diminishes when analyzing images of older adults [51].

Language is a critical component of many AAL technologies, particularly those involving voice-activated systems and communication aids. If these systems are primarily designed for certain dominant languages or dialects, non-native speakers or people who use regional dialects may find these technologies less responsive or accurate. This not only limits the usability of the device but can also isolate individuals linguistically, potentially exacerbating feelings of exclusion. Despite the recent expansion of research in NLP fairness, there has been little examination on how AI models represent disability [46], and age-related disability that can impact speech [34, 97]. Age influences user interactions with speech technology systems [14], differences which are not accounted for in the technology [82]. Research demonstrates that voice technologies exhibit unfairness due to disparities based on race and age. For instance, these technologies may show lower accuracy in recognizing the speech of Black older adults, highlighting biases in speech recognition systems [15, 44]. In addition to racial biases, studies also reveal gender biases in Automatic Speech Recognition technology, with female speakers being particularly affected [38, 98].

AAL technologies can also reflect and reinforce socioeconomic biases. High costs associated with the latest technologies can prevent lower-income individuals from accessing these potentially life-enhancing tools. Cost is among the main determinants and facilitators of older adults' adoption of technology [55, 86]. Additionally, designs that do not consider diverse living conditions may result in products that are less effective or irrelevant for those in different socioeconomic settings [57, 69].

Although technological solutions for elderly care are often praised as cost-efficient means to promote independence, safety, and health, research suggests that these positive views might ignore underlying issues of social inequality, ageism, and the exploitation of gendered care labor [33]. Dalmer et al. argue that technologies themselves are based on ageism, that the designers of Age Tech, frequently base their perceptions of aging on clichéd notions of frailty, disability, and decline, and tend to exhibit a restricted comprehension of older adults and their interactions with technology. They often fail to adequately account for how factors like gender, class, ethnicity, and ability can influence the usage of technologies—or whether they are used at all [33]. In the same article, together with other critical discourse, Dalmer et al. discuss that the success of smart home environments, residences, and private care settings often relies on the caregiving labor traditionally performed by women. This gendered labor, essential to the operation and maintenance of health and care technologies, is frequently overlooked.

Importantly, when we speak about audio- and video-based monitoring solutions with an emphasis on privacy protection, we can not omit the sociodemographic stance on privacy and the imbalances around it. Toward the close of the last century, Anita Allen was already making the case that privacy rights were originally designed with men in mind, not women, and in cyberspace, women do not experience the same degree or types of privacy as men [4]. Additionally, a systematic review of 37 studies found that women on social media sites exhibit greater concerns and behaviors regarding privacy compared to men [95]. Notably, studies have also highlighted the constrained privacy experienced by certain demographics; for example, people of color have historically been subjected to privacy infringements through surveillance practices [16], while those from lower socioeconomic backgrounds often face reduced privacy rights [43].

While AAL technologies hold significant promise for enhancing the lives of many, it is imperative to address the biases that may undermine their effectiveness and accessibility. By taking proactive steps towards inclusive design and evaluation, we can utilize the full potential of these technologies in a way that benefits all members of society. This requires ongoing research, diverse data representation, and collaborative efforts across disciplines to ensure that AAL solutions are equitable and responsive to the needs of all users.

13.4 Dataveillance and Normalization of Surveillance

In the literature on the social implications of Internet-of-things technologies, the increasing normalization of surveillance is sometimes mentioned as a social issue on the macro level. [39], for example, discuss such a risk in the context of smart connected toys (SCTs), which are targeted at children and thus address a particularly vulnerable and protected group. Empirical research on SCTs, for example by [78], problematizes how these products "introduce surveillance in playful and uncritical ways with potentially powerful, wide-ranging ramifications" [39, p. 138]. A similar issue emerges in the context of AAL. Given that AAL systems are frequently developed for vulnerable groups such as older adults or people with disabilities and mobility constraints, there tends to be a stark power imbalance between these groups and other individuals in their network such as caretakers and healthy friends or family members. Even if these other individuals have benign intentions, they still might see it as desirable to keep more control than needed, for example by engaging in intimate surveillance,[2] thus restricting the privacy or autonomy of the vulnerable users. Over time, a habituation to such intimate surveillance could lead to shifting norms around surveillance and lower the thresholds for practices we see as problematic today, for example watching live video streams or listening to live audio within a relative's or friends' home through AAL systems when someone gets unauthorized (or authorized) access.

An adjacent risk in that regard, which has received increasing attention in the privacy and surveillance literature [17, 18, 77, 90, 91], are chilling effects. They are defined as "the self-inhibition of (legitimate) behaviors, such as expressing one's opinion online [...] or searching the web for (sensitive) information" [17] due to surveillance—and in the digital age especially dataveillance. The literature on chilling effects stresses the democratic and participatory risks when chilling effects occur, but existing research in this area has focused more on government surveillance than corporate surveillance [17], despite important adjacent literature on surveillance capitalism [103] and dataveillance [96]. Thus, we have a limited understanding if and how sustained monitoring through AAL systems leads to behavioral change and chilling effects–and under what conditions.

13.5 Re-shaping of Care Relationships

As AAL technologies become more prevalent, they inevitably impact the roles, identities, tasks, and routines of healthcare professionals such as doctors and nurses, as well as the dynamics of care relationships between caregivers and care recipients. This transformation encompasses both opportunities and challenges for formal caregivers (e.g., doctors, nurses, personal support workers, rehabilitation specialists, etc.) [53, 58], informal caregivers (e.g., family members, relatives) and end users. This digital transformation, as observed by Colnar et al., could potentially also contribute toward the configuration of new care models more individual-centered "to move away from traditional hospital-centered systems to more desirable community based and integrated care structures" [28, p. 17133]. This section will present the challenges and opportunities of AAL technologies in the context of care relationships and how these technologies re-shape care relationships between caregivers and caretakers, as well as healthcare roles and tasks.

AAL technologies including sensors assist with the analysis of patient behaviors, help with early illness detection, prevent risks (e.g., falls), and support nursing

---

[2] The concept of intimate surveillance has been developed in the context of parenting in the digital age, describing how parents use technologies such as location-tracking, dedicated apps or security cameras in the children's room to monitor their children [62]. The key motive for this intimate surveillance is safety and security but it has been criticized as problematic because the children are often unaware of these practices, and if they are, they remain unable to consent or resist this surveillance due to the power imbalances at play.

decision-making in patient care. Following [23], Ahmad et al. argue that AAL technologies are already playing a key role in supporting caregivers, who mainly believe that "technology can help them to make care giving more efficient, effective, safer and less stressful" [1]. In particular, AAL technologies for people with dementia help nurses to reduce their worry and anxiety and increase the length of the rehabilitation activities [79]. AAL solutions, such as telehealth and remote activity monitoring, allow taking care of older adults, as well as an efficient communication between them and health care professionals and informal caregivers in a cost-effective way to enhance independence, security, and health [1, 33]. For instance, remote patient monitoring, as observed by [1], offer helpful alternatives to "track the user's healthcare conditions outside of traditional health care settings, such as hospitals and care units". These technologies can empower individuals to manage their own health and well-being more effectively, therefore, reducing their reliance on formal caregivers. For example, remote monitoring systems and wearable devices allow users to track vital signs, medication intake, and activity levels, enabling them to take a more proactive role in managing their health [5, 93].

Despite the identified benefits that AAL can provide to improve older adults' care, many professional caregivers are reluctant to the introduction of these technologies due to ethical considerations, fear that technology will have a negative impact on building relationships, as well as lack of skills to operate these devices [28, 32]. Chaharsoughi et al. explain that also formal carers, such as nurses, must catch up with the workings of AAL technologies adding more stress and workload, thereby decreasing job satisfaction, which limits the potential benefits these new technologies may bring to nursing practice and patient care [20]. As Crawford also discusses, AI may paradoxically involve an increased workload for humans as well as a restructuring of how the work is performed [31]. In addition, from a Feminist perspective, Dalmer et al. argue that use of AAL technologies also involve "social inequality, agist bias, and exploitative gendered care labour" [33, pp. 77–78]. According to them, informal carers, often women who "are already burdened with the bulk of caregiving", are now expected to operate and fulfill the competencies necessary to understand the workings of care technologies to track bodily activities (e.g., eating, sleeping, and medication schedules, bathroom use) "including discerning deviations in data patterns or moments and responding to emergency calls and alerts". Technologized gendered older age care labor is intertwined with the broader political economy of health, yet it remains largely invisible in the design of AAL technologies that claim to reduce the need for paid or unpaid care providers [33, 67, 80]. Milligan acknowledges that although AAL technologies are part of a strategy from Western governments to reduce the number of older adults entering residential care and hospitals, they also need resources to operate [67]. Despite AAL technologies being perceived as cost-efficient for society, they also involve (invisible) labor needed for tracking the routines of older people and managing the extensive data requiring interpretation, which pushes caregivers to integrate physical and online worlds, becoming on-call data intermediaries [33]. Building on [41]; Dalmer et al. argue that tracking actions or routines creates a situation that brings to light the myriad of actors and activities involved in care, often unnoticed, underscoring the need to consider the materiality of data, laboring bodies, and social relations involved in care practices [33].

The introduction of AAL technologies also transforms the tasks and routines performed by healthcare professionals in clinical and home-based care settings. In particular, remote patient monitoring (RPM) devices powered by AI allow doctors and nurses to track patients' health parameters in real-time and design of personalized care plans: "AI-enabled RPM architectures have transformed healthcare monitoring applications because of their ability to detect early deterioration in patients' health, personalize individual patient health parameter monitoring using federated learning, and learn human behavior patterns using techniques such as reinforcement learning" [83]. However, following [80], Dalmer et al. highlight that AAL technologies introduce an artificial division of care in three separate tasks: monitoring, physical care, and social-emotional care, thereby "undermining the complexities of care work and oversimplifying both the care experience and the complexities of social-spatial relations of care" [33, p. 88]. Moreover, AAL technologies imply that both formal and informal care providers are skillful in the use of these devices, therefore, intensifying inequalities between technically-skilled and "unskilled" non-technical labor. In order to face these challenges and prepare for the future, Chaharsoughi et al. suggest that "nursing must begin the immediate transformation into a digitally enabled profession that can respond to the complex global challenges facing health systems and society" [20, p. 149].

13.6 Trust in (AAL) Technologies and Barriers to Adoption

In 2016, Yusif and colleagues conducted a systematic literature review across disciplines and identified a set of potential barriers to the adoption of Assistive Technologies (AT) in domestic settings [102]. The most critical barriers were related to privacy concerns of the end-users (34% of surveyed articles). It was followed by factors linked to (the lack of) trust in AT as well as value-added functionality, with 27% and 25%, respectively, of the total examined empirical studies. Those concerns were followed by high costs of the deployment, maintenance, and use of the AT at home, as well as their ease of use and suitability for everyday tasks (23% each). The other factors were related to the perception of 'no need' for such technologies in domestic settings (20%), associated stigmas related to their use (18%), fears of dependence (16%) as well as limited opportunities for training, specially tailored to older learners (16%). Finally, the authors identified related feelings of embarrassment of using such technologies, loss of dignity and autonomy, and overall lack of accessibility and social inclusion as contributing factors that impede the adoption and use of AT at home.

When it comes to trust, it serves as the foundation for numerous human interactions and relationships [36, 59]. Furthermore, trust can be transferred to institutions, organizations, and technologies [11, 12]. Cheshire conceptualized this as "system trust" [22]. With the automation and complexity of digital technologies, trust is especially important as it is a prerequisite for successful technology use and adoption [42, 48]. Scholars examined the importance of trust in AAL technologies and their acceptance using various methodologies [88] and in the different contexts [10, 71, 72], including, most notably, medical applications [47, 75], advisory services [10], domestic technologies [27], and care institutions, such as AT centers (e.g., [69, 70]).

Leitner et al. [56] employed contextual design and technology acceptance modeling and evaluated 20 real-world household installations of their AAL prototype, and reported on the gender differences when it comes to access to AAL technology. In turn, Otten et al. [74] used a scenario-based approach to identify the acceptance criteria focusing on video-based AAL technologies. They have concluded that data protection, information, and communication flow, as well as associated trust criteria, consisting of health and emotional aspects, play a role in the acceptance of video-based AAL technologies. Additionally, they emphasized the role of context as a contributing factor for acceptance, specifically honoring interactions among technicians, caregivers, and caretakers. They concluded: "It is important to remember that people still place their trust to a large extent in humans and by extension, on their recommendations of said technologies" [74, p. 133].

Similarly to [74], Offermann-van Heek and Ziefle employed realistic case scenarios to identify perceived benefits and barriers to the adoption of AAL technologies at home surveying 140 individuals [71]. Potential users reported that privacy, perceived control, attitudes towards AAL, medical necessity, and the added value to their daily routines contribute to AAL acceptance. They have also highlighted the differences between those new to caregiving and those with caregiving experience in their reasons for using AAL technologies in the home setting. For the former group, the reasons to opt in for AAL technology are the increase in process efficiency and medical safety, while for the latter, the most important considerations are the emotional relief and the felt safety for a person in care. As for the barriers, they have examined the access to personal data from third parties and the handling of processed or recorded data as impeding factors for the adoption of AAL in the domestic context.

Human-computer interaction scholars have also investigated the aspects of trust and barriers to the adoption of AAL technologies, especially for older populations [87, 89, 101]. For example, Steinke et al. [87] conducted a survey among older adults aged between 60 and 90 years old in Germany and distinguished two stratification criteria, i.e., gender and housing situation, that influence trust within (sensor-based) AAL technologies. Specifically, the authors demonstrated that people living in a single household showed lower levels of trust in sensor technology than the ones who lived in a shared household. Furthermore, similarly to [56], gender played a role in forming trust in sensor technology: men had distinctly higher levels of trust than women. Finally, they have concluded that key factors to trust AAL systems among older adults are perceived reliability and ease of use (also corroborated in a subsequent experimental setup [89]); when it comes to the form factors of such technology, they deemed that stationary AAL setups (e.g., fixed sensors in the home environment) were more reliable than the wearable ones.

13.7 Conclusion

In this chapter, we discussed important social and societal issues in AAL, making sure to deal with implications that are as distinct as possible from the ethical and legal [19, 29] aspects. However, social, ethical and legal issues are intertwined and not always clearly separable. For example, privacy is a topic that can be approached from a social perspective [81], from a legal one [85] and from an ethical one [66]. Social and societal issues refer to the development and use of these technologies in context and in real-life settings, rather than in the lab. They also capture historical dynamics and cultural perceptions of the technology. As such, the social and societal issues in AAL are conducive to be approached from multiple disciplines spanning the humanities and social sciences and using different methods such as quantitative (e.g., surveys, experiments), qualitative (e.g., ethnographies, interviews, focus groups, discourse analysis), mixed methods (any combination and integration of qualitative and quantitative methods), as well as conceptual, archival and desk research approaches (e.g., scoping reviews, historical analysis of development and implementation of specific systems). Cross-disciplinary projects and a critical perspective, for example informed by science and technology studies [76] or critical data studies [8], are particularly conducive to studying the social and societal issues in AAL, because they allow for a holistic understanding of the underlying dynamics at play.

Specifically, we discussed five critical social or societal issues, dedicating a section to each. We first highlighted cultural adaptation and differences. The review showed how cultural factors such as country of residence can affect people's acceptance of and attitudes towards AAL solutions, but demographic aspects and physical status, for example disability, matter too. In a second step, we dealt with the key issue of socio-cultural, ethnic and linguistic biases. The overview of extant literature showed biases in terms of gender, age and race, as well as the importance of an intersectional perspective. Linguistic biases are a topic that requires further attention when systems are voice-activated. Large language models (LLMs) that are more and more incorporated into AI analysis pipelines are known to perpetuate systematic racial prejudices [49]. Then we described the issue of dataveillance and the potential for normalizing surveillance among vulnerable groups such as older adults or individuals with psychiatric disorders. AAL technologies rely on sensitive data, for example audio and video recordings of people in their private home, and the normalization of increasingly private data collection could carry risks such as power abuse, function creep or chilling effects, which we discussed.

A fourth social issue is the re-shaping of care relationships, with AAL systems re-configuring tasks and responsibilities in the care sector, for example for nurses. The literature shows both opportunities, where certain aspects of AAL systems are welcomed, but also challenges, for example additional burdens and responsibilities, especially for women, and a necessity for re-skilling. Finally, we looked into trust and barriers to AAL adoption. User-oriented research in the area shows the importance of privacy concerns and a lack of trust as barriers to adoption of AAL systems. Trust seems gendered, with men reporting higher levels of it.

Together, these five social and societal issues show the complexity of the technology and the plurality of stakeholders involved. Thus, approaching AAL technologies from an ecosystem perspective might prove fruitful, with actor-network theory as a promising theoretical lens to better grasp the social and societal issues and their interplay [65]. The issues discussed point to implications for different stakeholders, including developers, users (where different user groups have to be distinguished depending on the context and use case, for example patients vs. care personnel, see [2]), policymakers and researchers.

For *developers*, there is a need to design AAL systems in a way that minimizes social issues and societal harms. Of course, developers cannot foresee all the downstream consequences of the technology, but having a keen eye for these issues, including conversations with ethics experts and social scientists, as well as a strong consideration of user needs in the vein of participatory design, are good starting points. For *users*, it is advisable to develop a solid level of AAL literacy, which includes not only knowledge of technical aspects such as a basic understanding of how the technology works, but also contextual knowledge, for example about the benefits and risks and about the technological implications more broadly. However, such a literacy will not be developed on its own, so that institutions, including industry, civil society, academia and policy, are encouraged to come together to implement suitable literacy programs, for example through understandable info materials and targeted workshops. For *policymakers*, a strong awareness of the social and societal issues of AAL is necessary to appropriately govern this technology, so that regular consultation with technical and social AAL experts should take place.

In terms of existing regulatory tools, the European Union AI Act, which went into force recently, provides a comprehensive framework to regulate AI-based technologies such as AAL (see for example [29] in this volume). It uses a risk-based approach and classifies AI technologies into four risk groups with specific regulatory demands: unacceptable, high, limited, and minimal risk, respectively. Aiming to foster trustworthiness [92], the AI Act prohibits systems with unacceptable risks, while high-risk applications come with many obligations for developers, for example regarding risk management, cybersecurity, documentation and human oversight. AI technologies that process biometric data and use profiling are considered high-risk. Thus, many AAL systems (which need to identify a person in the care environment to monitor their data) are likely to fall within the high-risk category. Kuźmicz discusses the importance of balance in the governance of AAL, with both the AI Act and the General Data Protection Regulation (GDPR) referencing the concept [54]. He specifies that "to achieve balance, it is crucial to identify aspects or situations where one party is disadvantaged and empower more vulnerable stakeholders" (p. 22). Thus, law and policy, technology and user needs (see [94] in this volume) must go hand in hand for a socially-aware and successful implementation of AAL technologies. Finally, *researchers* should intensify the study of the social and societal issues of AAL.

Future research should study the social issues we discussed here empirically and through a range of social science methods, both quantitative and qualitative ones. Observational methods are fruitful to investigate, for example, the normalization of surveillance, chilling effects and issues of bias and trust. However, given the sensitivity of AAL data such methods are subject to higher ethical requirements and scrutiny than self-reported data from interviews, surveys or media coverage. Theoretical contributions that situate the social and societal issues we discussed within existing theories or develop new theories are also very much welcome.

Acknowledgements This publication is based upon work from COST Action GoodBrother—Network on Privacy-Aware Audio- and Video-Based Applications for Active and Assisted Living (CA19121), supported by COST (European Cooperation in Science and Technology). We would like to thank the editorial team, Albert Ali Salah, Liane Colonna and Francisco Florez-Revuelta, for their helpful feedback on our chapter and their tireless efforts that went into editing this book. Christoph Lutz was partly funded by the Research Council of Norway, project number 299178 "Algorithmic Accountability: Designing Governance for Responsible Digital Transformations", while writing the chapter. Rodrigo Perez-Vega dedicates this chapter to Sofia and never ending adventures.

References

1. Ahmad, I., Asghar, Z., Kumar, T., Li, G., Manzoor, A., Mikhaylov, K., Harjula, E.: Emerging technologies for next generation remote health care and assisted living. IEEE Access **10**, 56094–56132 (2022). https://doi.org/10.1109/ACCESS.2022.3177278
2. Ake-Kob, A., Aleksic, S., Alexin, Z., Blazeviciene, A., Cartolovni, A., Colonna, L., Dantas, C., Fedosov, A., Fosch-Villaronga, E., Florez-Revuelta, F., He, Z., Jevremovic, A., Adrzej, K., Lambrinos, L., Lutz, C., Malešević, A., Mekovec, R., Miguel, C., Mujirishvili, T., Pajalic, Z., Perez Vega, R., Pierscionek, B.K., Ravi, S., Sarf, P., Solanas, A., Tamò-Larrieux, A.: Position paper on ethical, legal and social challenges linked to audio- and video-based AAL solutions. SSRN Electron. J. (2022). https://doi.org/10.2139/ssrn.4282341
3. Ake-Kob, A., Blazeviciene, A., Colonna, L., Cartolovni, A., Dantas, C., Fedosov, A., Colantonio, S.: State of the art on ethical, legal, and social issues linked to audio-and video-based AAL solutions. SSRN Electron. J. (2021). https://doi.org/10.2139/ssrn.3994835
4. Allen, A.L.: Gender and privacy in cyberspace. Stanford Law Rev. 1175–1200 (2000)
5. Appelboom, G., Camacho, E., Abraham, M.E., Bruce, S.S., Dumont, E.L., Zacharia, B.E., Connolly, E.S.: Smart wearable body sensors for patient self-assessment and monitoring. Arch. Publ. Health **72**(1), 1–9 (2014). https://doi.org/10.1186/2049-3258-72-28
6. Awad, E., Dsouza, S., Kim, R., Schulz, J., Henrich, J., Shariff, A., Bonnefon, J.F., Rahwan, I.: The moral machine experiment. Nature **563**(7729), 59–64 (2018)
7. Bechtold, U., Stauder, N., Fieder, M.: Attitudes towards technology: insights on rarely discussed influences on older adults' willingness to adopt active assisted living (AAL). Int. J. Environ. Res. Public Health **21**(5), 628 (2024)
8. Berridge, C., Grigorovich, A.: Algorithmic harms and digital ageism in the use of surveillance technologies in nursing homes. Front. Sociol. **7**, 957,246 (2022)
9. Berry, J.W.: Acculturation and adaptation. In: Handbook of Cross-Cultural Psychology, 3rd edn., pp. 291–326. Allyn & Bacon (1997)
10. Bertel, D., Teles, S., Strohmeier, F., Vieira-Marques, P., Schmitter, P., Ruscher, S., Paúl, C., Kofler, A.C.: High tech, high touch: integrating digital and human AAL advisory services for

older adults. In: 4th International Conference on Information and Communication Technologies for Ageing Well and e-Health (ICT4AWE), Funchal, Portugal, 22–23 March 2018, pp. 241–249. SciTePress (2018)
11. Bodó, B.: Mediated trust: a theoretical framework to address the trustworthiness of technological trust mediators. New Med. Soc. **23**(9), 2668–2690 (2021)
12. Botsman, R.: Who can you trust?: How technology brought us together–and why it could drive us apart. Penguin, UK (2017)
13. Boujarwah, F.A., Riedl, M.O., Abowd, G.D., Arriaga, R.I.: React: intelligent authoring of social skills instructional modules for adolescents with high-functioning autism. ACM SIGACCESS Access. Comput. **99**, 13–23 (2011)
14. Brewer, R., Pierce, C., Upadhyay, P., Park, L.: An empirical study of older adult's voice assistant use for health information seeking. ACM Trans. Interact. Intell. Syst. (TiiS) **12**(2), 1–32 (2022)
15. Brewer, R.N., Harrington, C., Heldreth, C.: Envisioning equitable speech technologies for black older adults. In: Proceedings of the 2023 ACM Conference on Fairness, Accountability, and Transparency, pp. 379–388 (2023)
16. Browne, S.: Dark Matters: On the Surveillance of Blackness. Duke University Press (2015)
17. Büchi, M., Festic, N., Latzer, M.: The chilling effects of digital dataveillance: a theoretical model and an empirical research agenda. Big Data Soc. **9**(1), 1–14 (2022). https://doi.org/10.1177/20539517211065368
18. Büchi, M., Fosch-Villaronga, E., Lutz, C., Tamò-Larrieux, A., Velidi, S., Viljoen, S.: The chilling effects of algorithmic profiling: mapping the issues. Comput. Law Secur. Rev. **36**, 105,367 (2020). https://doi.org/10.1016/j.clsr.2019.105367
19. Čartolovni, A., Dantas, C., Malešević, A., Ilgaz, A.: Ethical issues in AAL. In: Salah, A.A., Colonna, L., Florez-Revuelta, F. (eds.) Privacy-Aware Monitoring for Assisted Living. Springer, Cham (2025)
20. Chaharsoughi, N.T., Ahmadifaraz, M., Kahangi, L.S.: The impact of digital technologies in nursing care and their application: a narrative review. J. Multidiscipl. Care **11**(3), 149–156 (2022). https://doi.org/10.34172/jmdc.2022.1127
21. Charpignon, M.L., Carrel, A., Jiang, Y., Kwaga, T., Cantada, B., Hyslop, T., Cox, C.E., Haines, K., Koomson, V., Dumas, G., et al.: Going beyond the means: exploring the role of bias from digital determinants of health in technologies. PLOS Digital Health **2**(10), e0000,244 (2023)
22. Cheshire, C.: Online trust, trustworthiness, or assurance? Daedalus **140**(4), 49–58 (2011). https://doi.org/10.1162/DAED_a_00114
23. Chi, N.C., Demiris, G.: A systematic review of telehealth tools and interventions to support family caregivers. J. Telemed. Telecare **21**(1), 37–44 (2015). https://doi.org/10.1177/1357633X14562734
24. Choy, T., Baker, E., Stavropoulos, K.: Systemic racism in EEG research: considerations and potential solutions. Affect. Sci. **3**(1), 14–20 (2022)
25. Chung, J., Thompson, H.J., Joe, J., Hall, A., Demiris, G.: Examining Korean and Korean American older adults' perceived acceptability of home-based monitoring technologies in the context of culture. Inform. Health Soc. Care **42**(1), 61–76 (2017)
26. Cirillo, D., Catuara-Solarz, S., Morey, C., Guney, E., Subirats, L., Mellino, S., Gigante, A., Valencia, A., Rementeria, M.J., Chadha, A.S., et al.: Sex and gender differences and biases in artificial intelligence for biomedicine and healthcare. NPJ Dig. Med. **3**(1), 1–11 (2020)
27. Claes, V., Devriendt, E., Tournoy, J., Milisen, K.: Attitudes and perceptions of adults of 60 years and older towards in-home monitoring of the activities of daily living with contactless sensors: an explorative study. Int. J. Nurs. Stud. **52**(1), 134–148 (2015)
28. Colnar, S., Penger, S., Grah, B., Dimovski, V.: Digital transformation of integrated care: literature review and research agenda. IFAC-PapersOnLine **53**(2), 16890–16895 (2020). https://doi.org/10.1016/j.ifacol.2020.12.1221
29. Colonna, L., Riva, G.M.: The legal and regulatory issues in AAL: the case of smart mirrors. In: Salah, A.A., Colonna, L., Florez-Revuelta, F. (eds.) Privacy-Aware Monitoring for Assisted Living. Springer, Cham (2025)

30. Courtney, K.L., Demeris, G., Rantz, M., Skubic, M.: Needing smart home technologies: the perspectives of older adults in continuing care retirement communities. J. Innov. Health Inform. **16**(3), 195–201 (2008)
31. Crawford, K.: The Atlas of AI: Power, Politics, and the Planetary Costs of Artificial Intelligence. Yale University Press (2021)
32. Cresswell, K., Sheikh, A.: Organizational issues in the implementation and adoption of health information technology innovations: an interpretative review. Int. J. Med. Inform. **82**(5), e73–e86 (2013). https://doi.org/10.1016/j.ijmedinf.2012.10.007
33. Dalmer, N., Ellison, K., Katz, S., Marshall, B.: Ageing, embodiment and datafication: dynamics of power in digital health and care technologies. Int. J. Ageing Later Life **15**(2), 77–101 (2022)
34. Dunlop, D.D., Song, J., Manheim, L.M., Daviglus, M.L., Chang, R.W.: Racial/ethnic differences in the development of disability among older adults. Am. J. Public Health **97**(12), 2209–2215 (2007)
35. European Commission: Final evaluation of the active and assisted living research and development programme. Technical report, European Commission, Brussels (2022). https://eur-lex.europa.eu/LexUriServ/LexUriServ.do?uri=SWD:2022:0404:FIN:EN:PDF
36. Fedosov, A., Zavolokina, L., Krumhard, S., Huang, E.M.: "This could be the day i die": unpacking interpersonal and systems trust in a local sharing economy community. In: Extended Abstracts of the 2023 CHI Conference on Human Factors in Computing Systems, CHI EA'23. Association for Computing Machinery, New York, NY, USA (2023). https://doi.org/10.1145/3544549.3585744
37. Feiner, J.R., Severinghaus, J.W., Bickler, P.E.: Dark skin decreases the accuracy of pulse oximeters at low oxygen saturation: the effects of oximeter probe type and gender. Anesth. Analg. **105**(6), S18–S23 (2007)
38. Fenu, G., Medda, G., Marras, M., Meloni, G.: Improving fairness in speaker recognition. In: Proceedings of the 2020 European Symposium on Software Engineering, pp. 129–136 (2020)
39. Fosch-Villaronga, E., Van der Hof, S., Lutz, C., Tamò-Larrieux, A.: Toy story or children story? Putting children and their rights at the forefront of the artificial intelligence revolution. AI Soc. **38**(1), 133–152 (2023). https://doi.org/10.1007/s00146-021-01295-w
40. Fosch-Villaronga, E., Lutz, C., Tamò-Larrieux, A.: Gathering expert opinions for social robots' ethical, legal, and societal concerns: findings from four international workshops. Int. J. Soc. Robot. **12**(2), 441–458 (2020). https://doi.org/10.1007/s12369-019-00605-z
41. Fotopoulou, A.: Understanding citizen data practices from a feminist perspective. In: Stephansen, H., Trere, E.(eds.) Citizen Media and Practice, pp. 227–242. Routledge (2019)
42. Gefen, D., Karahanna, E., Straub, D.W.: Trust and tam in online shopping: an integrated model. MIS Quart. 51–90 (2003)
43. Gilliom, J.: Overseers of the Poor: Surveillance, Resistance, and the Limits of Privacy. University of Chicago Press (2001)
44. Harrington, C.N., Garg, R., Woodward, A., Williams, D.: "It's kind of like code-switching": black older adults' experiences with a voice assistant for health information seeking. In: Proceedings of the 2022 CHI Conference on Human Factors in Computing Systems, pp. 1–15 (2022)
45. Harris, M.T., Rogers, W.A.: Developing a healthcare technology acceptance model (H-TAM) for older adults with hypertension. Ageing Soc. **43**(4), 814–834 (2023)
46. Herold, B., Waller, J., Kushalnagar, R.: Applying the stereotype content model to assess disability bias in popular pre-trained NLP models underlying AI-based assistive technologies. In: Ninth Workshop on Speech and Language Processing for Assistive Technologies (SLPAT-2022), pp. 58–65 (2022)
47. Hick, S., Biermann, H., Ziefle, M.: How deep is your trust? A comparative user requirements' analysis of automation in medical and mobility technologies. Humanit. Soc. Sci. Commun. **11**(1), 1–13 (2024)
48. Hoffmann, A., Hoffmann, H., Söllner, M.: Fostering initial trust in applications–developing and evaluating requirement patterns for application websites. In: 21st European Conference on Information Systems (ECIS), Utrecht, The Netherlands (2013)

49. Hofmann, V., Kalluri, P.R., Jurafsky, D., King, S.: AI generates covertly racist decisions about people based on their dialect. Nature 1–8 (2024)
50. Kilcullen, S., Heffernan, E., Hussey, P., Lee, H., Moran, K., Murphy, C., Smeaton, A.F., Timon, C.M., Gallagher, P., Hopper, L.: A theoretical domains framework (TDF) approach to the qualitative analysis of older adults' intentions to adopt assistive smart home technology. Gerontochnology **21**(1) (2022)
51. Kim, E., Bryant, D., Srikanth, D., Howard, A.: Age bias in emotion detection: an analysis of facial emotion recognition performance on young, middle-aged, and older adults. In: Proceedings of the 2021 AAAI/ACM Conference on AI, Ethics, and Society, pp. 638–644 (2021)
52. Koerber, D., Khan, S., Shamsheri, T., Kirubarajan, A., Mehta, S.: Accuracy of heart rate measurement with wrist-worn wearable devices in various skin tones: a systematic review. J. Racial Ethn. Health Disparities **10**(6), 2676–2684 (2023)
53. Ku, L., Liu, L.F., Wen, M.J.: Trends and determinants of informal and formal caregiving in the community for disabled elderly people in Taiwan. Arch. Gerontol. Geriatr. **56**(2), 370–376 (2013). https://doi.org/10.1016/j.archger.2012.11.005
54. Kuźmicz, M.M.: A concept of balance of interest in the context of active assisted living. Dig. Soc. **2**(3), 1–30 (2023)
55. Lee, C., Coughlin, J.F.: Perspective: older adults' adoption of technology: an integrated approach to identifying determinants and barriers. J. Prod. Innov. Manag. **32**(5), 747–759 (2015)
56. Leitner, G., Mitrea, O., Fercher, A.J.: Towards an acceptance model for AAL. In: Human Factors in Computing and Informatics: First International Conference, SouthCHI 2013, Maribor, Slovenia, July 1–3, 2013. Proceedings, pp. 672–679. Springer (2013)
57. Levasseur, M., Généreux, M., Bruneau, J.F., Vanasse, A., Chabot, É., Beaulac, C., Bédard, M.M.: Importance of proximity to resources, social support, transportation and neighborhood security for mobility and social participation in older adults: results from a scoping study. BMC Public Health **15**, 1–19 (2015)
58. Li, J., Song, Y.: Formal and informal care. In: Encyclopedia of Gerontology and Population Aging. Springer (2019)
59. Light, A.: Trust in collaborative economies and how to study it: relational assets and the making of more-than-strangers. In: Ethnographies of Collaborative Economies across Europe, vol. 13 (2022)
60. López, L., Green, A.R., Tan-McGrory, A., King, R.S., Betancourt, J.R.: Bridging the digital divide in health care: the role of health information technology in addressing racial and ethnic disparities. Joint Comm. J. Qual. Patient Safety **37**(10), 437–445 (2011)
61. Louie, W., McColl, D., Nejat, G.: Acceptance and attitudes toward a human-like socially assistive robot by older adults. Assist. Technol. **26**(3), 140–150 (2014)
62. Lupton, D., Williamson, B.: The datafied child: the dataveillance of children and implications for their rights. New Med. Soc. **19**(5), 780–794 (2017). https://doi.org/10.1177/1461444816686328
63. Lutz, C., Newlands, G.: Privacy and smart speakers: a multi-dimensional approach. Inf. Soc. **37**(3), 147–162 (2021). https://doi.org/10.1080/01972243.2021.1897914
64. Lutz, C., Schöttler, M., Hoffmann, C.P.: The privacy implications of social robots: scoping review and expert interviews. Mob. Med. Commun. **7**(3), 412–434 (2019). https://doi.org/10.1177/2050157919843961
65. Lutz, C., Tamò, A.: Communicating with robots: antalyzing the interaction between healthcare robots and humans with regards to privacy. In: Guzman, A. (ed.) Human-Machine Communication: Rethinking Communication, Technology, and Ourselves, pp. 145–165. Peter Lang (2018)
66. Martin, K.: Understanding privacy online: development of a social contract approach to privacy. J. Bus. Ethics **137**, 551–569 (2016)
67. Milligan, C.: There's no place like home: place and care in an ageing society. Ashgate (2009)

68. Mittelstadt, B.D., Allo, P., Taddeo, M., Wachter, S., Floridi, L.: The ethics of algorithms: mapping the debate. Big Data Soc. **3**(2) (2016). https://doi.org/10.1177/2053951716679679
69. Mujirishvili, T., Fedosov, A., Hashemifard, K., Climent-Pérez, P., Florez-Revuelta, F.: "I don't want to become a number": examining different stakeholder perspectives on a video-based monitoring system for senior care with inherent privacy protection (by design). In: Proceedings of the CHI Conference on Human Factors in Computing Systems, CHI'24. Association for Computing Machinery, New York, NY, USA (2024). https://doi.org/10.1145/3613904.3642164
70. Mujirishvili, T., Maidhof, C., Florez-Revuelta, F., Ziefle, M., Richart-Martinez, M., Cabrero-García, J.: Acceptance and privacy perceptions toward video-based active and assisted living technologies: scoping review. J. Med. Internet Res. **25**, e45,297 (2023)
71. Offermann-van Heek, J., Ziefle, M.: Nothing else matters! trade-offs between perceived benefits and barriers of AAL technology usage. Front. Public Health **7** (2019). https://doi.org/10.3389/fpubh.2019.00134
72. Olphert, W., Damodaran, L., Balatsoukas, P., Parkinson, C.: Process requirements for building sustainable digital assistive technology for older people. J. Assist. Technol. **3**(3), 4–13 (2009)
73. Orellano Colon, E.: Gender differences in the adoption and use of assistive technology (AT) among Hispanics. Am. J. Occup. Therapy **73**(4 Supp 1), 7311505,192p1 (2019)
74. Otten, S., Wilkowska, W., Offermann, J., Ziefle, M.: Trust in and acceptance of video-based AAL technologies. In: ICT4AWE, pp. 126–134 (2023)
75. Otten, S., Ziefle, M.: Exploring trust perceptions in the medical context: a qualitative approach to outlining determinants of trust in AAL technology. In: ICT4AWE, pp. 244–253 (2022)
76. Peine, A.: Technology and ageing—theoretical propositions from science and technology studies (STS). In: Neves, B.B., Vetere, F. (eds.) Ageing and Digital Technology, pp. 51–64. Springer (2019)
77. Penney, J.W.: Understanding chilling effects. Minn. Law Rev. **106**, 1451–1530 (2022)
78. Pinto, L., Nemorin, S.: Who is the boss? 'The elf on the shelf' and the normalization of surveillance. Canadian Centre for Policy Alternatives (2014). https://policyalternatives.ca/publications/commentary/whos-boss
79. Rantz, M.J., Alexander, G., Galambos, C., Flesner, M.K., Vogelsmeier, A., Hicks, L., Greenwald, L.: The use of bedside electronic medical record to improve quality of care in nursing facilities: a qualitative analysis. CIN: Comput. Inform. Nurs. **29**(3), 149–156 (2011). https://doi.org/10.1097/NCN.0b013e3181f9db79
80. Roberts, C., Mort, M.: Reshaping what counts as care: older people, work and new technologies. Alter **3**(2), 138–158 (2009). https://doi.org/10.1016/j.alter.2009.01.004
81. Roessler, B.J., Mokrosinska, D.: Social Dimensions of Privacy: Interdisciplinary Perspectives. Cambridge University Press (2015)
82. Sarı, L., Hasegawa-Johnson, M., Yoo, C.D.: Counterfactually fair automatic speech recognition. IEEE/ACM Trans. Audio, Speech, Lang. Process. **29**, 3515–3525 (2021)
83. Shaik, T., Tao, X., Higgins, N., Li, L., Gururajan, R., Zhou, X., Acharya, U.R.: Remote patient monitoring using artificial intelligence: current state, applications, and challenges. Wiley Interdiscipl Rev. Data Min. Knowl. Discov. **13**(2), e1485 (2023). https://doi.org/10.1002/widm.1485
84. Sharmila, C., Hameed, M.S.: Diaspora: exploring the use of affordances and mobile mediation among migrants' social connectedness. Migr. Lett. **20**(5), 122–144 (2023)
85. Solove, D.J., Schwartz, P.M.: Information Privacy Law. Aspen Publishing (2020)
86. Steele, R., Lo, A., Secombe, C., Wong, Y.K.: Elderly persons' perception and acceptance of using wireless sensor networks to assist healthcare. Int. J. Med. Inform. **78**(12), 788–801 (2009)
87. Steinke, F., Fritsch, T., Brem, D., Simonsen, S.: Requirement of AAL systems: older persons' trust in sensors and characteristics of AAL technologies. In: Proceedings of the 5th International Conference on Pervasive Technologies Related to Assistive Environments, PETRA'12. Association for Computing Machinery, New York, NY, USA (2012). https://doi.org/10.1145/2413097.2413116

88. Steinke, F., Fritsch, T., Silbermann, L.: Trust in ambient assisted living (AAL)-a systematic review of trust in automation and assistance systems. Int. J. Adv. Life Sci. **4**(3–4) (2012)
89. Steinke, F., Ingenhoff, A., Fritsch, T.: Personal remote assistance in ambient assisted living–experimental research of elderly people's trust and their intention to use. Int. J. Human-Comput. Interact. **30**(7), 560–574 (2014)
90. Strycharz, J., Segijn, C.M.: Chilling effects as a result of corporate surveillance in digital communication: a comparison between American and Dutch media users. Int. J. Commun. **18**, 320–343 (2023)
91. Strycharz, J., Segijn, C.M.: Ethical side-effect of dataveillance in advertising: impact of data collection, trust, privacy concerns and regulatory differences on chilling effects. J. Bus. Res. **173**, 114,490 (2024). https://doi.org/10.1016/j.jbusres.2023.114490
92. Tamò-Larrieux, A., Guitton, C., Mayer, S., Lutz, C.: Regulating for trust: can law establish trust in artificial intelligence? Regul. Gov. **18**(3), 780–801 (2024)
93. Tariq, M.U.: Advanced wearable medical devices and their role in transformative remote health monitoring. In: Transformative Approaches to Patient Literacy and Healthcare Innovation, pp. 308–326. IGI Global (2024)
94. Tellioglu, H.: Integrating ethics by design and co-design principles in the development of ambient assisted living technologies. In: Salah, A.A., Colonna, L., Florez-Revuelta, F. (eds.) Privacy-Aware Monitoring for Assisted Living. Springer, Cham (2025)
95. Tifferet, S.: Gender differences in privacy tendencies on social network sites: a meta-analysis. Comput. Hum. Behav. **93**, 1–12 (2019)
96. Van Dijck, J.: Datafication, dataism and dataveillance: big data between scientific paradigm and ideology. Surveill. Soc. **12**(2), 197–208 (2014)
97. Venkit, P.N., Wilson, S.: Identification of bias against people with disabilities in sentiment analysis and toxicity detection models. arXiv:2111.13259 (2021)
98. Walker, P., McClaran, N., Zheng, Z., Saxena, N., Gu, G.: BiasHacker: voice command disruption by exploiting speaker biases in automatic speech recognition. In: Proceedings of the 15th ACM Conference on Security and Privacy in Wireless and Mobile Networks, pp. 119–124 (2022)
99. Weck, M., Afanassieva, M.: Toward the adoption of digital assistive technology: factors affecting older people's initial trust formation. Telecommun. Policy **47**(2), 102,483 (2023)
100. Wilkowska, W., Offermann-van Heek, J., Florez-Revuelta, F., Ziefle, M.: Video cameras for lifelogging at home: preferred visualization modes, acceptance, and privacy perceptions among german and turkish participants. Int. J. Human-Comput. Interact. **37**(15), 1436–1454 (2021)
101. Wilkowska, W., Otten, S., Maidhof, C., Ziefle, M.: Trust conditions and privacy perceptions in the acceptance of ambient technologies for health-related purposes. Int. J. Human–Comput. Interact. 1–16 (2023)
102. Yusif, S., Soar, J., Hafeez-Baig, A.: Older people, assistive technologies, and the barriers to adoption: a systematic review. Int. J. Med. Inform. **94**, 112–116 (2016). https://doi.org/10.1016/j.ijmedinf.2016.07.004
103. Zuboff, S.: The Age of Surveillance Capitalism: The Fight for a Human Future at the New Frontier of Power. Profile Books (2019)

Open Access This chapter is licensed under the terms of the Creative Commons Attribution 4.0 International License (http://creativecommons.org/licenses/by/4.0/), which permits use, sharing, adaptation, distribution and reproduction in any medium or format, as long as you give appropriate credit to the original author(s) and the source, provide a link to the Creative Commons license and indicate if changes were made.

The images or other third party material in this chapter are included in the chapter's Creative Commons license, unless indicated otherwise in a credit line to the material. If material is not included in the chapter's Creative Commons license and your intended use is not permitted by statutory regulation or exceeds the permitted use, you will need to obtain permission directly from the copyright holder.

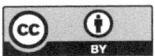

Chapter 14
Integrating Ethics by Design and Co-design Principles in the Development of Ambient Assisted Living Technologies

Hilda Tellioğlu

Abstract This chapter synthesizes the integration of ethics by design and co-design methodologies in the development of Ambient Assisted Living (AAL) technologies, addressing the ethical challenges posed by these innovations. After showing several notions of design and ethics, it underscores the necessity of embedding ethical considerations within the design phase of technology development and engaging stakeholders through co-design to align these technologies with users' needs and ethical values. It attempts to systematize the considerations in an initial framework of integration of ethics into design practice.

Keywords Ambient assisted living (AAL) · Design · Co-design · Ethics · Co-creation · Stakeholder engagement

14.1 Introduction

The advent of Ambient Assisted Living (AAL) technologies represents a significant evolution in the pursuit of enhancing the quality of life for older adults and individuals with disabilities. These technologies, designed to provide support, assistance, and monitoring within the living environment, promise not only to extend the time people can live in their preferred setting by increasing their autonomy and safety but also to alleviate the societal and economic burdens posed by ageing populations worldwide [9]. However, as with many technological advancements, the integration of AAL systems into daily life introduces a spectrum of ethical considerations that must be carefully navigated to ensure that these innovations serve to empower rather than diminish the dignity and rights of their users [7].

The growing need for AAL systems is underscored by demographic shifts towards older populations, with projections indicating that the global population aged 65

H. Tellioğlu (✉)
Faculty of Informatics, TU Wien, Vienna, Austria
e-mail: hilda.tellioglu@tuwien.ac.at

© The Author(s) 2025
A. A. Salah et al. (eds.), *Privacy-Aware Monitoring for Assisted Living*,
Intelligent Systems Reference Library 270,
https://doi.org/10.1007/978-3-031-84158-3_14

and over will double by 2050 [21]. This demographic transition is accompanied by an increased prevalence of chronic conditions, mobility issues, and cognitive impairments, highlighting the critical role of AAL technologies in supporting ageing-in-place strategies. Moreover, the COVID-19 pandemic has further accentuated the importance of such technologies in enabling remote care and reducing the strain on healthcare facilities [10].

Yet, the deployment of AAL technologies raises significant ethical concerns, notably regarding privacy, autonomy, consent, and the risk of social isolation. Privacy concerns emerge from the continuous monitoring inherent in many AAL systems, raising questions about who has access to sensitive data and how it is used [6]. Autonomy and consent are challenged by technologies that make decisions on behalf of users or limit their freedom under the guise of safety [18]. Furthermore, the substitution of human care with technological solutions risks exacerbating social isolation among older adults, a group already vulnerable to loneliness [14].

Addressing these ethical challenges necessitates a thoughtful integration of ethical considerations into the design and deployment of AAL systems. This paper posits that ethics by design and co-design methodologies offer robust frameworks for embedding ethical principles into the fabric of AAL technologies. Ethics by design involves the proactive incorporation of ethical considerations at each stage of the technology design process, ensuring that ethical safeguards are built into AAL systems from the outset [8]. Co-design, involving stakeholders—particularly end-users—in the design process, ensures that AAL technologies are not only ethically sound but also aligned with the needs, preferences, and values of those they intend to serve [22].

The literature already establishes the role of co-design in ethical technology development. A number of studies have pointed out how this approach offers very specific benefits for increasing technology acceptance, usability, and ethical conformism. For instance, [11] discusses how co-design may involve ethical dimensions—say, privacy and autonomy—in digital health technologies.

While the literature on ethics by design and, in particular, co-design methodologies is increasingly available, some gaps remain. First, there is a need for more empirical research on how ethics by design principles are applied in AAL system development. Again, while the theoretical frameworks are very well-articulated, case studies and applications that describe the practical application within the domain of AAL are limited. Second, much of the earlier literature on co-design has been strongly focused on process, and relatively little on how such co-design practices actually address ethical concerns explicitly in technology development. Last but not least, only a few studies have focused on the intersection of ethics by design and co-design methodologies. Of central interest for future research is how these approaches can synergistically be applied within an AAL systems context.

Gaps of this kind will be addressed in the paper by putting forward a research perspective based on the application of ethics by design and co-design methodologies in the development of AAL systems. The paper has two objectives: the analysis of ethical concerns with AAL technologies and the delineation of a comprehensive framework that would serve all needs in meeting the challenges; to shed some light on how ethics by design and co-design can be operationalized in the process of AAL system development. In particular, the objective of this paper is to contribute to the debate on the ethical development of technologies by synthesizing and analyzing the literature for delivery concerning sets of points that are actionable by researchers, designers, and policymakers involved in creating AAL technologies and actually putting them into practice. Firstly, it identifies terms, notions, and (design) approaches connected to the ethical design of AAL technologies. Secondly, it relates properties of ethical aspects into the identified terms, notions, and approaches to emphasize the ways of dealing with ethical requirements in systems design and development, especially by considering AAL technologies.

14.2 Research Setting

Before presenting and discussing the framework for integrating ethical values into co-design practices, it's crucial to first define key concepts such as ethical values, co-design, and integration. A foundational understanding of these terms is essential to create the setting for the considerations. This semantic groundwork will enable a better understanding of how to effectively embed ethical values into the co-design practices, especially from a cooperation perspective.

14.2.1 Ambient Assisted Technologies

Ambient Assisted Technologies (AAT) refer to systems and devices integrated into living environments that are targeted for care recipients, especially older adults and those living with disabilities [5]. Such technologies aim at enhancing an intelligent, adaptive, and responsive environment for quality of life, independent living, and safety and well-being.

Smart home AATs are generally integrated with automated lighting and climate control technologies, to security systems. These help create a living environment that is both comfortable for the user and secure [4]. *Health monitoring technologies* often incorporate sensors and wearables that monitor proven health parameters, e.g., heart rate, blood pressure, glucose levels, etc. Continuous monitoring allows potential health-related problems to be caught early and an intervention applied on time if necessary [13]. AAT encompasses a range of *assistive devices* that are used to help in mobility, communication, and daily activities, such as smart wheelchairs, voice-activated personal assistants, or automated medication dispensers [16]. Special to most AAT systems, there is a *rescue operation* having some features like fall detection and automatic alert systems, which, on sensing any emergency, produce vibrations to warn guardians or even the related responsible department. AAT uses *context-aware computing* to adapt to the needs and preferences of an individual in real time. The systems use the afforded data, including that on the environment and the user, in making personalized assistance and giving recommendations [1]. This adaptation of features in AAT would hence, help in the overall development of autonomy and safety status of the individual, hence improving the quality of life.

14.2.2 Co-design Practices

Another key issue that needs to be introduced is the term participatory design or co-design practice, defined as a collaborative process in which the end-users, the designers, and any other concerned actor participate in the making of design and development of products, services, or systems. The approach applies to the consideration and solution created jointly so that the result will match the actual needs and preferences of the user. The core objective of this kind of approach is that the co-designed results become more effective, user-centred, and innovative through collaboration and shared decision-making among stakeholders.

The generic process of collaborative designing with requirements among the actors in ensuring success can be described as follows (see Fig. 14.1): The initiation and alignment, which will have a clear objective setting and role and responsibilities definition; research and exploration as information sourcing and collective share and synthesis; ideation and conceptualization, by use of a brainstorming and co-creation workshop; prototyping and testing through the development of prototypes with iterative feedback. This follows the finalization of design and refinishing of development, which follows the assessment of the outcomes and planning of how best to improve in the future.

In design collaborations with vulnerable groups, the described collaboration situation is a little bit more challenging. Even if one can argue that the collaboration with end users should happen on an equal footing, if the end users are people with special mental or physical needs, designers have to consider several collaboration aspects and to prepare the base for a smoother and easier cooperation.

The key to co-design practices is *stakeholder engagement* which encourages a wide range of parameters to be included in the co-design, including end-users, who provide valuable insights into their needs and experiences, together with other relevant parties, like designers, developers, and domain experts [17]. Normally, co-design is an *iterative process* that allows multiple cycles of prototyping, testing,

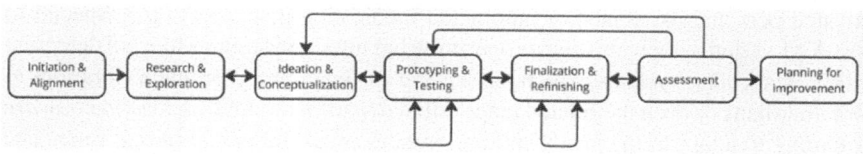

Fig. 14.1 The process of collaborative design

and obtaining feedback. Through an iterative approach, therefore, it becomes certain that design will evolve through continuous input and refinement into stronger and much more user-friendly solutions [2]. Co-Design practices call for *empathy* with a deep *understanding* of user contexts, challenges, and aspirations. Techniques like user interviews, ethnographic studies, and empathy mapping are regular means through which an understanding of the lives of the users is gained to set the design course [19]. Effective co-designing relies on *collaboration* and *co-creation*, making it most successful when stakeholders are actively involved in generating ideas, solving problems, and making decisions together. Workshops, co-creation sessions, and collaborative prototyping are typical means used to ease the collaborative process taking place [23]. Involvement of stakeholders in an actual design process empowers them to feel *ownership* of the outcome. That *empowerment* is bound to increase acceptance, adoption, and satisfaction of the designed solutions.

The fundamental notion behind co-design, co-production, and co-creation is that of involving stakeholders through collaborative design in products, services, or systems. Though these three terms have often been used and interchanged, one could say that this hides aspects making them quite different from each other, thus giving a more complex meaning to the conceptualization of practices of participation in design and innovation.

Co-design refers to the integration of end-users and other stakeholders in the process of designing. The purpose of the process is to make sure that the end product is as near as possible to what the user needs and prefers in a way that involves people bringing many perspectives and expertise from all participants to yield results that are more centred on users and innovative [17]. Throughout the co-designing process, there should be iterations of prototyping and testing, and feedback can be gained for continuous improvement and making it easier to revise the work one has done on the new design [2].

Co-design methodologies are major guarantees of the inclusiveness and effectiveness of AAL technologies' development. This methodology ensures that technologies developed by relying on it would not only be technically rigorous but also ethically sensitive, oriented to the needs of their end-users, with an inclusive spectrum of stakeholders: end-users, caregivers, and healthcare professionals. [17] argue for this participatory approach and underline its role in the creation of solutions deeply informed by those they are meant to serve. According to [20] co-designing is supposed to ensure an inclusive, ethically attuned technology development process. In any case, this will protect autonomy, independence, privacy, and safety—high-stake factors—and underpin due process amidst attacks on some very basic principles of human dignity.

An important example concerning the real effectiveness of co-design is represented by a project aimed at engaging patients with dementia, informal caregivers, and healthcare professionals in developing an AAL system targeted at promoting users' independence while ensuring their safety. This collaboration resulted in a system not only addressing practical needs but also linking these to ethical principles. In essence, this highlights the profound potential of co-design to bridge the gap between technological innovation and ethical considerations. The case epitomizes how co-design can work in achieving the alignment of AAL technologies with nuanced users' needs and ethical concerns and can serve as a model for further technology development efforts that target sensitive and complex care environments.

Co-production extends the principles of co-design beyond the design phase into the complete lifecycle of a product or service. This includes not only the creation but also the delivery and evaluation stages. The central emphasis behind co-production lies in shared responsibility between service providers and users leading to partnership, which in turn enhances the relevance and effectiveness of service [3]. This orientation is especially strong in public services and healthcare, where outcomes can be substantially improved with user engagement.

Co-creation is a more elaborate concept wherein stakeholders work together to generate value through the joint development process. It means making use of co-design, co-production, and another level deeper to co-create new insights, solutions, and experiences. Co-creation is aimed at the creation of mutual value through collaboration—a collective exchange of creativity and input from the very compilation of ideas to the final realization process.

In reality, these concepts are intertwined because they emphasize active and collaborative engagement with stakeholders. The three approaches are very important for the engagement of many stakeholders, cutting across the end users and designers, among others. This ensures that a wide range of ideas is brought to bear for more holistic and effective solutions [17]. Co-design, co-production, and co-creation can be described as an iterative and collaborative process. The methods rely on systematic feedback and improvement in a manner that the outcomes are always up-to-date in relation to the needs and preferences of the stakeholders at the point of delivery [2]. While co-designing addresses the design phase and co-production the delivery phase, co-creation reflects the entirety of the value generation spectrum. It is holistic in the sense that stakeholder input and collaboration should benefit all stages of development [15]. Involvement in the design, production, and creation processes by the stakeholders directly places them in a situation involving empowerment and ownership of the final product. Acceptance, adoption, and satisfaction with whatever is finally being implemented are further raised with empowerment.

14.2.3 Example PHOBILITYaktiv

PHOBILITYaktiv was a research project between 2018 and 2020. In the following, such co-design practices should be illustrated to create a concrete context for the approaches described.

An open traffic system, enabling equal mobility to all social groups is a fundamental prerequisite of democratic societies. The preceding project, PHOBILITY (FFG project number 849032), investigated the traffic participation of road users who suffered from fears, compulsory disorders, or phobias for the first time. Research estimated that the lifetime prevalence of persons among the population who suffer

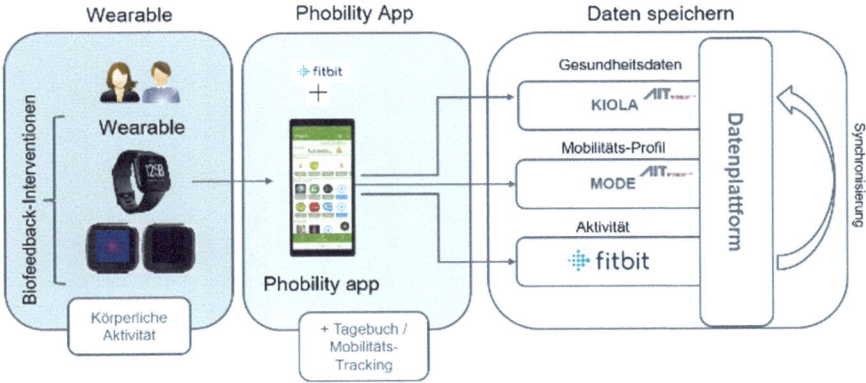

Fig. 14.2 The system architecture of the PHOBILITYaktiv system developed in the project

from fears, phobias, and compulsory disorders was 10–25%. Situational conditions, psychic barriers, and lack of information made persons affected believe that they are unable to control the routine situations of their daily lives. A precondition of full traffic participation was the ability to control fears that are related to this situation to a sufficient degree. In the worst case, affected persons withdraw completely from social and occupational life. These persons themselves, as well as traffic- and health experts, reported that one of the most important supportive measures are tools for self-distraction, self-calming, and self-manipulation, as well as information for traveling and planning trips. These tools help reduce anxieties if they are combined with therapeutic principles. Knowledge derived from the PHOBILITY project was the basis for its successor, PHOBILITYaktiv which aimed at developing and testing these solutions.

The aim of PHOBILITYaktiv was to enable equal mobility for persons who suffer from anxieties, phobias, and compulsory disorders which also implied equal participation in social life. It helped them to regain and maintain their usual forms of mobility and their active participation in public transport as long as possible. In order to achieve this aim, recent developments in the field of mental health apps and cognitive therapy have been combined (see Fig. 14.2).

Figure 14.3 shows some illustrations of the Phobility App[1] we have designed and developed together with the users.

---

[1] https://apkcombo.com/phobility-aktiv/at.ac.ait.phobility/, Accessed 25 September 2024.

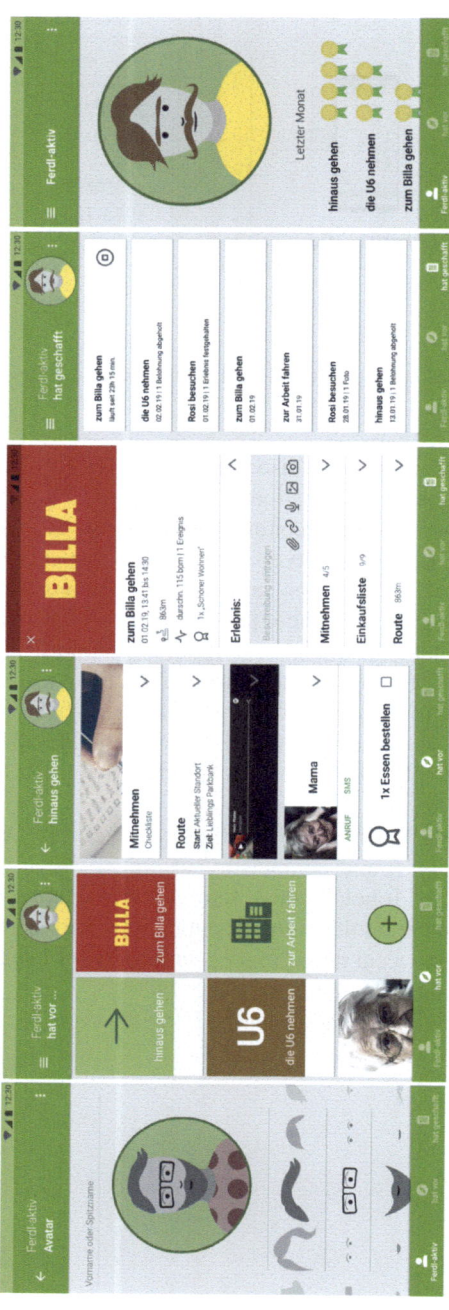

Fig. 14.3 Illustrations of the Phobility App developed collaboratively with the end users in the project

14.2.4 Ethics by Design

The inclusion of ethical considerations at the design stage in AAL technologies is paramount if such innovations can respond to the challenges of sustaining autonomy, privacy, dignity, and well-being. For instance, an "ethics by design" approach for AAL multidimensionally means a strategy to have technologies align with ethical principles right from the outset. Such an approach gives a theoretical underpinning of ethics by design in AAL technologies and applies principles of ethics, given concrete case studies successfully implemented.

Ethics by design in AAL technologies entails that, at every respective stage of their development life cycle, from ideation through deployment and beyond, ethical reflection should be integrated. The approach should include anticipatory ethics, the identification of possible or retrospective moral issues prior to their emergence, and the setting of mechanisms of prevention or mitigation of the said issues. This also emphasizes that ongoing ethical reflection and modification should accompany the development of the technology over time, such that the ethical standards are fitting to the value of society and the necessities of vulnerable populations. Proactive ethical engagement is, therefore, much more than a mere trust-building activity; it also intensifies the general impact and acceptability of AAL technologies.

Applied ethical principles relevant to AAL include respect for autonomy, beneficence, non-maleficence, and justice. Respect for autonomy guides that AAL technologies secure the potential of users to make informed decisions regarding themselves. Beneficence demands that these technologies guarantee improvements in the well-being of users while bringing minimal harm—that is, non-maleficence. Finally, justice means equal opportunities within different population groups to enjoy the benefits secured by AAL technologies. These ethical principles can be anchored within the design phase by various strategies, such as stakeholder engagement, ethical impact assessment, and iterative evaluation of the technology in a real-world setting. The end-user engagement, to be more precise, stakeholder engagement, would be very important in understanding the values of all those interacting with the AAL system and all its needs and concerns identified therein.

Ethical impact assessments are tools for reviewing in a reasoned way the possible ethical implications of AAL technologies and providing guidelines about design decisions in line with ethical principles. Iterative evaluation provides repeated assessment of the ethical implications of technology in development and deployment, thus keeping pace with emerging ethical challenges.

The "ethics by design" framework is pivotal for embedding ethical principles—respect for autonomy, beneficence, non-maleficence, and justice—within the lifecycle of AAL technologies [8]. It anticipates ethical issues, advocating for their early identification and integration into design solutions, thereby promoting technologies that respect users' dignity and rights. This approach is illustrated through case studies, such as the incorporation of privacy-enhancing technologies in health monitoring systems, showcasing the method's effectiveness in addressing privacy and autonomy concerns [24].

14.3 Ethical AAL Technologies

Co-designing is a participative strategy in which all stakeholders related to the process are actively involved in the development of technology. They include the end-user, care-givers, professionals, and members of the community. This collaborative approach is of added importance within the sphere of AAL technologies, in which design outcomes must be aligned with ethical values, needs, and user preferences. Co-design practice in AAL technologies can address ethical concerns. Indeed, only those systems that are user-centred, respect citizens' rights and dignity, and are context-aware will be considered.

The ethical imperatives with regards to a stakeholders' involvement in the design of AAL technologies are part of, among others, respect for autonomy, beneficence, non-maleficence, and justice. Co-design methodologies operationalize these ethical principles within an inclusive environment wherein stakeholders' voices are heard and acknowledged for their contribution. In this way, AAL technologies will not only be technically feasible but also socially accepted and ethically justifiable.

Co-designing enhances respect for autonomy by giving end-users the possibility to articulate their needs and preferences and influence the functionality and usability of AAL systems. It represents a form of empowerment that underpins the independence and self-determination of any person concerned with ethics in technologies for AAL. Beneficence and non-maleficence are addressed by making sure that the design process is active in seeking to maximize gains while minimizing potential harms—for instance, privacy breaches or undue reliance on technology—by prioritizing user well-being. Lastly, justice is rendered by the inclusive co-design approach, whereby it was taken to see an equal distribution of access to technological gains by different categories of users, hence, bridging disparities in the adoption and outcomes of technology [25].

Figure 14.4 shows the interrelationship of stakeholder management to design practice in a collaboration framework, which consists of co-design, co-production, and co-creation practices, by emphasizing the relation to a potential outcome of "ethical AAL technologies". On the one side, it shows the design practice; on the other, the outcome. Stakeholder management has an impact on the ways of shaping and carrying out the design and development of technologies. The design process has to be seen as a whole containing implementation methods of ideas and strategies developed through collaborative efforts.

Three key processes—co-design, co-production, and co-creation—are bridges between stakeholder management and design practice. Co-design takes place at the very early stages of a project, involving stakeholders in design conceptualization. Co-production involves stakeholders during creation and development to ensure that their input finds its shape in the final outcome. Co-creation shows continuous collaboration between stakeholders and designers throughout the project for an ongoing partnership.

The activity "(qualitative) evaluation and update" from the right-hand side of the illustration to the left part tells that the process and its outcome are under constant appraisal. In other words, the project remains flexible and open to stakeholder requirements and feedback in this repetitive cycle of evaluation. Thus, one could say that the illustration depicts a spiral-like approach where stakeholder management and design practice are very closely connected and nurtured by constant evaluation and improvement.

Figure 14.4 expresses the junction between ethics and the emerging field of AAL technologies. It brings an important message: that progress in the area of AAL technologies, designed for supporting vulnerable populations such as older adults or disabled persons, must proceed with a stringent ethical framework. This is not a wish but an exigency if these technologies are to develop in a responsible manner.

AAL technologies must be able to go beyond their technical functionality. Although the innovation in the domain of AAL is focused/targeted on increasing quality of life and easing independence and safety, without an ethical commitment, these benefits could not be realized. Thus, the illustration indicates that ethics should inform from the very beginning, right through deployment and realisation.

The ethical framework highlighted by the figure emphasizes some important elements, such as consent: users should be free to make informed decisions about engaging with AAL technologies. Further, data protection is essential because personal and sensitive information captured through these technologies should be handled safely and not exploited. It respects the autonomy of the user in the centre, acknowledging that although these technologies aid, they need not harm the control by users on their lives. Transparency in how these technologies work and their effects on users comes next in importance, allowing for trust to be built between developers, users, and caregivers.

Figure 14.4 also highlights the wider social dimensions of AAL technologies. The more integrated such tools are to be within the lives of users, the greater will be their bearing on societal norms and structures beyond individual interactions. Ethical AAL technologies should, therefore, add to the common good by diminishing inequalities and increasing inclusiveness; otherwise, they might exaggerate existing disparities.

Essentially, Fig. 14.4 presents the guide and serves as a caution simultaneously. This requires strengthening the call for AAL research and development to be carried out within an ethical frame, with advanced yet fair, equitable, and values-based innovations toward human dignity and respect. In this regard, ethical underpinning is very important to make sure that technologies belonging to AAL genuinely uplift human life, more particularly those who are vulnerable without affecting their fundamental rights. It thus serves as a graphic manifesto for an ethical stewardship of technology at the service of humanity.

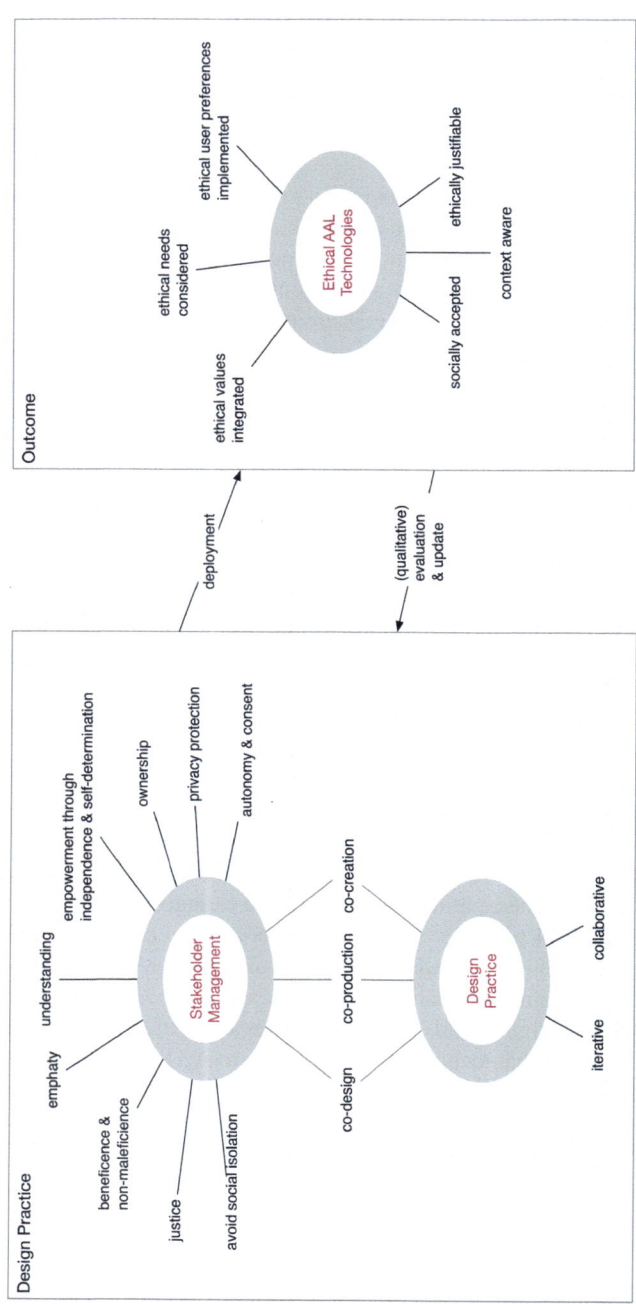

Fig. 14.4 Research and design aspects to consider while developing ethical AAL technologies

14.4 Discussion

The findings from the literature review affirm that ethics by design and co-design can significantly mitigate ethical concerns in AAL technologies. These methodologies enhance ethical alignment and user acceptance and address critical issues such as privacy, autonomy, independence, and social inclusion (also see [12] in this volume). However, challenges such as the complexity of ethical decision-making, unequal stakeholder participation, and resource constraints necessitate further research and innovative solutions [22].

Ethics by design and co-designing methodologies give very strong tools for answering ethical issues arising in the development of AAL technologies. These methods contribute to raising ethical consistency in AAL systems and improving their social acceptance through the specific embedding of ethical considerations within the designing process and involving all relevant stakeholders in meaningful cooperation. Indeed, there are several challenges and limitations connected with ethics by design and co-designing approaches that underline the necessity of further research and development in this field. Such challenges will be overcome by new solutions to ethical decision-making, stakeholder involvement, and resource distribution. Commitment to ethics by design and co-design in further development within the area of AAL technologies will ensure that such technologies, in their developments and applications, increase the quality of life for users in an ethically responsible manner.

While ethics by design and co-design add advantages in the mitigation of ethical issues within AAL technologies, there exist challenges and limitations to their implementation. One such kind of grand challenge is the complexity characterizing the ethical decision-making for technology design, often marked by conflicting values and interests. For example, finding an adequate equilibrium between the highest level of privacy and the benefits of monitoring and intervention in AAL systems is challenging and has to consider severe ethical principles and the urgent perspectives of stakeholders.

A further challenge is related to uneven participation in co-design processes. Ensuring that all stakeholders, in particular those with any kind of cognitive impairment or other vulnerabilities, can meaningfully contribute to the design process lies at the heart of ethical integrity for co-design. Optimizing the likelihood of this happening can be very challenging and requires specialized knowledge and resources to facilitate inclusive and accessible co-design activities. There are several ways to address this challenge:

Open communication about the issues of design is important to provide effective channels and regular schedules for communication to ensure everyone is updated and misunderstandings are minimized. In the case of cooperation with a vulnerable group, the ways of open communication need to be considered each time carefully in order not to promise too much about the features or possibilities in interaction with the system-in-development.

A successful collaboration is based on the trust vested in the abilities and inputs of each of the collaborators and respect for their differing perspectives and expertise.

One can, in a manner either consciously or unconsciously, underestimate the abilities and inputs of participants with disabilities. This will not be due to a scrutiny of the actual abilities and capabilities but a preconceived notion of their limitations. For example, they could communicate in a different way. For instance, one is bound to meet a participant who has a cognitive disability that is unable to articulate ideas in usual ways, a participant who has a speech impairment that is not understandable during spoken conversations, among others, and other communication variations that can constrict views. The last group of people may not express or have their views supported well. Disabled participants can be perceived differently and can be treated in a certain way by other team members. The stigma of biases related to disabilities can reflect how other team members perceive and act toward the disabled participants. It can create a feeling of disesteem or lower self-confidence in professional capabilities.

A shared vision and mutual goals permit a common view of what the project is supposed to achieve and are therefore used to direct all the effort toward these common goals. The format and language for these visions and goals may differ. All these translations must ferret out concerns being expressed by participants on some matter or value, out of which an effective design solution could be derived for system design. This might take some time, but the result is very worthwhile.

Working with people with special needs requires an appreciation of different opinions and backgrounds in a bid to foster creativity and innovation. There are several challenges to the appreciation of such diversity. It is often challenging to ensure proper integration of the different insights due to the possible barriers in communication, accessibility, and under-representation. Such challenges would work against a group benefiting fully from unique perspectives that enhance creative outcomes.

Moreover, ethics by design and co-design are time-consuming, expertise- and money-demanding activities. This makes them a barrier to their uptake, mostly in small-scale or low-capacity projects and organizations. If technology continues changing dynamically with society, so will the ethical concerns raised over time, therefore requiring continued follow-up on ethics begun during the initial designing phase of such works.

14.5 Conclusions

This research shows that technology-competent, ethical-responsible, and user-centred AAL is only feasible through ethics-by-designing and co-designed technologies. Participatory design by diverse stakeholders is a way through which the AAL technologies can be made ready to answer, in a more appropriate way, the complex needs and ethical considerations of users, which can then enhance their independence, safety, and quality of life. The findings point to further research related to the application and outcomes of these methodologies. There is an exhortation to embrace these approaches in the design/approach practice to ensure ethical innovation in AAL technology development. Future research requires full-scale empirical studies to document whether these methodologies are effective and to find strategies for overcoming the difficulty of implementation while reviewing the evolving ethical considerations in response to new technological and social changes.

Acknowledgements The project PHOBILITYAktiv described in this paper is supported by the Austrian Research Promotion Agency (FFG) in the name of Federal Ministry Republic of Austria, Climate Action, Environment, Energy, Mobility, Innovation and Technology (BMVIT). This publication is based upon work from COST Action GoodBrother—Network on Privacy-Aware Audio- and Video-Based Applications for Active and Assisted Living (CA19121), supported by COST (European Cooperation in Science and Technology).

References

1. Augusto, J., McCullagh, P.: Ambient intelligence: concepts and applications. Int. J. Comput. Sci. Inf. Syst. **4**(1), 1–28 (2007)
2. Björgvinsson, E., Ehn, P., Hillgren, P.A.: Design things and design thinking: contemporary participatory design challenges. Des. Issues **28**, 101–116 (2012)
3. Bovaird, T.: Beyond engagement and participation: user and community coproduction of public services. Public Adm. Rev. **67**, 846–860 (2007)
4. Chan, R., Shum, D., Toulopoulou, T., Chen, E.: Assessment of executive functions: review of instruments and identification of critical issues. Arch. Clin. Neuropsychol. Off. J. Natl. Acad. Neuropsychol. **23**, 201–16 (2008)
5. Cicirelli, G., Marani, R., Petitti, A., Milella, A., D'Orazio, T.: Ambient assisted living: a review of technologies, methodologies and future perspectives for healthy aging of population. Sensors (Basel) **21**(10), 3549 (2021). https://doi.org/10.3390/s21103549
6. Essén, A.: The two facets of electronic care surveillance: an exploration of the views of older people who live with monitoring devices. Soc. Sci. Med. **67**(1), 128–136 (2008)
7. Floridi, L., Sanders, J.W.: On the morality of artificial agents. Mind. Mach. **14**, 349–379 (2004)
8. Friedman, B., Kahn, P.H., Borning, A.: Value sensitive design and information systems. In: Zhang, P., Galletta, D. (eds.) Human-Computer Interaction and Management Information Systems: Foundations, pp. 348–372. M.E. Sharpe (2008)
9. van Hoof, J., Demiris, G., Wouters, E.J.M.: Handbook of Smart Homes, Health Care and Well-Being. Springer International Publishing, Cham, Switzerland (2017)
10. Ienca, M., Fabrice, J., Elger, B., Caon, M., Scoccia Pappagallo, A., Kressig, R.W., Wangmo, T.: Intelligent assistive technology for Alzheimer's disease and other dementias: a systematic review. J. Alzheimers Dis. **65**(2), 455–484 (2020)
11. Lindsay, S., Jackson, D., Schofield, G., Olivier, P.: Engaging older people using participatory design. In: Proceedings of the SIGCHI Conference on Human Factors in Computing Systems, pp. 1199–1208 (2012)
12. Lutz, C., Miguel, C., Mujirishvili, T., Perez-Vega, R., Fedosov, A.: Social and societal issues in AAL. In: Salah, A.A., Colonna, L., Florez-Revuelta, F. (eds.) Privacy-Aware Monitoring for Assisted Living. Springer, Cham (2025)
13. Marschollek, M., Gietzelt, M., Schulze, M., Kohlmann, M., Song, B., Wolf, K.H.: Wearable sensors in healthcare and sensor-enhanced health information systems: all our tomorrows? Healthc. Informat. Res. **18**, 97–104 (2012)
14. Oinas-Kukkonen, H., Harjumaa, M.: Persuasive systems design: key issues, process model, and system features. Commun. Assoc. Inf. Syst. **24** (2009)
15. Prahalad, C., Ramaswamy, V.: Co-creation experiences: the next practice in value creation. J. Interact. Mark. **18**(3), 5–14 (2004)

16. Rashidi, P., Mihailidis, A.: A survey on ambient-assisted living tools for older adults. IEEE J. Biomed. Health Inform. **17**(3), 579–590 (2013)
17. Sanders, E.B.N., Stappers, P.J.: Co-creation and the new landscapes of design. CoDesign **4**(1), 5–18 (2008)
18. Spiekermann, S., Pallas, F.: Technology paternalism—wider implications of ubiquitous computing. Poiesis Prax. **4**(1), 6–18 (2006)
19. Steen, M., Manschot, M., De Koning, N.: Benefits of co-design in service design projects. Int. J. Des. **5**(2), 53–60 (2011)
20. Tellioğlu, H.: User-centered design. In: Xiang, Z., Fuchs, M., Gretzel, U., Höpken, W. (eds.) Handbook of e-Tourism. Springer, Cham (2022)
21. United Nations: World Population Prospects, The 2019 Revision - Volume I: Comprehensive Tables. United Nations (2019)
22. Vines, J., Clarke, R., Wright, P., McCarthy, J., Olivier, P.: Configuring participation: on how we involve people in design. In: Proceedings of the SIGCHI Conference on Human Factors in Computing Systems, pp. 429–438. ACM (2013)
23. Visser, F.S., Stappers, P.J., van der Lugt, R., Sanders, E.B.N.: Contextmapping: experiences from practice. CoDesign **1**(2), 119–149 (2005)
24. Ziefle, M., Röcker, C., Holzinger, A.: Medical technology in smart homes: exploring the user's perspective on privacy, intimacy, and trust. In: Proceedings of the 7th International Conference on Smart Homes and Health Telematics, pp. 312–319 (2011)
25. Zwijsen, S.A., Niemeijer, A.R., Hertogh, C.M.P.M.: Ethics of using assistive technology in the care for community-dwelling elderly people: an overview of the literature. Aging Mental Health **15**(4), 419–427 (2011)

Open Access This chapter is licensed under the terms of the Creative Commons Attribution 4.0 International License (http://creativecommons.org/licenses/by/4.0/), which permits use, sharing, adaptation, distribution and reproduction in any medium or format, as long as you give appropriate credit to the original author(s) and the source, provide a link to the Creative Commons license and indicate if changes were made.

The images or other third party material in this chapter are included in the chapter's Creative Commons license, unless indicated otherwise in a credit line to the material. If material is not included in the chapter's Creative Commons license and your intended use is not permitted by statutory regulation or exceeds the permitted use, you will need to obtain permission directly from the copyright holder.

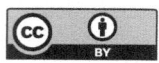

Index

Symbols
0-day exploit, 115

A
AAL Products Catalogue, 10, 13
Acceptance of assistive technology, 316
Accumulation of deficits, 160
Acoustic event detection, 197
Acoustic scene classification, 197
Action spotting, 202
Active sensors, 195
Activities of Daily Living (ADL), 17, 188, 224
Advanced Encryption Algorithm (AES), 110

Affine invariance, 193
AI Act, 174, 240, 249, 250, 324
Alarm fatigue, 61, 149, 204
Alzheimer's Disease (AD), 167, 168
Ambient Assisted Technologies (AAT), 335

Ambient intelligence, 8
Amyotrophic Lateral Sclerosis (ALS), 171
Anonymization, 306
Anthropomorphism, 261
Anxiety, 339
Artificial Intelligence of Things (AIoT), 103, 104
Assistive devices, 335
Augmented Reality, 293
Authorization, 123
Automated individual decision making, 298

Automatic Speech Recognition (ASR), 266, 267, 317

Autonomy, 334
Avatars, 260

B
Balanced accuracy, 56
Bayes' Theorem, 31
Beamforming, 86
Bias, 172, 226, 295, 316, 317, 323, 346
  ageism, 317, 320, 323
  audio systems, 317
  demographic, 142, 316, 317
  linguistic, 323
  majority class, 65, 244, 297
  mitigation, 49
  socioeconomic, 317
  training data, 297
Biometric data, 148, 168, 174, 230, 250, 300

  gait, 156, 167–170, 175
Black-box medicine, 297
Black box models, 33
BlindSpot system, 88
Body skeleton, 193
Bucinator, 145

C
Camera
  depth, 192
  infrared, 140, 144, 148
  near-infrared, 192, 221, 227
  omni-directional, 19, 144
  RGB-D, 169
  security camera, 294
  thermal, 142, 221, 231

© The Editor(s) (if applicable) and The Author(s) 2025
A. A. Salah et al. (eds.), *Privacy-Aware Monitoring for Assisted Living*,
Intelligent Systems Reference Library 270,
https://doi.org/10.1007/978-3-031-84158-3

visible light, 191, 221
wearable, 148
Canadian Community Health Survey, 134
Cardiovascular Health Study (CHS), 161
Care work, 321
Chatbots, 260
Checksum, 109
Chilling effects, 319
Circumplex model, 241
Cloud computing, 102
Co-creation, 338
Co-design, 334, 336, 337
Cognitive disability, 346
Cognitive games, 164
CogvisAI system, 140, 149
Cohen's kappa, 163
Cold mirror, 148
Comprehensive Geriatric Assessment (CGA), 160, 162
Confusion matrix, 56
Context-aware computing, 335
Co-production, 338
COVID-19 pandemic, 228
Cross-validation, 48
Crypto API, 116
Cryptographic key, 101
Cyber Resilience Act (CRA), 122

D
Dark patterns, 80
Data
  anonymization, 100
  augmentation, 232
  authenticity, 100
  availability, 100, 101
  confidentiality, 100, 101, 123
  controllers, 299–301, 304, 305
  encryption, 306
  heart sound datasets, 228
  imputation, 49
  integrity, 100, 105, 109
  joint-controllers, 305
  leakage, 111
  management, 280
  meta data, 305
  minimization, 123, 280
  non-repudiation, 105
  obfuscation, 82, 158, 175
  portability, 123
  protection, 100, 102, 104, 105, 176, 230, 231, 280, 292, 343
  respiratory sound datasets, 227
  security, 105
  video datasets, 226
Data protection by design, 292
Data protection impact assessment, 299
Dataveillance, 315, 318
Dementia, 279, 282, 320
Demographic parity, 248
Denial of Service (DoS), 101, 124
Design practice, 343
Differential privacy, 68, 82
Digital Operation Resilience Act (DORA), 122
Digital signature, 108
Dimensioning, 104
Discrete Wavelet Transform (DWT), 196
Disentanglement, 82, 85
Distributive justice, 281
Doppler sensors, 137
Doppler signature, 35
Dual obfuscation, 175
Dynamic consent, 279
Dysarthria, 266

E
EarBit system, 198
Ecological Momentary Assessment (EMA), 156, 171
Edge computing, 11, 104
Egocentric vision, 26
Egovision, *see* First-person video (FPV)
Electrocardiogram (ECG), 220
Electromyogram (EMG), 171
EMA-based frailty recognition systems, 175

Emotion recognition, 250, 293
  facial affect, 241–243, 317
  multimodal, 244
  physiological signals, 243
  speech affect, 244
  text affect, 244
Equalized odds, 248
E-skin, 221
Ethical impact assessments, 341
Ethical principles, 281, 342, 344
  accountability, 247
  autonomy, 248, 281, 341, 342
  beneficence, 247, 282
  consent, 279, 292, 334
  fairness, 248, 281, 317
  fidelity, 284
  informed consent, 279
  justice, 247, 283, 341, 342

Index   351

non-maleficence, 247, 282, 283
principlism, 247
Ethics by design, 334
Eulerian Video Magnification (EMV), 222, 223
European Active and Assisted Living Research and Development Programme (AAL2), 314
European Next Generation Ambient Assisted Living Innovation Alliance (AALIANCE2), 132
European Union acquis, 308
European Union Agency for Cybersecurity (ENISA), 122
Explainability, *see* Explainable AI
Explainable AI, 33, 297
Exploitable vulnerability, 124

F
Facial landmarking, 223
Fail-secure system, 119
Fall
    definition, 132
    getup events, 144
    prevention, 144
    risk factors, 133
    statistics, 132
False alarms, 149
Fast Fourier Transformation (FFT), 142
Fault-Containment Region (FCR), 118
Fault hypothesis, 118
First-Person Video (FPV), 25
Fog computing, 104
Frailty, 156, 168
    frailty index (FI), 160, 162
    metrics, 163
    short physical performance battery (SPPB), 162
Function creep, 240
Fundamental Human Rights Impact Assessment (FHRIA), 307

G
Gammatone spectogram, 196
General Data Protection Regulation (GDPR), 81, 120, 157, 206, 240, 280
Ground truth, 226

H
Health monitoring technologies, 335
Histogram of Optical Flow (HOF), 193

Histogram of Oriented Gradients (HOG), 142, 143, 147, 193
Homomorphic encryption, 85, 90, 113
Human Activity Recognition (HAR), 27, 166, 187, 196
Human dignity, 286, 321
Huntington's disease, 171

I
Identity management systems, 123
Image processing
    background subtraction, 193
    bandpass filtering, 222
    blurring, 91
    cartooning, 92
    depth image, 140, 173, 193
    false colouring, 92
    infrared image, 140, 143
    IUV image, 21
    Kanade-Lucas-Tomasi algorithm, 222
    mean shift, 92
    morphing, 92
    pixelation, 91
    registration, 223
    RGB image, 138
    steganography, 90
    thresholding, 193
    warping, 92
Independent Component Analysis (ICA), 193, 198
Inertial Magnetic Unit (IMU), 167
Information isolation, 83
Infrastructure as a Service (IaaS), 102
Internet of Health Things (IoHT), 7, 11
Internet of Things (IoT), 11, 27, 102, 103
Internet Protocol Security (IPsec), 116
Interpretability, 248

L
Large Language Model (LLM), 323
LifeAlert system, 9
Lifelogging, 7
LiShield system, 88
Local Binary Pattern (LBP), 142, 143
Loneliness, 164

M
Machine Learning (ML)
    adversarial learning, 83–85
    artificial neural network (ANN), 31, 51
    autoencoder, 52, 54, 83, 142, 169, 199

bagging, 67
boosting, 67
clustering, 51
conditional random field (CRF), 196
convolutional neural network (CNN), 31, 142, 194, 199, 222
decision tree (DT), 50
deep learning (DL), 10, 32, 51, 54, 64, 92, 157–159, 169, 170, 174, 197, 199, 202, 205, 228, 232, 243
dynamic Bayesian network (DBN), 196
end-to-end learning, 194
end-to-end training, 243
federated learning, 68
Gaussian mixture model (GMM), 52
generative adversarial network (GAN), 53, 92, 202
gradient boosting, 196
graph convolutional network (GCN), 170
hidden Markov model (HMM), 193, 196
hierarchical clustering, 52
isolation forest, 52
k-means clustering, 51
k-nearest neighbor (KNN), 51
Kernel discriminant analysis (KDA), 193
long short-term memory (LSTM), 170, 194, 199
machine unlearning, 299
model evaluation, 55
multi-dimensional scaling (MDS), 241
multimodality, 33, 47, 69, 225
Naive Bayes (NB), 51
overfitting, 49, 232
random forest (RF), 50, 196
recurrent neural network (RNN), 169, 170, 194, 199
reinforcement learning, 53
semi-supervised learning, 52
stacking, 67
supervised learning, 50
support vector machine (SVM), 50, 141, 196
transfer learning, 194, 197, 224, 243
transformer model, 197, 222
unsupervised learning, 51
MagicMirror system, 263
Maleficence, 341
Mel-Frequency Cepstral Coefficients (MFCC), 196, 224
Microphone
  array, 28
  condenser, 27
  polar pattern, 28

Miratar project, 262
Mist computing, 104
Mobile Health (mHealth), 7
Monitoring, 278, 345
Multidimensionality, 341
Multiple encryption, 113
Multiple Sclerosis (MS), 170

N
Never Give Up (NGU) strategy, 119
Non-interference, 281

O
Obtrusiveness, 148
Ocuvera system, 147
Open communication, 345
Open source, 116

P
Parkinson's Disease (PD), 167, 168, 170, 171
  MDS-Unified Parkinson's Disease Rating Scale (MDS-UPDRS), 169
Partial Occlusion by Background Alignment (POBA), 201
Participatory design, 336
People with special needs, 217, 346
Performance-Oriented Mobility Assessment (POMA), 160, 162
Pernicious memory, 296
PHOBILITYaktiv project, 338
Photoplethysmography, 227
Phyx.io system, 269
PinePhone system, 88
Platform as a Service (PaaS), 102
Podiatry, 167
Precision, 56
Principal Component Analysis (PCA), 193
Privacy by Design (PbD), 306
Privacy Enhancing Technologies (PETs), 306
Private Content-based Image Retrieval (PCBIR), 90
Product lifecycle, 118
Product support, 124
Public key model, 106, 107
Publicly accessible space, 250

Q
Quadruple helix model, 285
Quantified Self movement, 7

Index

R
Ransomware, 101
Recall, 56
Remote Patient Monitoring (RPM), 321
Rescue operation, 335
Re-skilling, 315
Resource distribution, 345
Risk management, 306
Rome Declaration, The, 278
RSA algorithm, 107
R transform, 193

S
SafeLife system, 9
San Diego County Elderly Falls Report, 134

Secret key model, 106
Secure by default configuration, 123
Secure Multi-party Computation (SMC), 89

Security by design, 120, 122, 123
Self-driving cars, 315
SEMEOTICONS project, 264
Sensors, 14, 156
  accelerometer, 135, 137, 166, 294
  acoustic, 27, 29, 137, 148, 195
  ASUS Xtion, 20, 169
  barometric altimeter, 136
  camera, *see* Camera
  dynamometer, 166
  electronic compass, 137
  electronic stethoscope, 228
  finger pulse oximeter, 226
  floor sensors, 29
  force sensing resistor (FSR), 168
  global positioning system (GPS), 89
  gyroscope, 139, 294
  inertial magnetic unit (IMU), 168, 170
  infrared, 19
  Intel RealSense, 22
  laryngophone, 29
  medical, 11
  microphone, *see* Microphone
  Microsoft Kinect, 22, 141, 142, 146, 147, 169
  motion capture (MoCap), 157, 167
  Orbbec Astra, 20, 142
  passive, 195
  passive infrared (PIR), 137
  piezoelectric chest belt, 228
  pressure, 137
  saturation, 88
  ultrasonic, 29, 195
  wearable, 231
  wristband, 166
Sequential Forward Floating Selection (SFFS), 198
Service provider status, 304
Signal processing, 10, 28
  blind source separation, 195
  denoising, 223
  filtering, 223, 225
  frequency-domain features, 196
  segmentation, 223
  spectral filtering, 230
  time-domain features, 196
  white noise, 225
Silhouette detection, 141
Silhouette images, 193
Skinned Multi-Person Linear Model (SMPL), 21
Sleep, 224
Smart Connected Toys (SCTs), 318
Smart devices, 11
  smart dynamometer, 166
  smart fabrics, 221
  smart home, 14, 335
  smart mats, 145, 164
  smart mirror, 263–265, 292, 293
  smartphones, 166
  smart pressure balls, 166
  smart sleep monitors, 166
  smart speakers, 294
  smart TVs, 295
  smart walkways, 164
  smart watch, 166, 294
  smart weighing scales, 164
Smart objects, *see* Smart devices
Social inequality, 317, 320
Social isolation, 334
Software as a Service (SaaS), 102
Software backdoor, 101
Software Bill of Materials (SBOMs), 122, 125
Sound source separation, 86
Sound zones, 87
Stakeholder engagement, 13, 117, 239, 240, 284–286, 306, 307, 316, 324, 336, 337, 345
Stereoscopic computer vision, 20
Stigmatization, 279, 321, 346
Stratified sampling, 48
Stream encryption, 110
Study of Osteoporotic Fractures (SOF), 161

Surveillance, 278, 296
Surveillance capitalism, 319
Survey of Health, Ageing and Retirement in Europe (SHARE) project, 160
Synthetic Minority Over-sampling (SMOTE), 65
System trust, 321

T
TAALXONOMY project, 13
Time synchronization, 202
Transparency, 297
  prospective, 298
  retrospective, 298
Trust, 321

U
Uncanny valley, 260
Uneven participation, 345
Upper respiratory condition, 224
Use context, 304
User authentication, 101
User compliance, 221, 230
User empowerment, 342
User privacy, 100
User safety, 117
User status, 304

V
Video-based monitoring systems, 307
Video preprocessing, 193
Virtual Private Networks (VPN), 112
Vital sign monitoring
  blood oxygenation, 218, 220, 223
  blood pressure, 220, 223
  body temperature, 220, 223
  ECG, *see* Electrocardiogram (ECG)
  heart rate, 218, 219, 222, 224, 228
  respiratory function, 219, 222, 224, 227
Vital signs, 218
Voice recognition, 293
Vulnerability reporting, 122, 124

W
Warmth-competence model, 261
Wearable devices, 156, 164, 231
Weighted Error Rate (WER), 56
Welfare, 280
Wi-tracker system, 225
Wize Mirror system, 264
World Health Organization (WHO), 133

Y
Yale Precipitating Events Project, 160

The manufacturer's authorised representative in the EU is Springer Nature Customer Service Centre GmbH, Europaplatz 3, 69115 Heidelberg, Germany. If you have any concerns regarding our products, please contact ProductSafety@springernature.com

Printed and bound by CPI Group (UK) Ltd, Croydon, CR0 4YY

26/03/2026

02078974-0004